Dedicated to Bill Veis

I would like to dedicate this book to my father Bill Veis. Bill founded Space Maintainers Laboratory almost fifty years ago and some of my fondest memories are of the days I would go to work with him. I watched him build his business from a one-man lab into one of the most respected companies in the industry. He did this by never forgetting to help his clients out in any way that he could. In particular my father was always dedicated to helping the young dentist and over the years many aspiring dentists have worked their way through school by being technicians at the lab.

Because of his example, I knew from the age of eight that I wanted to be a dentist. I have now been practicing dentistry for twenty years. My hope is that this book will continue my father's life work of helping dentists to provide their patients with the best care possible.

Principles of Appliance Therapy for Adults and Children

TABLE OF CONTENTS

Anatomy of An Appliance	1
Space Maintenance	2
Habits	3
Regaining Space	4
Closing Space	5
Individual Tooth Movement	6
Crossbites	7
Arch Development	8
Functional Orthopedics	9
Orthodontics	10
Finishing / Maintaining	11
Mouthguards	12
Splints	13
Restorative Enhancements	14
Interim Partials / Bridges	15
Implant Services	16
Periodontal Services	17
Obstructive Sleep Apnea & Snoring	18
General Index	
References	

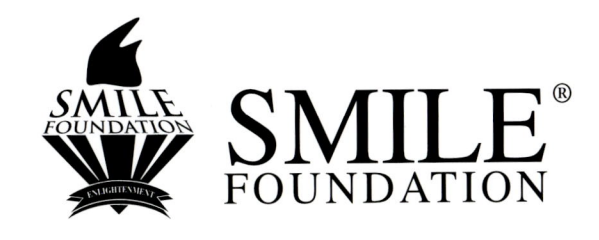

SMILE FOUNDATION
SMILE® FOUNDATION

USING THIS TEXT

The Principles of Appliance Therapy for Adults and Children is an encyclopedic resource for Appliance Therapy procedures. It describes treatment philosophy and possibilities, diagnostic procedures and descriptions for more than 300 appliances. It will provide you with the basic knowledge and appliance designs needed to incorporate appliance therapy into your practice.

These techniques described in this textbook range from minor interceptive orthodontics and cosmetic tooth movement procedures through much more comprehensive treatment plans requiring specialized qualifications. By carefully studying the designs and recommended treatment criteria on the following pages, you will be able to proceed with confidence and obtain predictable results for your patients while adding a new dimension to your practice.

Our goal in writing this text was to create a tool that would help you provide the best care possible for your patients. We know that there is more to appliance therapy than just selecting an appliance out of a book.

FOR OPTIMUM RESULTS

- Read through the entire text for an overview of our treatment philosophy, diagnostic procedures, and treatment possibilities.
- Study the sections that seem to have the most relevance for the patients in your practice and your style of dentistry.
- Begin to identify the candidates for possible treatment in your practice.
- Take all the records necessary to create a treatment plan. This may include some or all of the following: study models, a construction bite, intraoral and extraoral photographs, full mouth X-rays, a panorex, a lateral cephalometric film, and TM joint films.
- Identify the needed treatment procedures and possible appliance designs by turning to the appropriate section of this book.
- Have a consultation with your patient (or with the parents of the underage patient).
- Once your patient has agreed to your treatment plan, prepare an informed consent form and have the patient or parent sign it.

OF SPECIAL NOTE

Library of Congress Cataloguing-in-Publication Data
Rob W. Veis, D.D.S. and John C. Christian III, C.D.T.
Principles of appliance therapy for adults and children
ISBN 0-9749-8560-0   2004101954

Authors: Rob W. Veis, D.D.S.
                  John C. Christian III, C.D.T.

Editor: Susan Wilkinson

Photographer: Steve Gross, C.D.T.
                  All appliances/models fabricated

Publisher: Smile Foundation
                  A Member of the Appliance Therapy Group
                  Chatsworth, California 91311

Principles of Appliance Therapy for Adults and Children

Copyright © 2004 by Selane Products, Inc.

Permission to reproduce or transmit in any form or by any means, electronic or mechanical, including photocopying and recording, or by an information storage and retrieval system, with the exception of forms and questionnaires meant to be copied, must be obtained by writing to:

Smile Foundation
9129 Lurline Avenue
Chatsworth, CA 91311

Library of Congress Control Number: 2004101954
Printed in Hong Kong

ANATOMY OF AN APPLIANCE

an overview: ANATOMY OF AN APPLIANCE

Chapter 1

FIXED OR REMOVABLE APPLIANCE?

Many of the tooth movements in the following pages can be treated with either fixed or removable appliances. In cases where either appliance will accomplish the same results, the following check list is provided to help you decide which approach may be best suited for your patient.

FIXED

- Bodily movements of teeth are needed.
- Anterior bands, brackets, and wires are acceptable to the patient.
- The teeth to be banded have the clinical crown fully exposed.
- The patient has excellent oral hygiene, making the possibility of decay minimal.
- Patient cooperation in wearing a removable appliance is doubtful.

REMOVABLE

- Bodily movements of the teeth are not required as removable appliances mainly provide a tipping action.
- Esthetics are important. The patient needs an inconspicuous appliance.
- Enough teeth are present and sufficiently erupted for anchorage of the appliance.
- The patient requires an appliance that does not interfere with proper oral hygiene.
- The patient is cooperative and responsible, i.e. they will wear an appliance as prescribed and will guard against loss or breakage.
- There are economic considerations. Removable appliances require less chair time.

All appliances and models contributed by:

SPACE MAINTAINERS LABORATORY

ANATOMY OF AN APPLIANCE

Clasps

Adams Clasp

The Adams clasp can be used on both molars and bicuspids. It gains its retention by engaging the mesial and distal undercuts of these teeth. Therefore, it is essential that the tooth being clasped be sufficiently erupted so that the mesial and distal undercuts are fully exposed. Another consideration when using this clasp is to place it only where it will not create an occlusal interference. An occlusal interference can cause a functional shift of the patient's mandible.

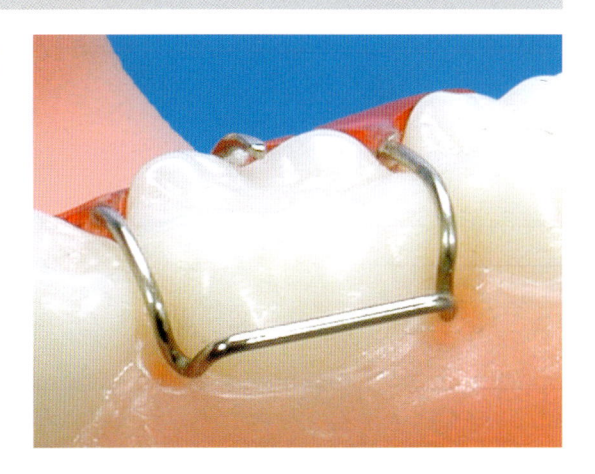

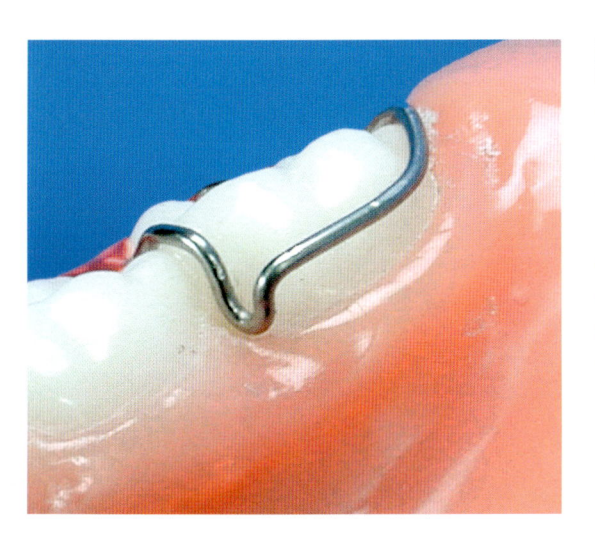

Half Adams

When the distal-buccal undercut of the tooth being clasped is too far sub-gingival to use a standard Adams clasp, the half Adams clasp is an effective clasp to use. As illustrated, the "arrow-point" is placed accurately to engage the mesial-buccal undercut of the molar while the distal portion of the clasp is adapted tightly around the rest of the molar. This clasp is very stable as it still has two anchor points into the lingual acrylic. Again, care should be taken to select those teeth where the possibility of occlusal interference will not be an issue.

"C" Clasp

"C" clasps are most commonly used where the use of another type of clasp would create a significant occlusal interference. Eliminating an unwanted occlusal interference is important for two reasons. In children, an occlusal interference can cause them to abnormally shift their mandible. In adults, these interferences usually lead to poor compliance as biting on the clasps is very uncomfortable. To make this clasp more retentive, it is usually used in conjunction with a composite buccal button. This composite undercut will allow the clasp to snap into position.

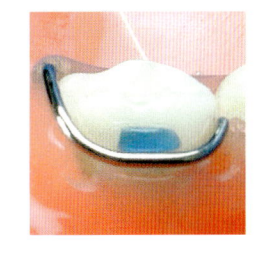

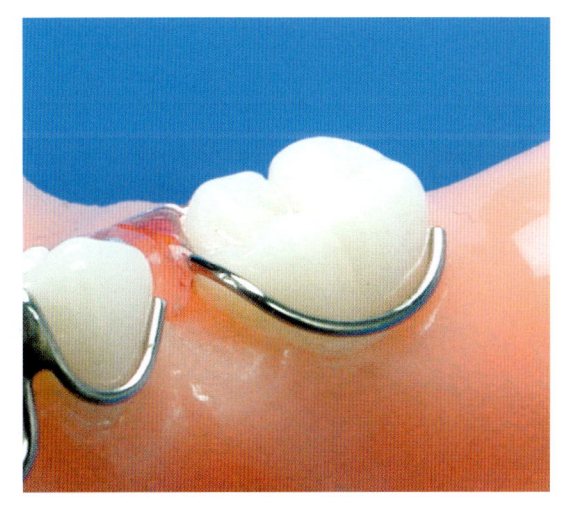

1.1

ANATOMY OF AN APPLIANCE

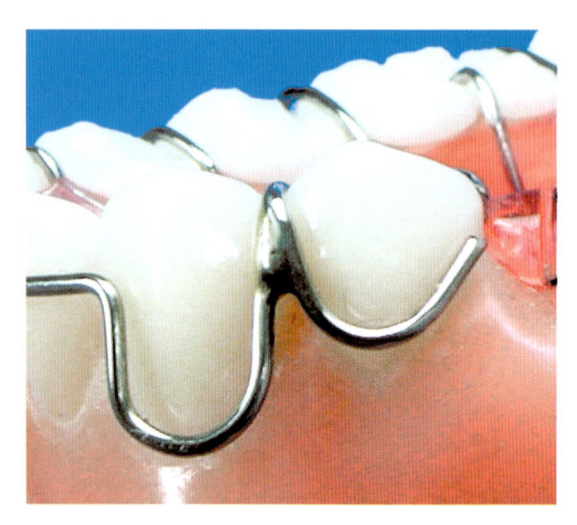

Soldered "C" Clasp

A "C" clasp can be soldered to a labial bow to create extra anterior retention. This is often done when moving anterior teeth. To make this clasp more retentive, it is usually used in conjunction with a composite buccal button. This composite undercut will allow the clasp to snap into position. All soldered clasps need extra care when adjusting them, as the solder joint when handled improperly is a potential point of breakage.

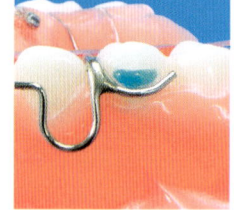

Delta Clasp

The Delta clasp is a derivation of the Adams clasp. Its name comes from the shape of its retentive portion. It is commonly used with the Clark Twin-Block because, with this appliance, occlusal interferences are not an issue and an extremely retentive clasp is needed. Like the Adams clasp, the tooth to be clasped must be erupted enough to expose the buccal undercuts.

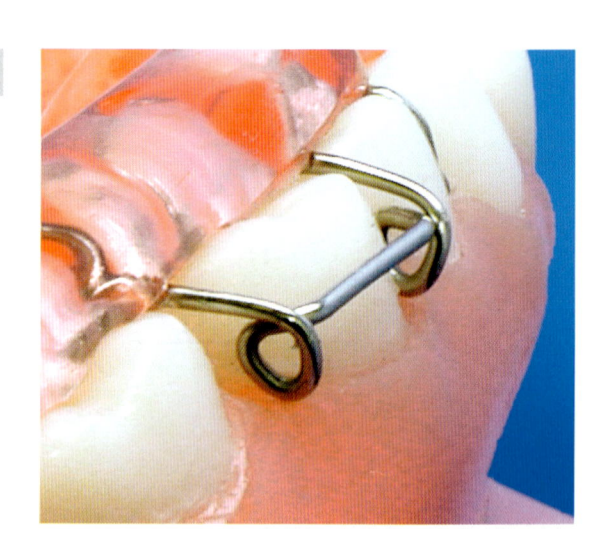

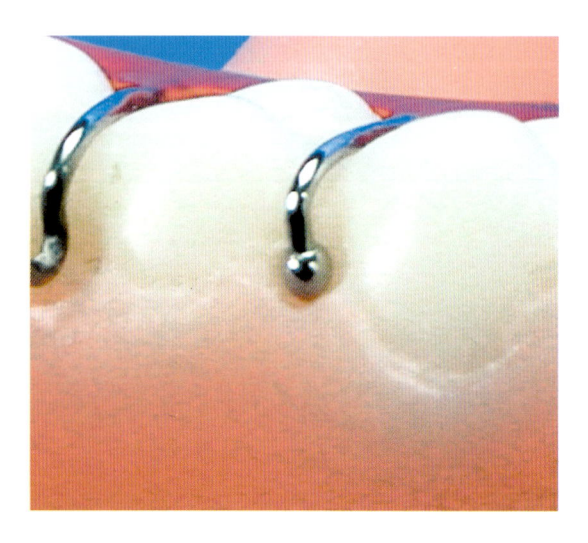

Ball Clasp

Ball clasps are typically used as auxiliary retention in conjunction with other clasps. They are usually placed tightly into the interproximal embrasure between two posterior teeth. This is usually sufficient to create the retention needed, however it can also be adjusted mesially or distally to engage the undercut of either tooth. This is particularly useful during the exfoliation stage of the mixed dentition. When one primary molar is lost, a simple adjustment will allow you to regain the retention needed to continue on with treatment.

ANATOMY OF AN APPLIANCE

Finger Clasps

Finger clasps are typically used as auxiliary retention in conjunction with other clasps in the primary and mixed dentition when 6-year molars are not sufficiently erupted to be clasped. The clasps are usually placed tightly between two posterior teeth and locked into the mesial or distal buccal undercut of one of them. Because the end of the wire is left sharp to increase retention, some patients complain that the clasp causes their tissue to become irritated.

This clasp is also particularly useful during the exfoliation stage of the mixed dentition. When one primary molar is lost, a simple adjustment towards the undercut of the remaining tooth will allow you to regain the retention needed to continue on with treatment.

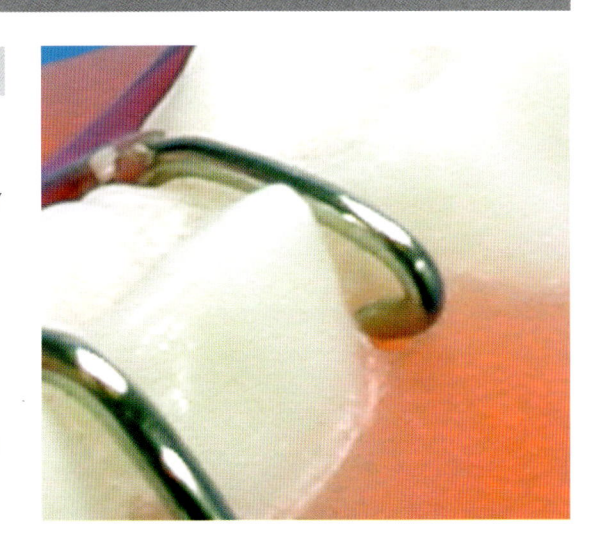

Buccal Bond "C" Clasp

When a buccal undercut needs to be created for retention of a clasp, composite can be easily bonded to the tooth. This composite ledge is usually placed after the appliance is fabricated. However, if you prefer, you can place the appropriate composite ledge(s) prior to taking the impression for appliance fabrication.

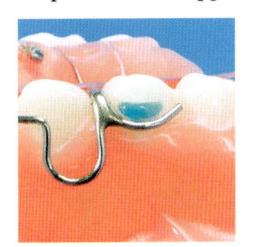

Lingual Sage Clasp

The Lingual Sage clasp is used on molars and bicuspids when they are fully erupted. It gains its retention by engaging the undercuts of the proximal surfaces and the lingual contour to the center of the tooth. Because this clasp does not have any part crossing the occlusion, it is often used in situations where the occlusion is extremely tight and any wire crossing over it would create an occlusal interference. It is mainly used as part of a final retainer and is not recommended for active appliances as it may not provide sufficient retention once the appliance is activated.

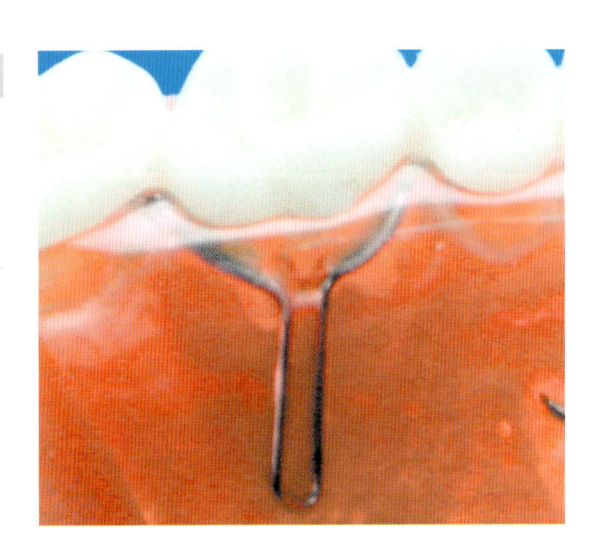

1.3

ANATOMY OF AN APPLIANCE

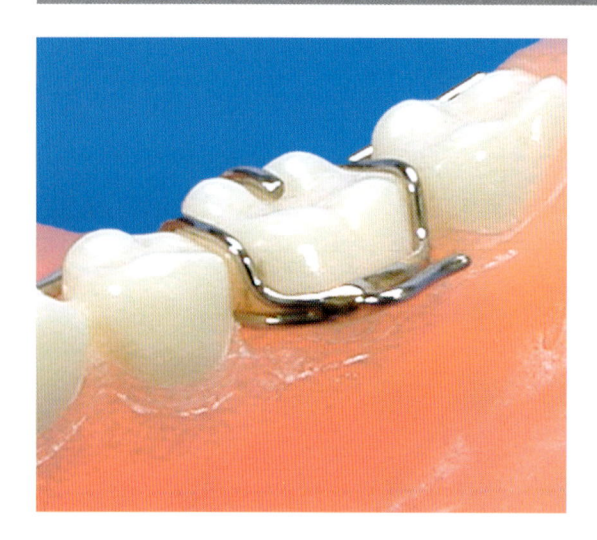

Crozat Clasp

Crozat clasps are typically used on first permanent molars as part of a Crozat appliance. They consist of three parts. The main body of the clasp, called *the crib*, is formed from one piece of wire and is tightly adapted around the entire tooth. The second wire, called *the crescent*, provides the retention by engaging the undercuts of the proximal surfaces. The third part of the clasp is *the occlusal rest*. It passes through the lingual groove and rests tightly on the occlusal surface.

"C" Clasp/Ball Clasp Combo

This double clasp design is quite effective in primary or mixed dentition cases when permanent molars are not adequately erupted for standard Adams clasps. As shown, it consists of a "C" clasp typically contoured to the second primary molar and a Ball clasp placed at the distal lingual undercut of the first primary molar. A composite ledge can be added to the buccal of the primary second molar to increase retention.

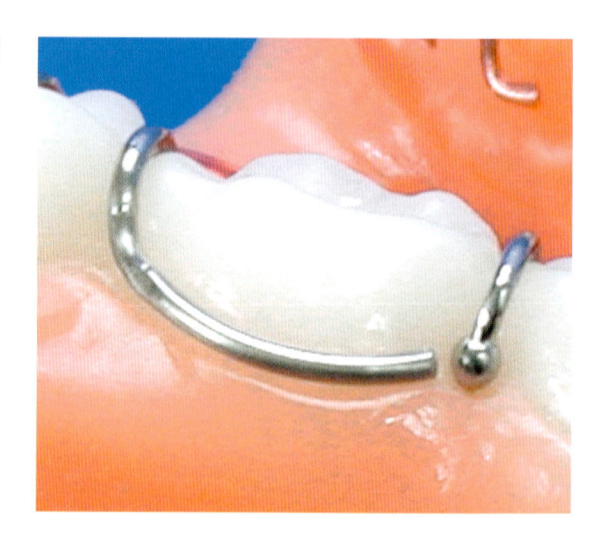

Design Notes:

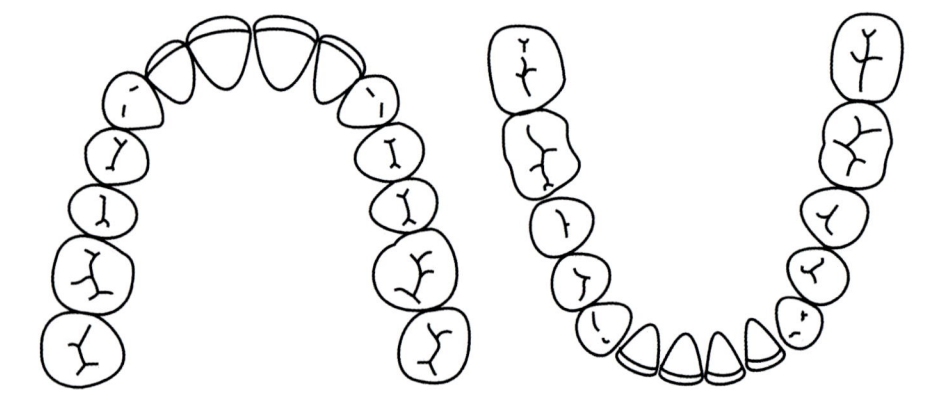

ANATOMY OF AN APPLIANCE

Labial Arch Wires

Labial arch wires can be used to create added retention. When an arch wire is being used in this manner, it will generally embrace the six anterior teeth and join the acrylic between the canine and the first premolar. However, the arch wire may be restricted to any part of the anterior region, or extended as far distally as the first molar. The numerous design modifications available are outlined here.

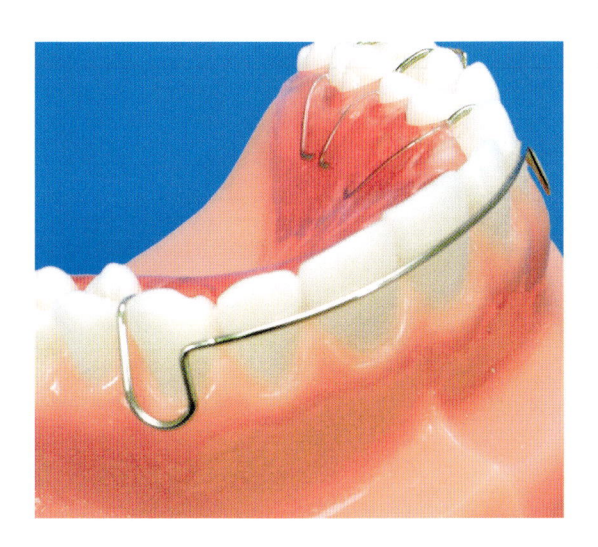

Standard

The most common arch wire design is shown here. The labial bow will generally embrace the six anterior teeth and join the acrylic between the canine and the first premolar. However, the labial portion may be restricted to any part of the anterior region, or extended as far distally as the first molar.

Round Contoured

A Round Contoured arch wire is bent to closely fit against the labial surface of the anteriors. It is used to securely hold the teeth in their final position after active treatment is completed.

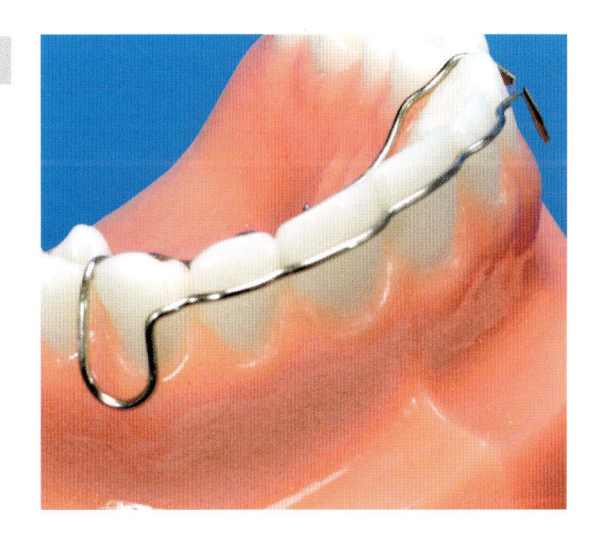

ANATOMY OF AN APPLIANCE

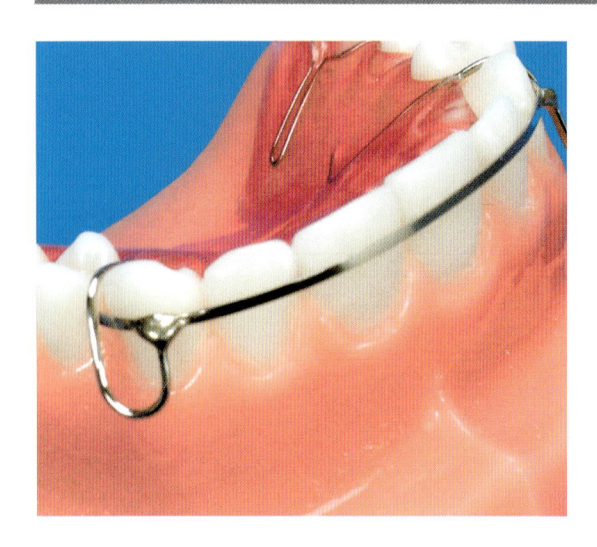

Flat Hawley

A Flat Hawley arch wire is often used in final retainers. It is chosen over a round wire because its flat surface provides more contact with the labial surface of the anterior teeth. The flat part of this wire is then soldered to the adjustment loops at the cuspids. Added retention to stabilize the cuspids after tooth movement can also be accomplished by contouring the flat wire back to the distal of the cuspids. (See "Contoured-Flat Hawley")

Contoured-Flat Hawley

Using the same wire as the Flat Hawley, the Contoured-Flat Hawley is individually contoured to the entire labial and interproximal surfaces of the incisors. Intimate contact like this is often preferred after significant rotations are corrected during active treatment to align the incisors.

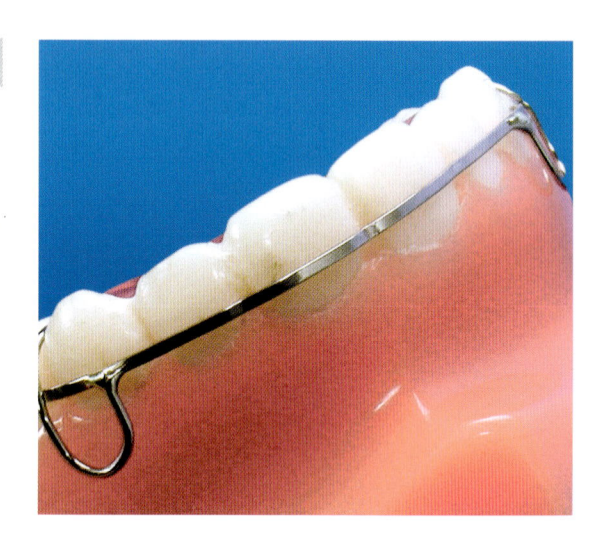

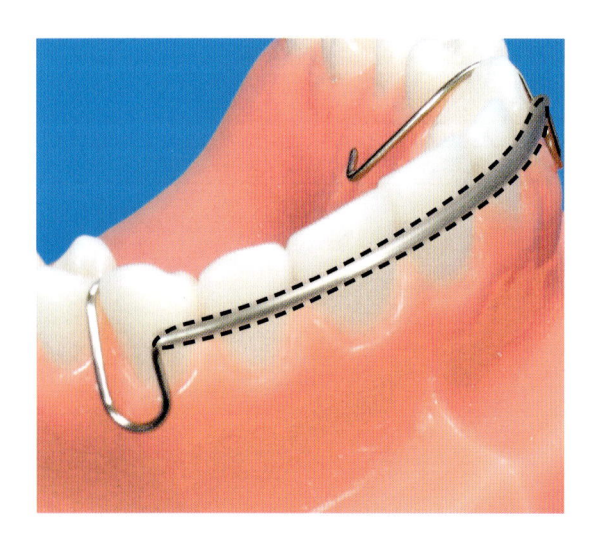

Plastic Coated Hawley

When anterior teeth have been restored with porcelain restorations such as veneers, a plastic coated labial wire is often preferred. This plastic coating protects the porcelain surfaces from possible abrasion from the wire.

ANATOMY OF AN APPLIANCE

Acrylic Arch Wire

This design gains superior anterior retention through the use of clear acrylic that tightly conforms to the labial and interproximal surfaces of the incisors. This prevents any movement of these teeth. It is often used on "wrap-around" labial wires because the intimate contact it creates stabilizes this long wire.

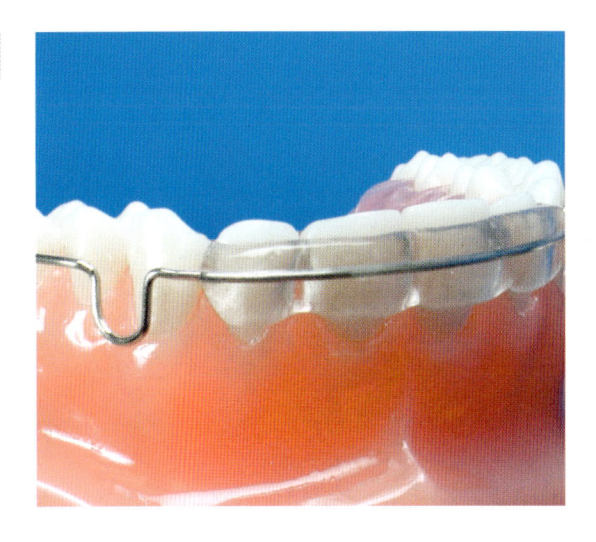

Reverse Hawley

The Reverse Hawley labial wire is fabricated with the adjustment loop running from the mesial to the distal of the cuspid. This design is chosen when you do not want any wire in the embrasure distal to the cuspids. A typical scenario requiring this design is when positive cuspid control is needed, particularly if the cuspid has been rotated significantly during orthodontic therapy.

Ricketts Arch Wire

The Ricketts arch wire, like the Reverse Hawley, crosses the dentition through the embrasures interproximal to the laterals and cuspids. The "U" loops are placed on the laterals and the distal recurved arms are contoured to the cuspids. These distal recurves can be used to increase retention and can help stabilize cuspids that may have required rotation during active treatment. If carefully activated, they can be used to effect minor lingual rotation of the cuspids, unilaterally or bilaterally.

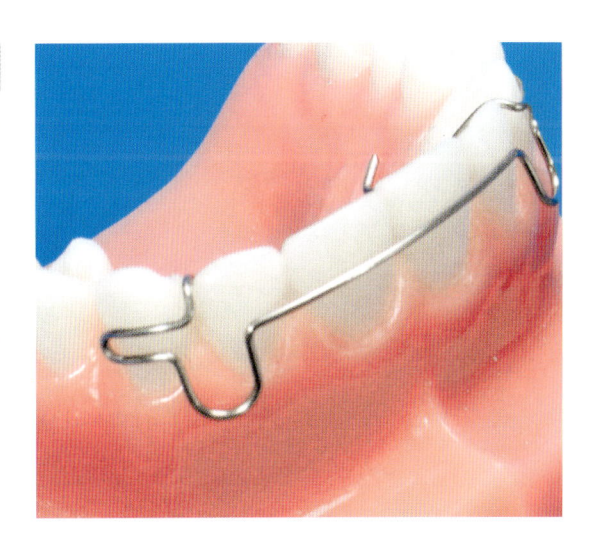

ANATOMY OF AN APPLIANCE

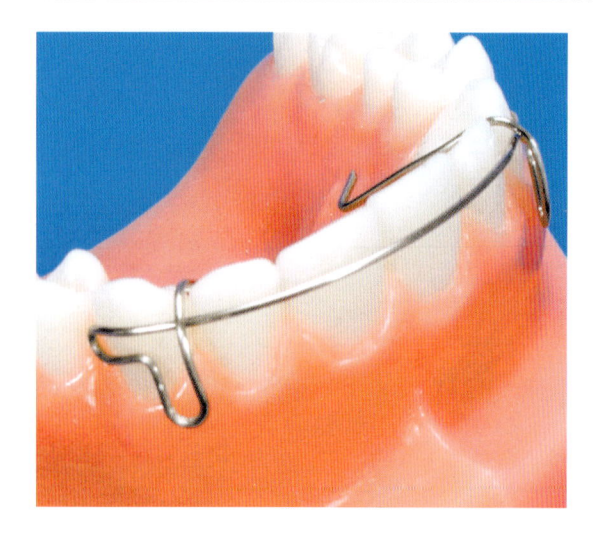

Witzig Double Loop

This labial arch wire is a modification of the Ricketts arch wire using a narrow vertical loop. This design is excellent for final stability of the anterior segment but only allows for very minor adjustments during retention. It is typically used only as part of a removable final retainer when orthodontic therapy is complete.

Wrap-Around

The Wrap-Around labial is excellent for final retention. It is usually soldered to the buccal bar of the Adams clasp or to "C" clasps. Retention wires are usually placed between the laterals and cuspids to help stabilize the long labial. Wrapping around in this manner eliminates the possibility of occlusal interferences or opening interproximal contacts.

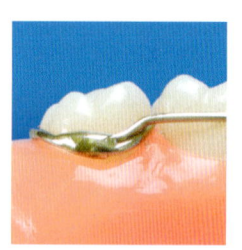

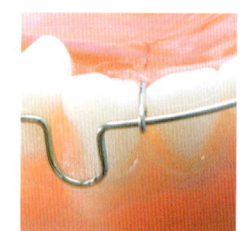

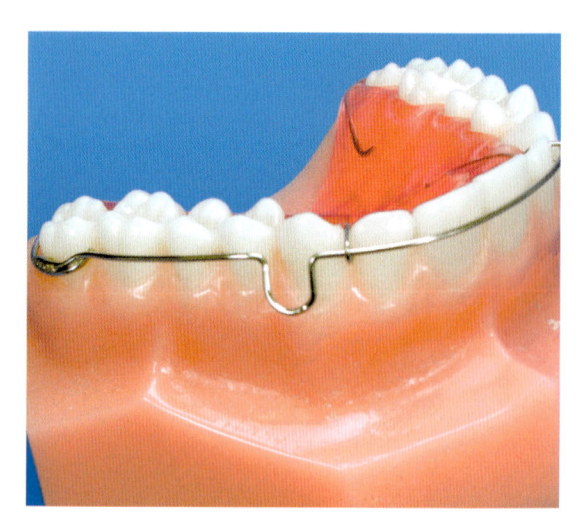

Design Notes:

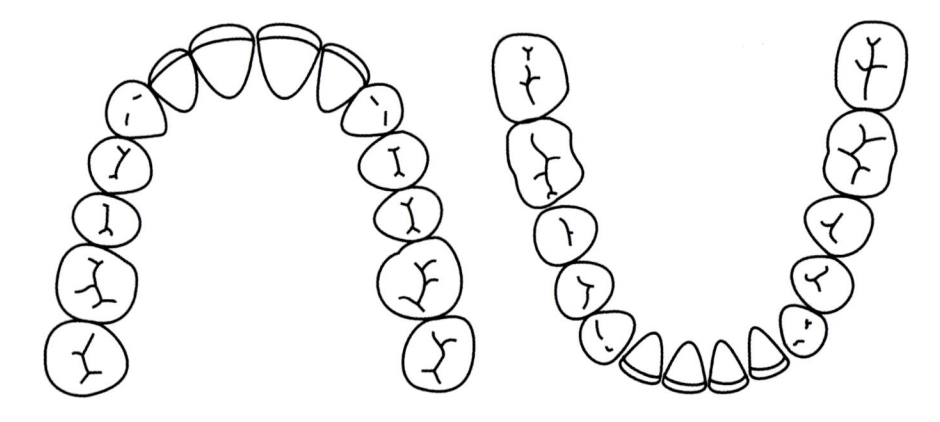

1.8

ANATOMY OF AN APPLIANCE

Acrylic

Acrylics are available in a wide variety of colors and designs. This is popular with adults as well as children and has proven to be an additional motivator resulting in successful treatment with removable appliance therapy. Colored acrylic appliances are rarely lost or abused by the patients.

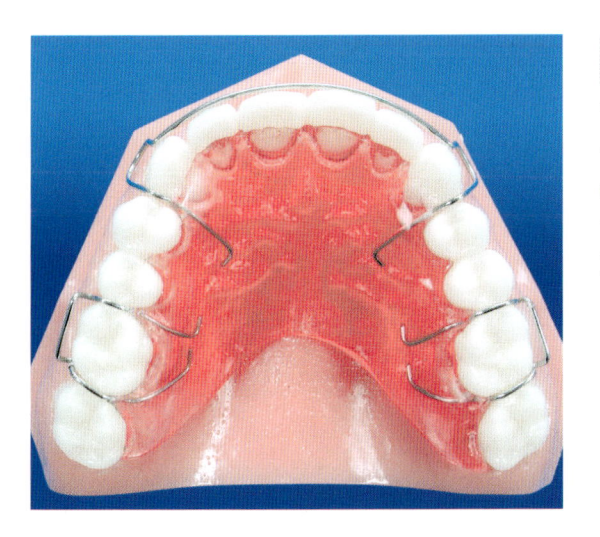

Full Palate

When extra anchorage is needed, a full acrylic palate can be used. In this design, the acrylic covers the entire hard palate and extends distally to the most posterior tooth in the arch. The acrylic rests intimately against the palate and lingual aspect of the teeth to provide extra stabilization and support.

Horseshoe

Although full palatal acrylic coverage provides the greatest amount of support, it can affect a patient's speech and, on occasion, trigger a gag response. To eliminate these negative effects, the palatal coverage can be cleared away from the soft palate. If you suspect that the patient may have a problem, ask the laboratory to horseshoe the palate.

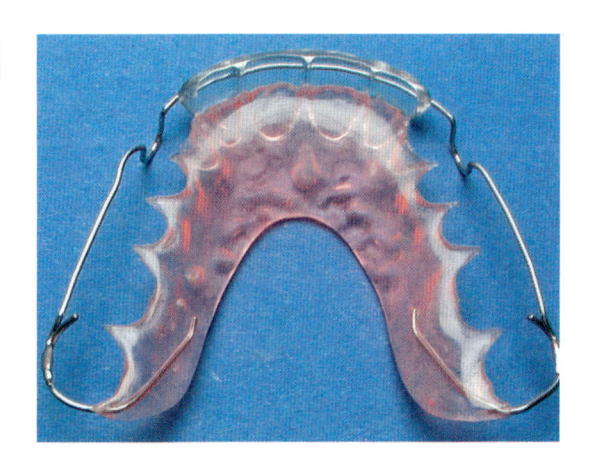

ANATOMY OF AN APPLIANCE

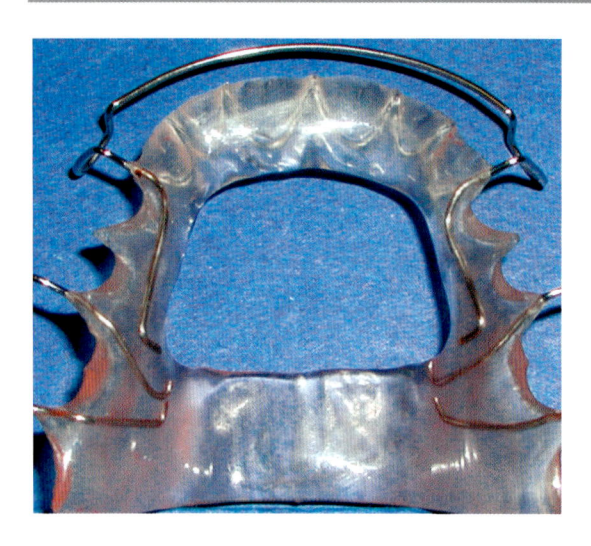

Speech Relief

By designing a final retainer with an open palate, the patient can wear the appliance 24-hours a day without being concerned that his or her speech will be affected. This is accomplished by placing a posterior palatal strap and lingual acrylic band that supports the anterior teeth. Kevlar fiber is usually added to the acrylic to provide added strength. This open palate design keeps the rugae area open to improve tongue position during speech.

Posterior Occlusal Coverage

A posterior occlusal acrylic bite plane is mainly used to open the vertical dimension sufficiently to correct a crossbite. However, by simply engaging the occlusal surface, extra retention for the appliance can be created.

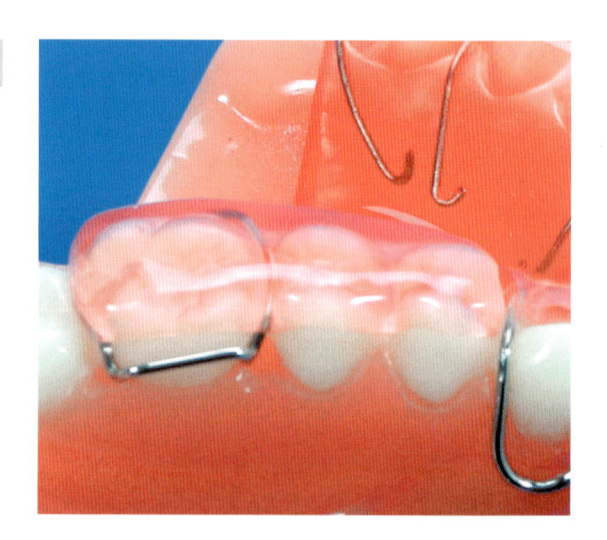

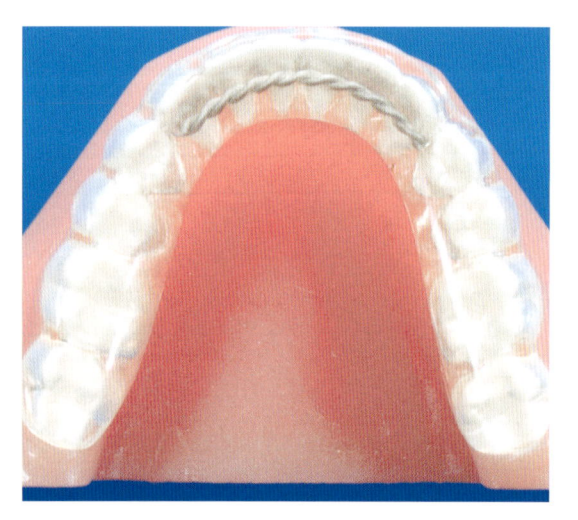

Complete Occlusal Coverage

Complete occlusal coverage is used to stabilize the occlusion, control the vertical dimension and establish the vertical and horizontal relationship between the mandible and maxilla. It can be designed to be fully intercuspated or flat planed.

ANATOMY OF AN APPLIANCE

Tooth Movement Components

The active components of removable appliances come in a wide variety of designs. Because each appliance is custom made, the various wires and mechanical screws can be configured in ways seemingly limited only by the imagination of the designer. However, there are several important rules that must be observed to maintain the optimum effectiveness of the appliance.

1. **Maintain anchorage.** Although we can build a large number of movements into an appliance, only one component should be adjusted at a time, in a logical sequence. Activating too many things at a time will create too much pressure and prevent the appliance from staying in place.

   Note - One of the advantages of removable appliances is this built-in safety valve. If you over adjust the appliance, it will not stay in place.

2. **Use light steady force.** Remember, when moving teeth, the harder you push, the slower they move. Light, continuous force will give you the optimum tooth movement.

3. **Adjust wires with care.** Breakage of wires from incorrect adjustment technique is one of the most common problems with removable appliances. Care must be taken not to stress or nick finger springs, arch wires, or clasps. An Appliance Adjustment Video/CD showing you every adjustment in a step-by-step approach is available for you and your staff.

Springs

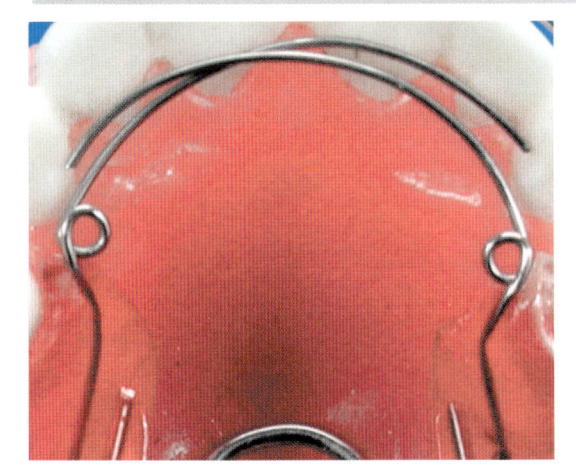

Lap Springs

Lap springs provide a gentle sweeping action against the lingual aspect of the upper and lower anteriors. These springs are most often used in conjunction with lateral developing appliances. Once there is enough space for the teeth, the lap springs can provide enough force to move them into alignment. A labial bow that has been pre-bent into the ideal arch form is usually used to prevent these springs from moving the anteriors too far labially.

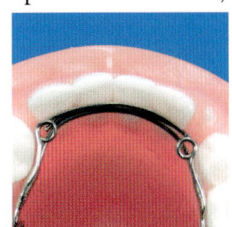

Recurved Springs

Recurved springs are designed to move an individual tooth in a labial or buccal direction. However, by altering the length and direction of the open end, it can also be used to help rotate the tooth. These springs can be made with or without helical coils.

Note - To prevent the activated spring from riding up the cingulum, a composite ledge is commonly placed on the lingual aspect of the tooth.

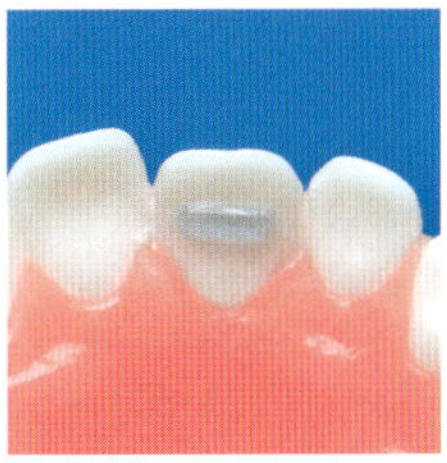

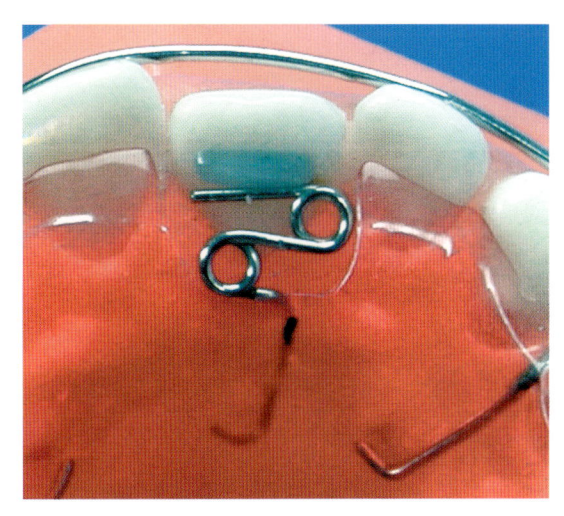

1.11

ANATOMY OF AN APPLIANCE

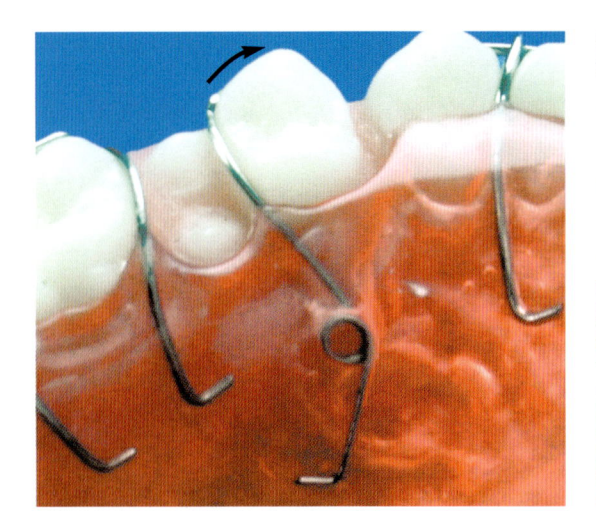

Mesial/Distal Kickers

Mesial and Distal Kicker springs are most commonly used to open or close space in the anterior region by engaging a single tooth. However, they can also be used to guide a bicuspid into a more ideal position. These kickers are placed in the lingual aspect of the appliance and are easily adjusted with finger pressure in the direction of the desired tooth movement.

Direct Pressure Springs

Direct Pressure springs are soldered to the labial arch wire and can provide a direct lingual movement, a rotation force, or an occlusal force depending upon their placement and adjustment. Three different design modifications are shown here.

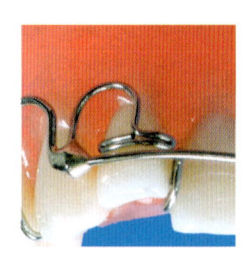

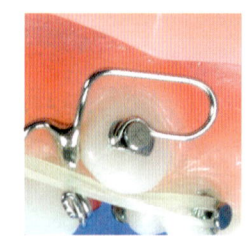

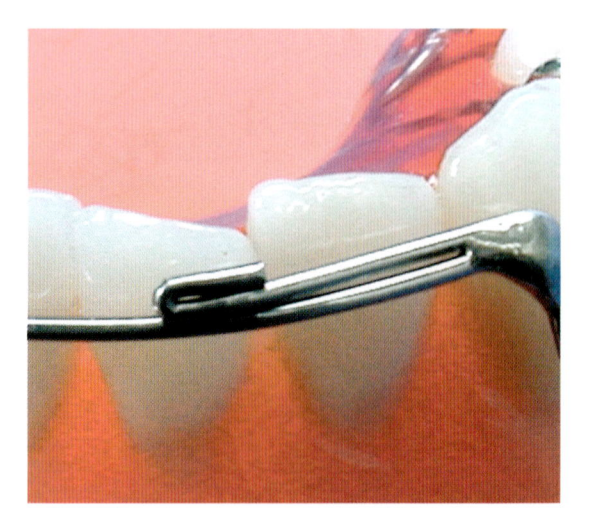

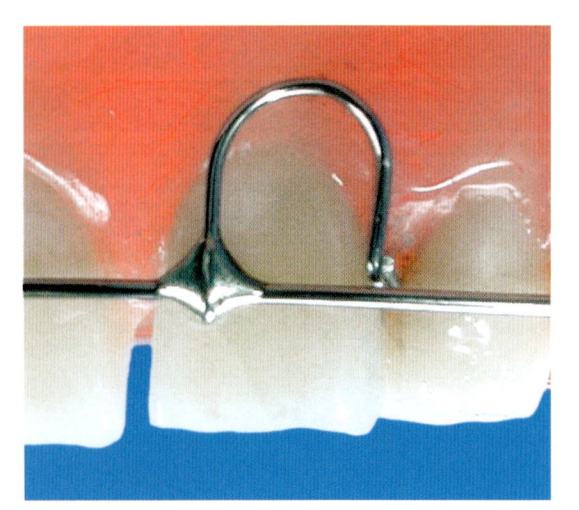

Mesial/Distal Labial Springs

Like Mesial and Distal Kickers, these springs are most commonly used to open or close space in the anterior region. Usually soldered to the labial arch wire, a simple adjustment can engage a single tooth and provide a tipping movement along the arch wire.

ANATOMY OF AN APPLIANCE

Cuspid Retraction Springs

Cuspid Retraction springs provide a positive force to tip a mesially inclined cuspid distally. The most effective design uses a coil that should be opened during activation. However, in cases with a shallow sulcus, the inverted coil design can be used to protect the tissue from irritation. In situations where the mesial aspect of the cuspid is not well exposed, the use of a bonded button or bracket will provide a positive contact point for the spring.

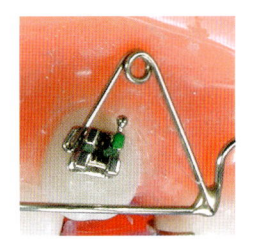

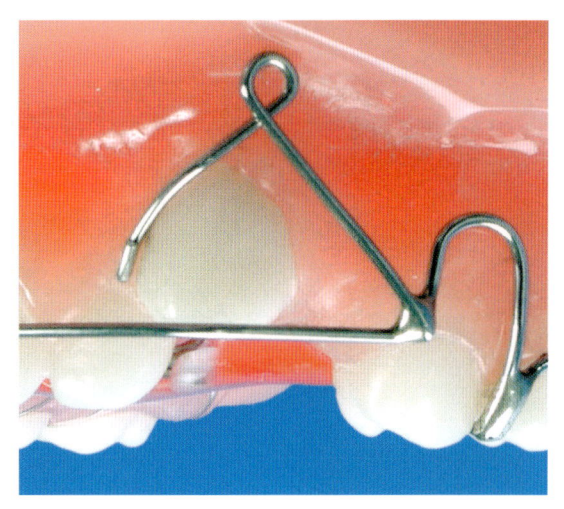

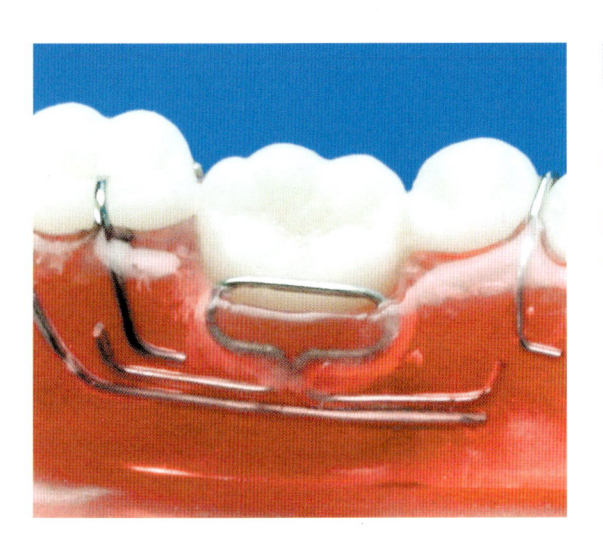

Lingual Mushroom Spring

Lingual Mushroom springs are used to upright any single lower posterior tooth with the exception of the distal-most tooth in the arch. They are often preferred over a micro-screw or mini-screw, because they are less bulky and less likely to irritate the patient's tongue.

Distal Recurved Spring

A Distal Recurved spring is used to upright a lingually tipped molar. This spring is easy to adjust and can effectively upright a molar with only a few adjustments. Placing a rest aids in controlling any super-eruption of the molar as it is being uprighted.

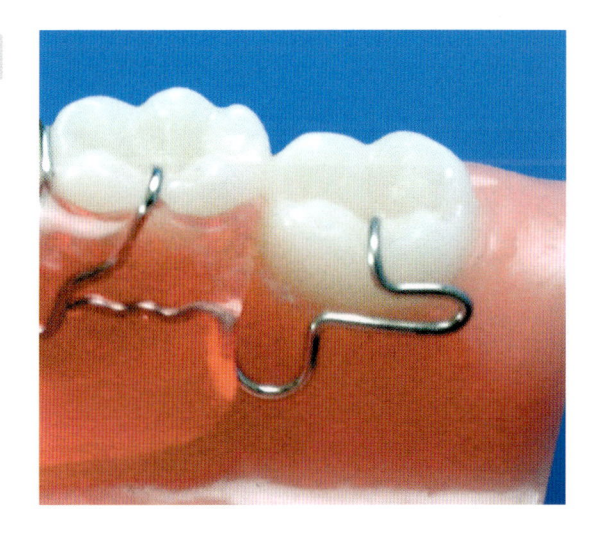

1.13

ANATOMY OF AN APPLIANCE

Screws

Stainless steel screws are threaded mechanical devices used in tooth movement procedures. They come in a variety of different sizes and designs. With the exception of the rapid palatal screws, they are usually activated with either wire keys or small screwdrivers at a rate that allows for approximately 1mm of movement a month. This is considered the optimum rate of movement and is what the operator should expect from most designs.

Palatal screw   Super screw 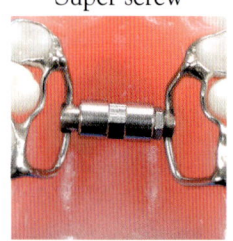   Micro-screw 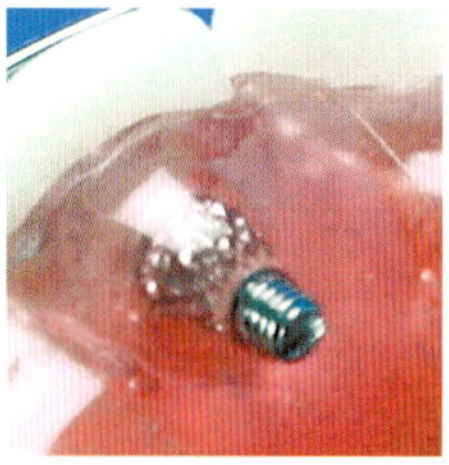   Wipla expansion screw

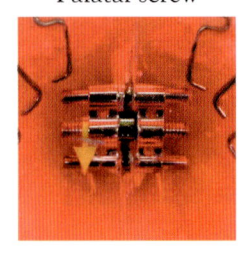

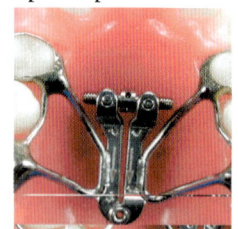

Palatal Screw

The Palatal screws can be used for either transverse or sagittal development. They are available in a variety of shapes and sizes, making them suitable for different arch forms. Smaller sizes may also be used for individual tooth movements or for unilateral crossbites.

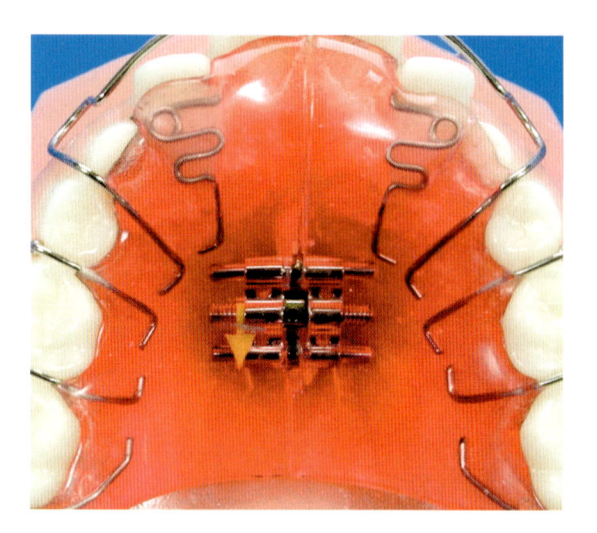

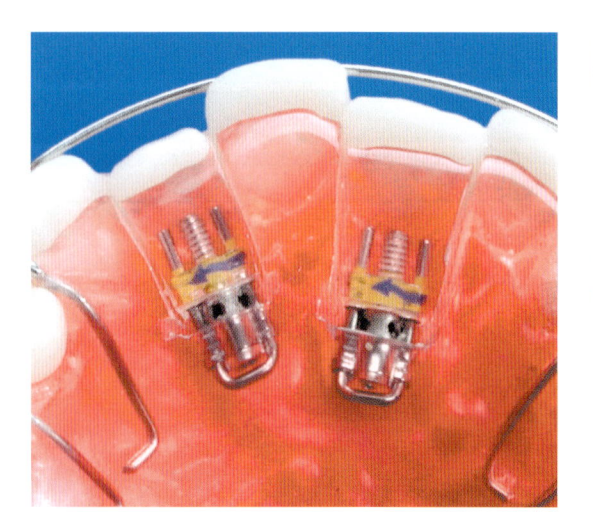

Mini-Screw

A Mini-screw is similar to the palatal screw in design and function. This "mini" version is used effectively for single tooth movement. Although this screw adds additional bulk to the appliance in the area of the expansion screw itself, it is typically preferred over a micro-screw as it is not as fragile and provides more surface contact with the tooth needing movement.

ANATOMY OF AN APPLIANCE

Micro-Screw

Micro-screws are used for individual tooth movement in a direct labial or buccal direction. When placed ideally they can also be used to rotate a tooth, however this movement is more easily accomplished with a recurved spring. Just a simple 180° turn of the screw with a screwdriver is all that is needed to activate the spring plunger mechanism. Many practitioners like this screw because it is easy to adjust. However, care must be taken not to over tighten the screw as it will cause the mechanism to lock up.

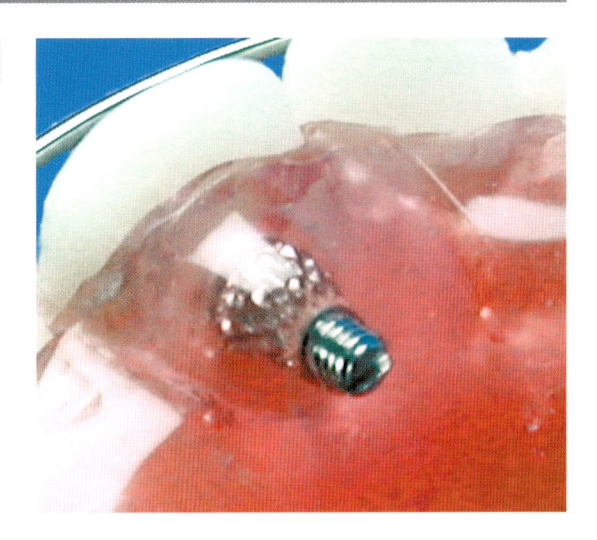

Molar Uprighting

This Molar Uprighting screw is specifically designed to buccally upright the most distally placed molar in the lower arch. Turning the screw applies a direct force on the lingually tipped molar in a buccal direction. In order for this screw to work, proper anchorage on the adjacent teeth is a must.

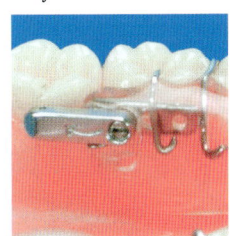

Three-Way

This unique device features three independently expanding sections in one housing for transverse as well as sagittal development. Each section can be independently activated.

When an equal amount of lateral development is desired, turn the two lateral sections at the same time. If a differential amount of lateral development is needed, by turning one of the lateral sections you can get unilateral movement. This is an excellent screw when the size of the palate is large enough to handle its considerable bulk. It is not suited for narrow palates or younger patients.

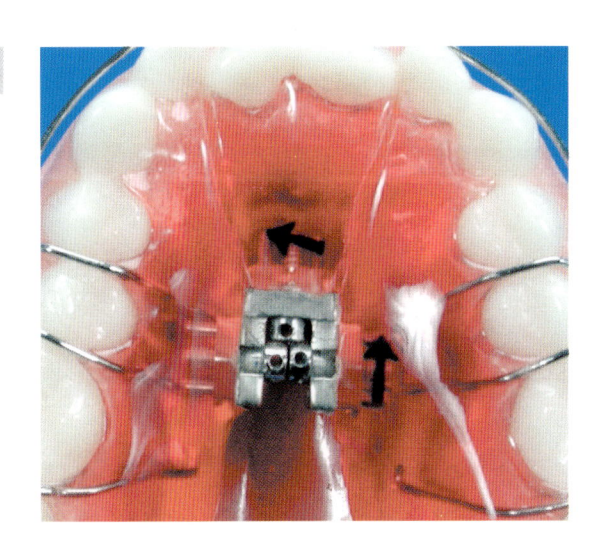

1.15

ANATOMY OF AN APPLIANCE

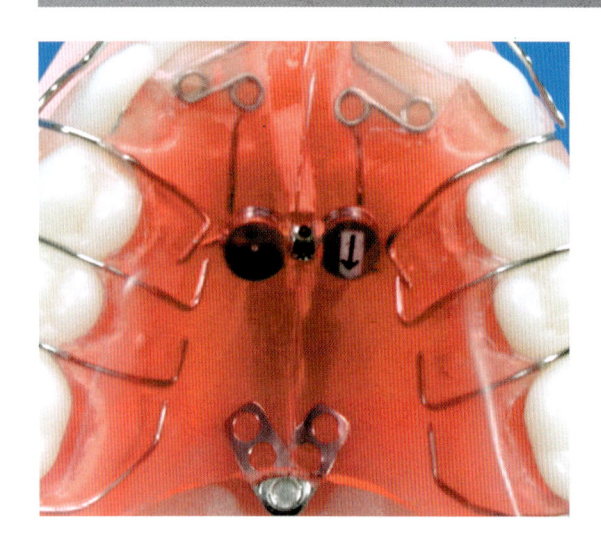

Swing Lock Expander

When a patient exhibits a V-shaped or Gothic arch form and is only narrow in the anterior region, an expansion appliance that expands equally in the posterior and anterior region would be contraindicated. To overcome this problem, a screw with a posterior hinge has been designed that allows you to gain anterior space without disturbing the posterior bite relationship. Since the expansion screw and the hinge are separate pieces, the palatal acrylic can be kept to a minimal thickness. This design is only effective for a limited amount of expansion (up to 4mm).

Wipla Expansion Screw

The Wipla expansion screw allows you to gain anterior space without disturbing the posterior bite relationship. It offers the same development as provided by the swing lock expansion screw; however, it is accomplished within a one-piece design. It is typically the preferred design in that it is extremely strong and provides up to 8mm of anterior lateral development. This screw can also be integrated into a fixed appliance.

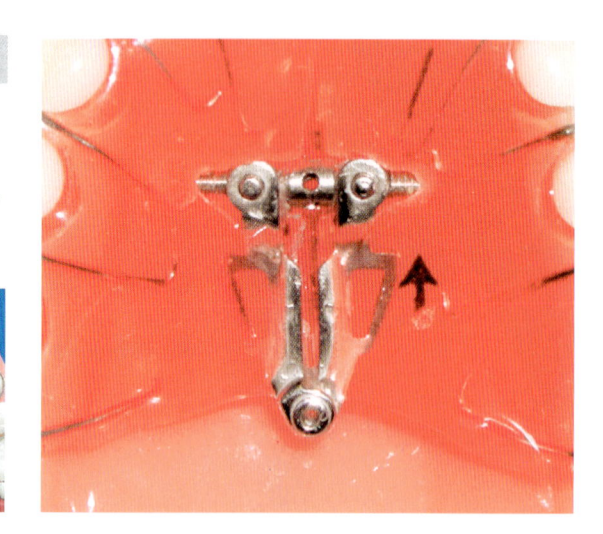

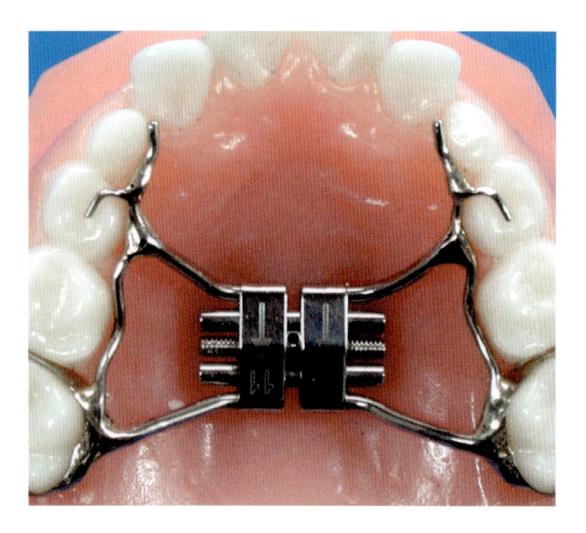

Rapid Palatal Expander

Rapid Palatal Expander (RPE) screws were designed to be used for rapid expansion and separation of the mid-palatal suture. To be effective, they must always be used in a fixed approach, either banded or bonded. These screws are available in a variety of sizes and configurations, offering a large range in the amount of lateral expansion that can be accomplished. Although designed for rapid palatal expansion, these screws are frequently used as part of a fixed appliance that applies gentle forces for slow development.

ANATOMY OF AN APPLIANCE

The Super-Screw

When a significant amount of lateral development is needed, even a standard RPE screw is sometimes not enough. When this happens, a second appliance frequently needs to be placed. Using a Super-screw will allow you to avoid having to place a second appliance. Available in two sizes, this screw offers between 12mm and 18mm of lateral arch width development. The Super-screw is easy to adjust from the front of the mouth with a small hex wrench. It has a clearly visible graduated scale milled into the body of the screw, making it very easy to monitor the amount of lateral development achieved, and it is quite comfortable due to its smooth rounded shape.

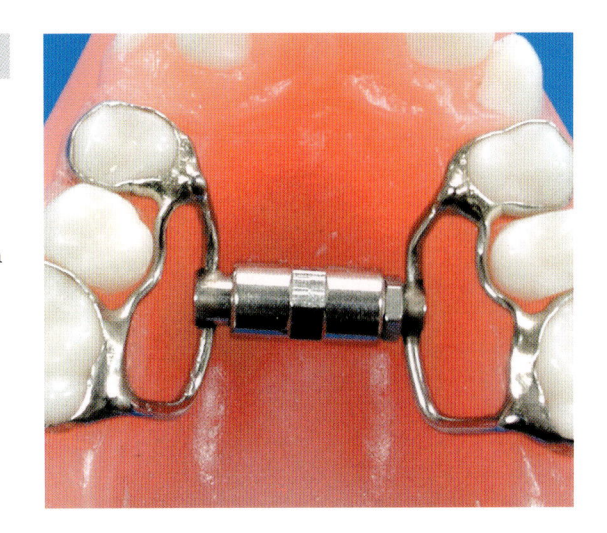

Memory Expansion Screw

The Memory Expansion screw has an internal NiTi coil spring that, when adjusted, supplies a continuous positive biologic force of about 500g over a distance of 0.8mm to 1mm. Adjustment typically involves placing three 90° turns once every three days. Many practitioners prefer this appliance over the open coil-spring RPEs.

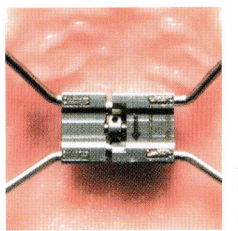

Note - The Memory Expansion screw is also available in a hyrax design.

Fixed Unilateral Developer

This unique expansion screw, when incorporated into a fixed anchorage system, will allow you to move a single molar distally on only one side of the arch. So, when space has been lost unilaterally you can easily distalize the offending molar up to 8mm.

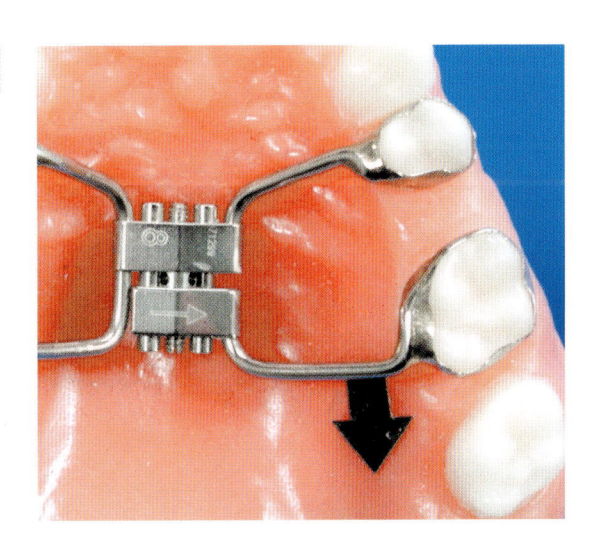

1.17

ANATOMY OF AN APPLIANCE

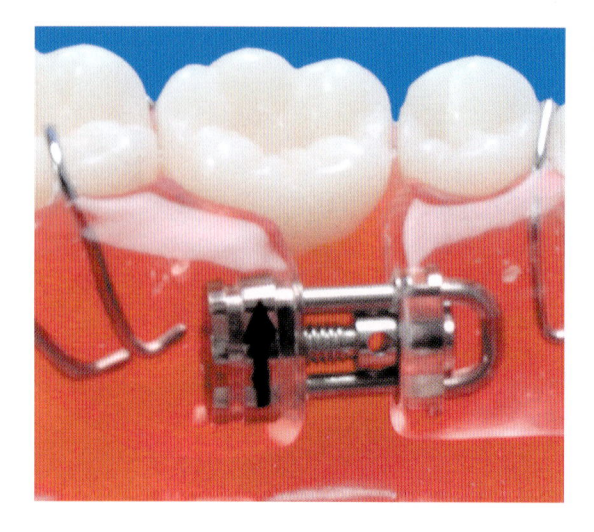

Retraction Screw

This screw is placed between two sections of acrylic in the "open" position. When activated, it then draws the two sections together to help in closing or reducing any interproximal spaces. It is commonly used for reducing modest anterior flaring or to close slight posterior interproximal spaces.

Sagittal Screw

This sectional expansion screw with its "U" shaped guide pin is used primarily to gain anterior/posterior arch length. It is available in a variety of sizes.

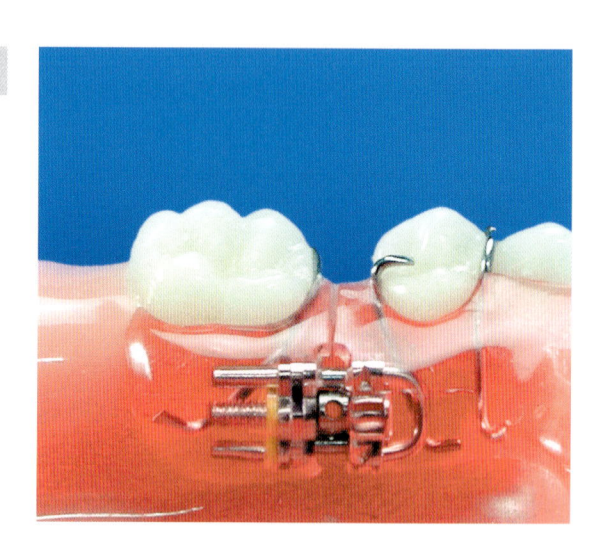

Design Notes:

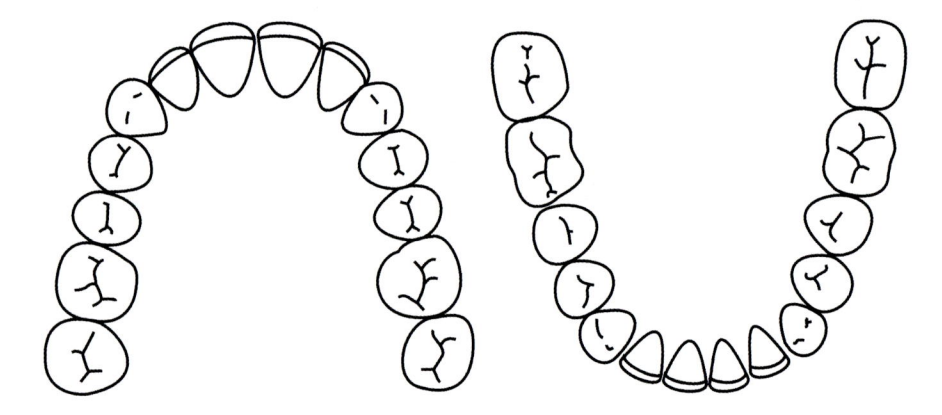

1.18

ANATOMY OF AN APPLIANCE

Active Labial Arch Wires

Although arch wires are mainly used for retention, any arch wire can be adjusted to apply enough force to cause tooth movement. This can be accomplished by retracting the whole wire or by placing a bend in a specific area to move a single tooth. Some arch wires, however, have been designed specifically to create an active force.

Apron Spring Labial (Roberts Retraction Arch Wire)

The Apron spring is an active labial arch wire that is primarily used to retract severely flared anteriors. It features two spring coils for light, continuous lingual movement and is easily activated with finger pressure.

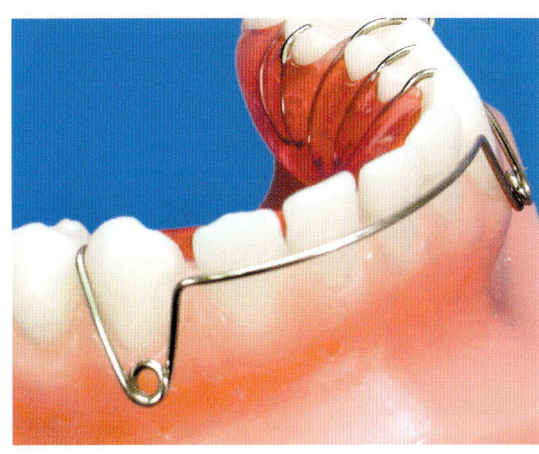

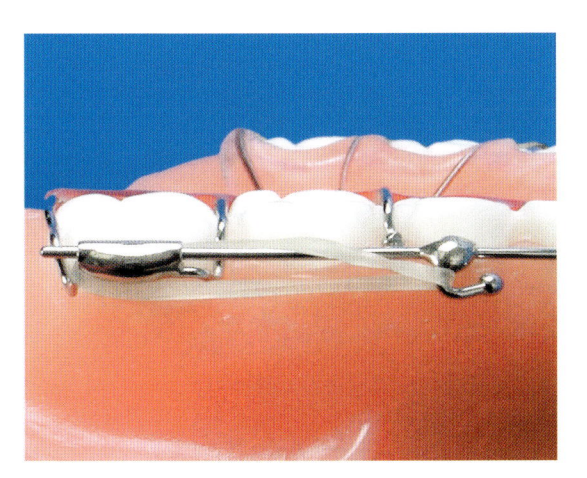

Sliding Labial

When the anteriors are not severely proclined, a sliding labial arch wire can provide a constant light lingual pressure sufficient to retract the anteriors and close up a small amount of excess space.

The amount of force is controlled by the size of the elastic stretched between the hooks on the labial wire and the tube soldered to the Adams clasps, through which it slides.

Ricketts Arch

The Ricketts arch, like the Reverse Hawley, crosses the dentition through the embrasures interproximal to the laterals and cuspids. The "U" loops are placed on the laterals and the distal recurved arms are contoured to the cuspids. These distal recurves can be used to affect minor lingual rotation of the cuspids, unilaterally or bilaterally.

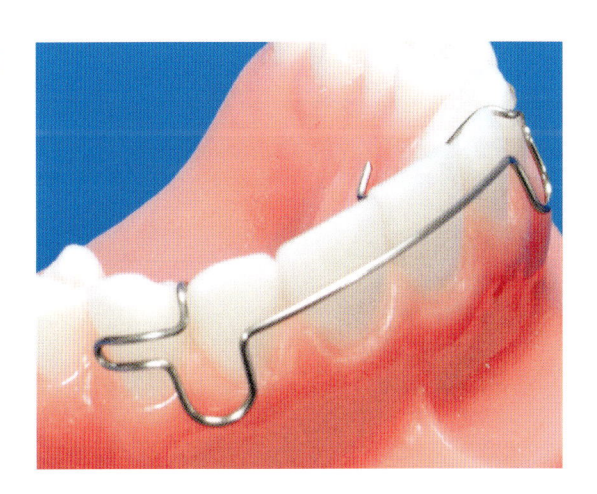

ANATOMY OF AN APPLIANCE

Acrylic Used for Active Movement

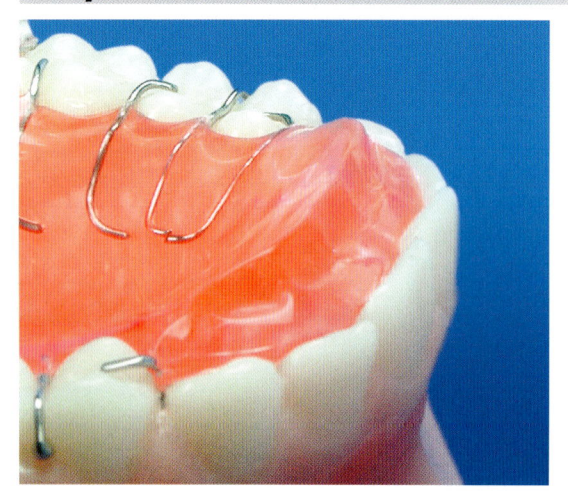

Incline Plane

An anterior incline plane is usually added to the acrylic when one wants to actively guide and maintain the mandible in a forward postured position. It is typically used when a minor skeletal correction is needed or as part of a support phase appliance during Class II treatment.

Anterior Bite Plane

Thickening the lingual acrylic behind the upper anteriors creates an anterior bite plane. This bite plane can open the vertical dimension by allowing the posterior teeth to erupt, provide clearance to correct teeth in a locked lingual crossbite, take pressure off of the anteriors in severely closed bite cases and clear the occlusion sufficiently to allow for the placement of brackets on the lower anteriors.

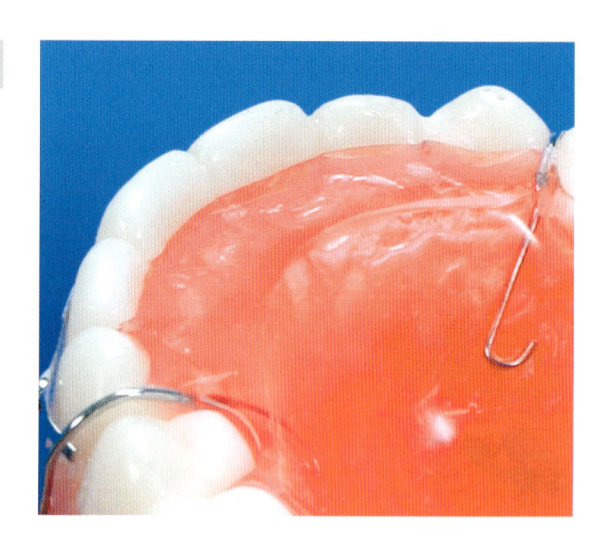

Posterior Occlusal Coverage

Posterior occlusal bite planes are mainly used to open the vertical dimension sufficiently to correct crossbites. When jumping an anterior crossbite, posterior coverage will prevent the eruption of the posterior segments controlling the development of an open bite. During the correction of a posterior crossbite, posterior coverage will allow the upper arch to be developed without dragging the lower arch along with it. By intercuspating one side, an anchorage unit can be set up that facilitates a unilateral crossbite correction.

ANATOMY OF AN APPLIANCE

Bands

A band is a thin metal strip of stainless steel that has been contoured to fit tightly around a tooth. They are usually made for molars and bicuspids and are cemented in place with a band cement. These bands are used to provide a means to attach a wire, bracket, or other auxiliary device to that tooth for anchorage or active tooth movement. There are two types of bands: custom bands and preformed bands.

Custom Bands

Your Laboratory can provide you with excellent custom fabricated bands for your fixed appliances. Using the laboratory for the indirect construction of bands affords several advantages. First, you don't have to maintain an expensive inventory of preformed bands. Second, but equally important, is the tight fit consistently obtained when bands are custom made. Bands coming loose cost you additional chair time and can extend treatment time significantly. There is also a very real probability of decay under poorly fitted bands. Well-adapted custom bands keep this problem to a minimum.

Important - In order for the laboratory to provide an excellent fitting band, it is **essential** that they receive the following:

1. An accurate model of the entire arch involved in the fixed appliance.

2. The tooth/teeth to be banded must be adequately erupted - i.e. **the clinical crown must be exposed, and the distal contour must be well defined and clearly above the tissue.** A tissue flap left over the distal occlusal surface of a tooth requires that we estimate the overall size and shape of the tooth. This may compromise the final band fit.

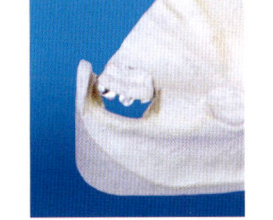

Note - The standard thickness of band material is .005". Band material is also available in .003", .004" and .006" upon request.

Preformed Bands

You are welcome to supply the lab with your own preformed bands. To use this approach, you must purchase a kit of bands with a selection of at least five sizes for each tooth you may need banded. A band is then selected and pre-fit directly on the patient, being sure to adapt it accurately and tightly.

Once this is accomplished, the band, or bands should be removed, appropriately identified and placed in a protective box or envelope prior to taking the impression. The impression should then be taken, poured immediately, allowed to set up completely, checked for accuracy, and then sent to the lab along with the Rx slip and bands.

DO NOT pour up the bands in place. Experience has shown there is a very high margin for error in this procedure. In fact, it is almost impossible to maintain the exact band position in the impression while pouring it up. If there is even the slightest movement, it is extremely hard to detect and difficult to correct in the laboratory. This will cause the appliance not to fit and you'll need to start over with new impressions.

Although it is more work, the lab would much rather take the time to accurately seat your preformed bands on your well-defined working model, thereby ensuring an excellent fit for your finished appliance.

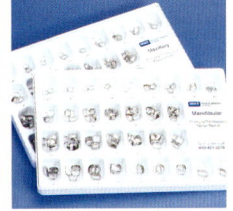

1.21

ANATOMY OF AN APPLIANCE

Brackets

A bracket is a small mechanical device that is attached to a band or direct bonded to a tooth and designed to hold an arch wire, elastic, or other auxiliary for anchorage or tooth movement. Brackets are available in stainless steel, ceramic, or plastic.

A wide variety of brackets and attachments are available that can either be spot welded to stainless steel bands or placed on metal mesh pads for direct bonding to the teeth.

The most popular varieties of the "straight-wire" (pre-torqued, pre-tipped, and pre-angulated) brackets are manufactured with the bonded base as an integral part of the bracket itself. However, should there be a need, the lab can custom make any bracket so that it is bondable directly to the tooth. Metal mesh pads are custom formed to individual teeth prior to attaching the brackets so that maximum adhesion is guaranteed.

Some examples of common brackets systems are straight wire brackets, standard edgewise brackets, Begg brackets, twin-wire brackets, molar hooks, buttons, buccal tubes, and horizontal or vertical lingual slot brackets for arch wires.

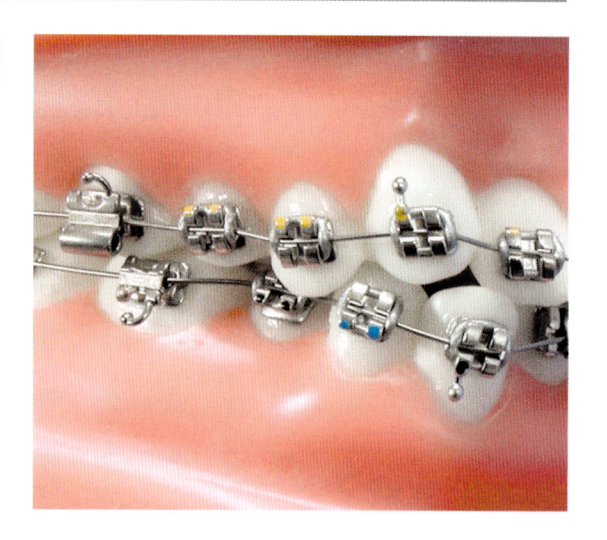

Design Notes:

1.22

ANATOMY OF AN APPLIANCE

Arch Wires

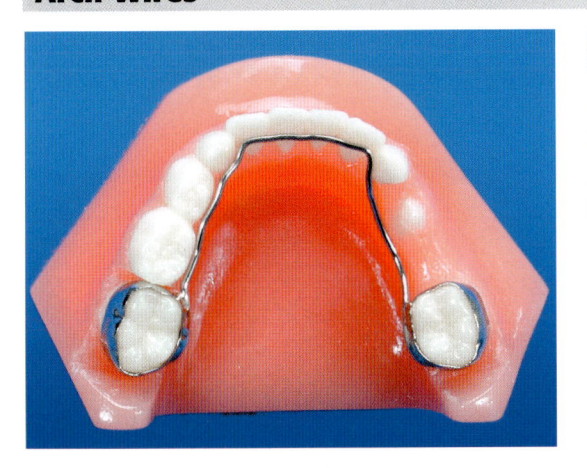

Lingual Arches

A lingual arch is a stainless steel wire that usually fits closely to the lingual surface of the teeth and is held in place by bands on the molars, bicuspids, or cuspids. Lingual arch wires can be attached to the bands in several ways:

1) For simple space maintaining devices, the arch wire can be soldered directly to the bands.

2) If the arch wire has adjustment loops, or soldered lingual lap springs, the arch wire can be attached to the molar bands with either horizontal or vertical lingual sheaths. This allows the arch wire to easily be removed and replaced when adjustments are necessary.

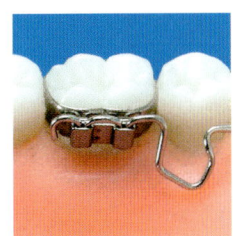

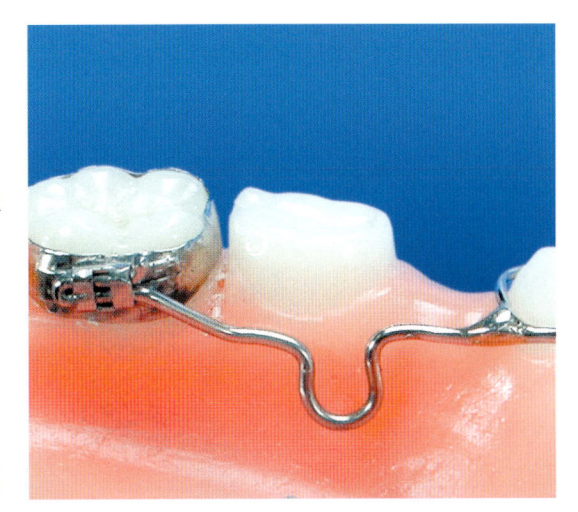

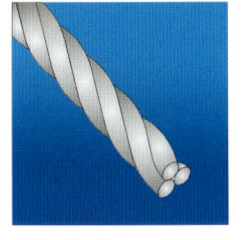

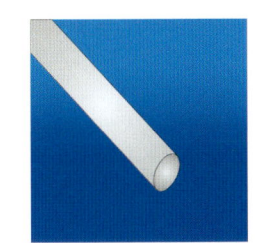

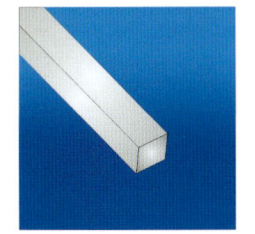

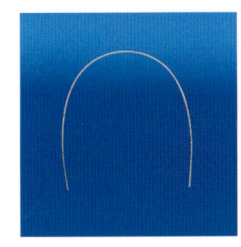

Buccal/Labial Arch Wires

Arch wires come in a variety of preformed sizes and arch forms. Selecting the appropriate type, size and arch form for each patient is a critical step for success when using fixed mechanics. Some of the factors that need to be considered when choosing an arch wire are listed here:
 1. Materials:
     Stainless steel
     Standard and heat activated nickel titanium (NiTi)
 2. Sizes:
     Range from .014mm to .022mm in round, braided, square and rectangular wire
 3. Forms: (with separate wires for the upper and lower arches)
     Tapered, Square and Ovoid

Your Laboratory should stock a complete range of arch wires for all the major techniques currently in use. They can be ordered on a per patient basis. Since new designs and improvements in performance are a common occurrence in these wires, it is usually not desirable to maintain a large inventory in the general practice.

1.23

ANATOMY OF AN APPLIANCE

Auxiliary Attachments

Several auxiliary attachments can be added to a simple fixed appliance in order to provide a variety of options as treatment progresses. In fact, almost every auxiliary that can be added to a removable appliance can be added to a fixed appliance.

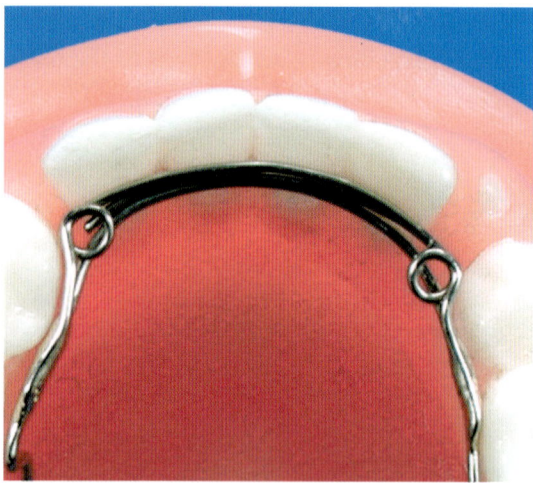

Lingual Lap Springs

Lingual lap springs can be added to align anteriors as they erupt into position.

Mesial/Distal Kicker

Mesial or distal individual kicker-springs can be added to guide teeth into their proper position as they erupt, or to tighten contacts between teeth when drifting occurs due to adjacent tooth loss.

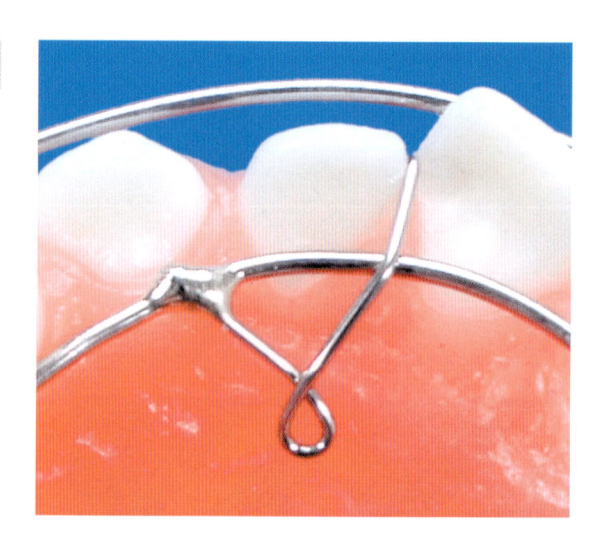

Stops

Stops, mesial or distal, can be added to a tooth to hold its position when an adjacent tooth is lost or not yet erupted. This will prevent drifting of the teeth into the edentulous space.

1.24

ANATOMY OF AN APPLIANCE

Fixed Recurve Pushers

Recurved pushers can be used for labial or buccal movements. These springs can be made with or without helical coils.

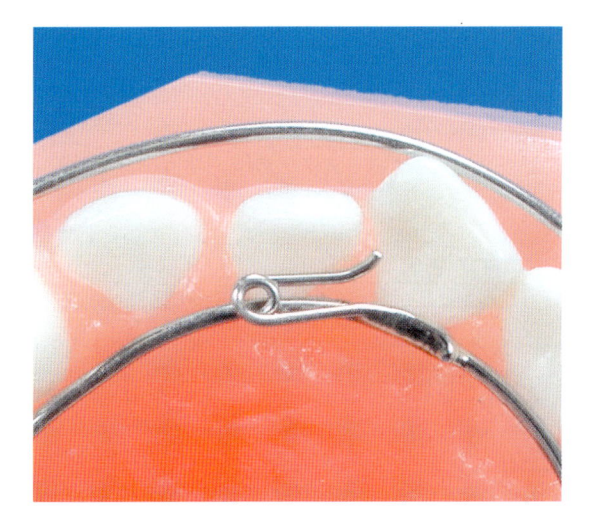

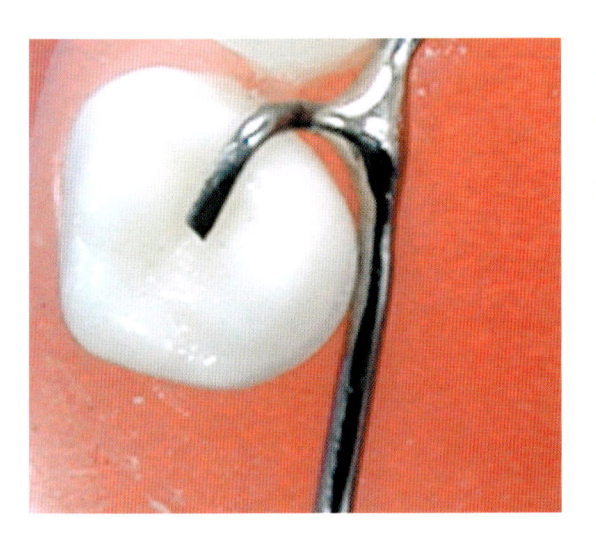

Occlusal Rest

Occlusal rests can be added to stabilize the arch wire when several edentulous areas are present. The occlusal rest can be covered with bonding material, to maximize retention of the entire appliance.

Cements

A wide variety of cements and direct-bond composites are available today. The key to success with these materials is in the application technique. In other words, for best results follow the directions exactly!

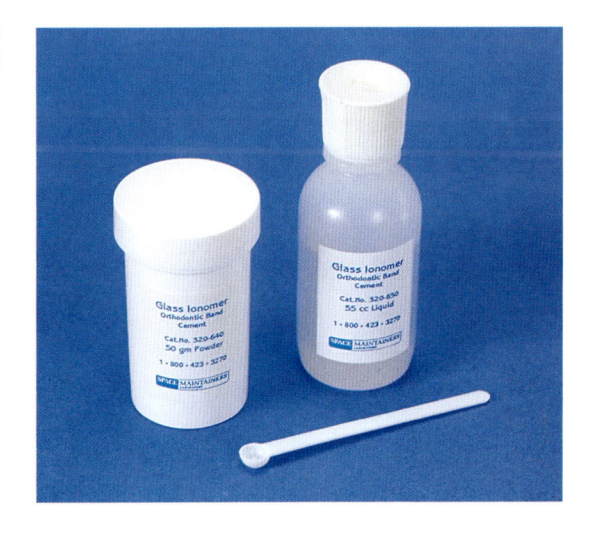

1.25

Design Notes

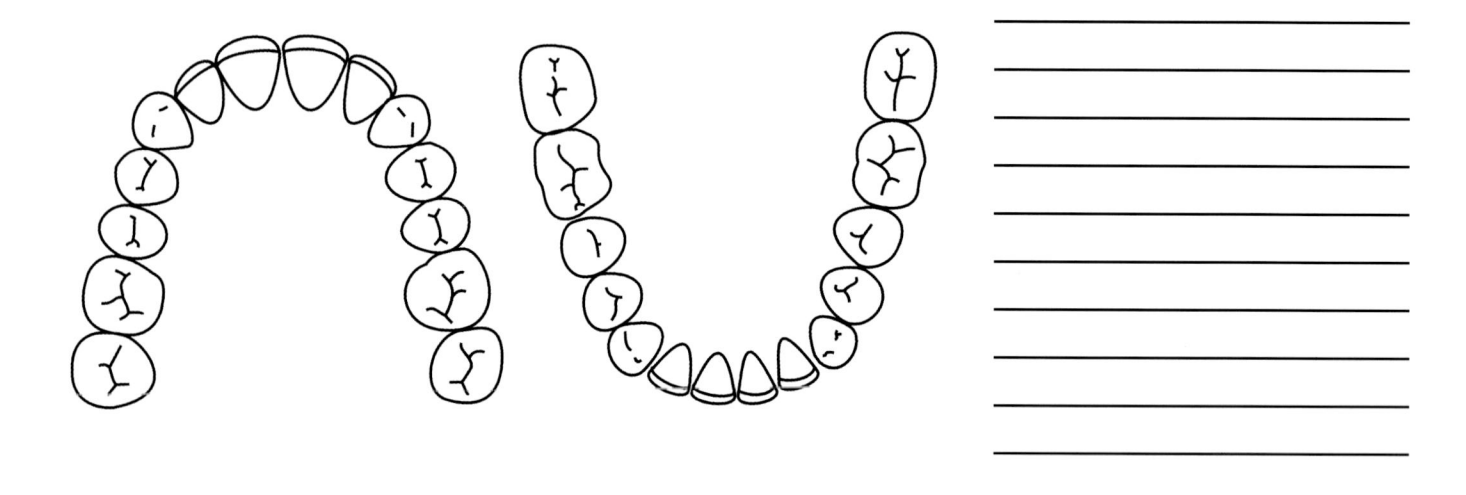

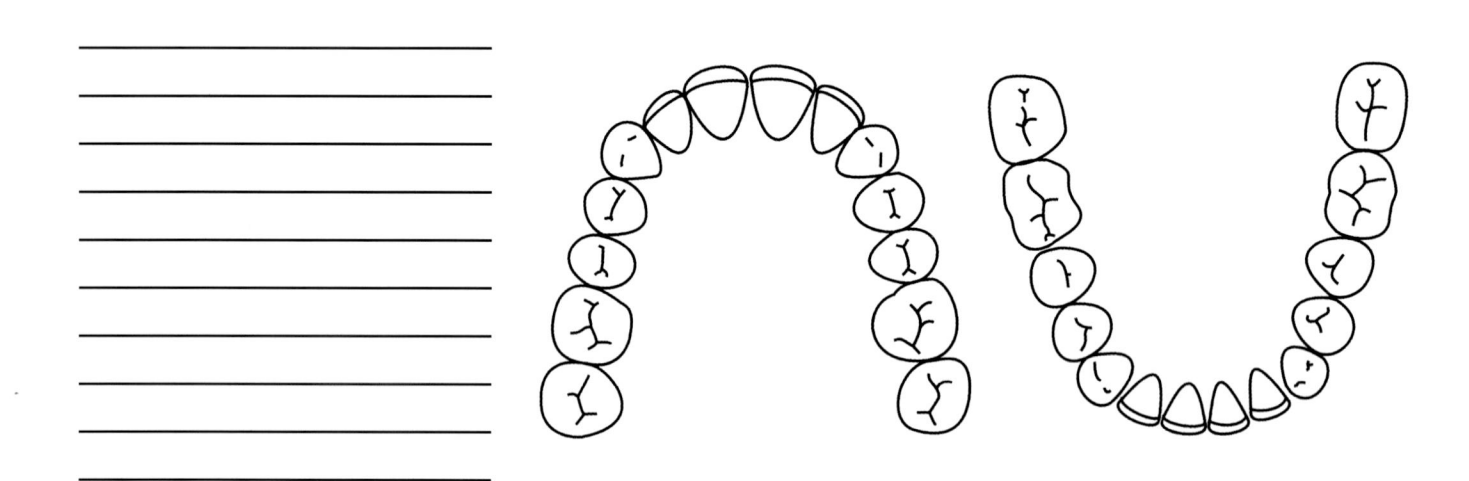

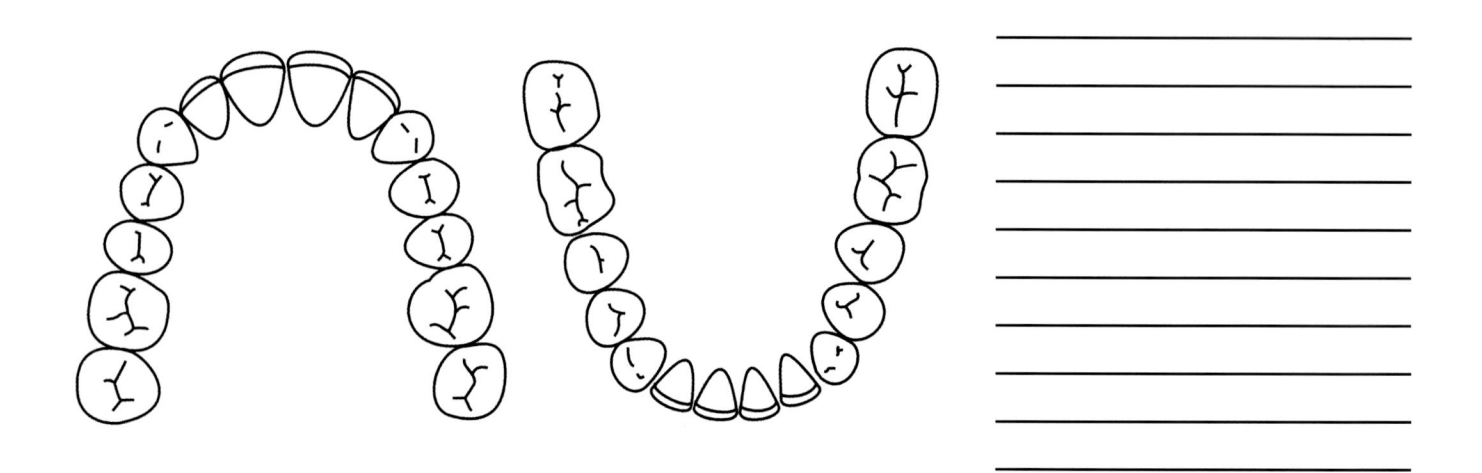

SPACE MAINTENANCE

an overview: SPACE MAINTENANCE

Chapter 2

GENERAL CONSIDERATIONS

Children

Most orthodontic problems begin during the period of time when the development of the entire masticatory apparatus, including the dental arch and occlusion, proceeds from the primary to the permanent dentition. Unfortunately, many patients do not see the orthodontic specialist during this time. This occurs because the orthodontist usually has to depend upon a referral from the general dentist.

Because the general dentist is the one who cares for the dental needs of the vast majority of growing children, it is imperative that they be able recognize growth problems as they occur. This will allow them to either actively intervene or immediately refer these patients to the orthodontist.

Although the dentition changes associated with growth and development are continuous, it is clinically very helpful to be able to classify these changes into several stages. Barnett classified the stages of occlusal development as follows:

Stages	Ages in Years	Characteristics
First stage	3	Primary dentition
Second stage	6	Eruption of the first permanent molars
Third stage	6 - 9	Exchange of the incisors
Fourth stage	9 - 12	Eruption of the cuspids and bicuspids
Fifth stage	12	Eruption of the second molars

For a smooth transition through these stages the following events must occur:

1. The eruption of the first permanent molar will be guided by the distal surface of the second primary molar. The location and arrangement of the permanent incisors will be guided by the mesial surface of the primary canine.

2. Once the permanent first molar and incisors are in the arch, (The Mixed Dentition Stage) the canine and two premolars will then erupt into the limited space between the mesial surface of the first permanent molar and the distal surface of the lateral incisor. This exchange takes about one and a half years to complete.

3. The sum of the mesio-distal widths of the primary cuspid and first and second primary molars is generally larger than that of the permanent cuspid and premolars by about 1mm per quadrant in the maxilla and about 2mm per quadrant in the mandible. This difference is called the leeway space. The leeway or extra space is a fundamental factor in allowing for an easy exchange of these teeth.

Chapter 2

4. A normal eruption sequence of the succedaneous teeth must take place in both the mandible and maxilla. In the mandible, the most frequent eruption sequence is the cuspid, first bicuspid, and second bicuspid. In the maxilla, the sequence of eruption typically seen is either the first bicuspid, second bicuspid and cuspid or first bicuspid, cuspid and second bicuspid.

5. When the second molars begin to erupt, the distal surface of the first permanent molar will guide them into the arch. In most cases, the eruptive force of the second molar will cause a reduction in the dental arch length using up the leeway space. In fact, the arch circumference of the permanent dentition may become shorter than that of the primary dental arch.

Unfortunately, a smooth transition through these stages is often disrupted by the premature loss of teeth. Tooth decay, trauma from a fall, or some other accidental injury are just some of the common reasons teeth are lost early. When this occurs, pediatric space management is the key to preventing a serious malocclusion in the permanent dentition. In the posterior quadrants, the early loss of primary teeth often results in a reduction of arch length. This change can directly affect the normal eruption of the adult teeth. If space loss has not already occurred, rapid intervention with a space-maintaining appliance is of utmost importance. In the anterior region space maintenance is important to maintain normal speech, function, and esthetics.

Adults

Proper space management is important for the adult patient in a variety of situations. During active restorative treatment, there is often a need for an interim appliance to maintain space. For example, an interim space maintainer is often used in young patients who, because of an accident, rampant caries, or hereditary partial anodontia, are missing either anterior or posterior teeth. Other indications for an interim space maintainer seen in the general practice on a daily basis are:

- to maintain space.
- to re-establish occlusion.
- to replace visible missing teeth while definitive restorative procedures are being accomplished.
- to serve while the patient is undergoing periodontal or other prolonged treatment.
- when healing is progressing after an extraction or a traumatic injury.
- to maintain function while accomplishing minor tooth movement.

These are covered in detail in the sections on partials/bridges and restorative enhancement appliances.

Design Notes

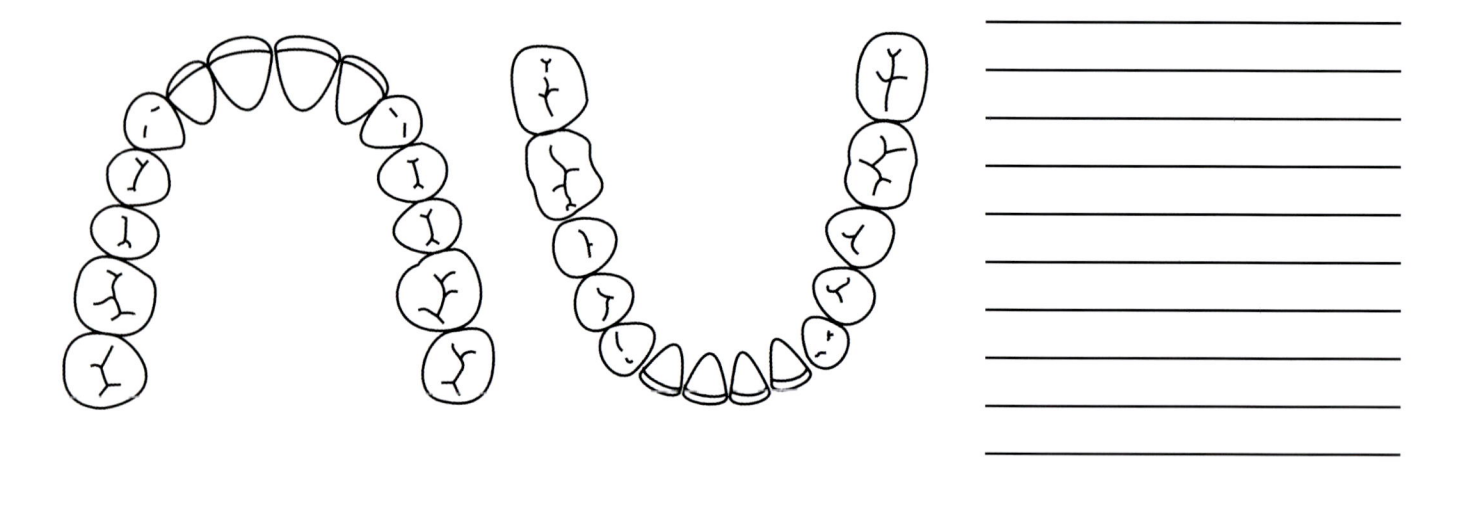

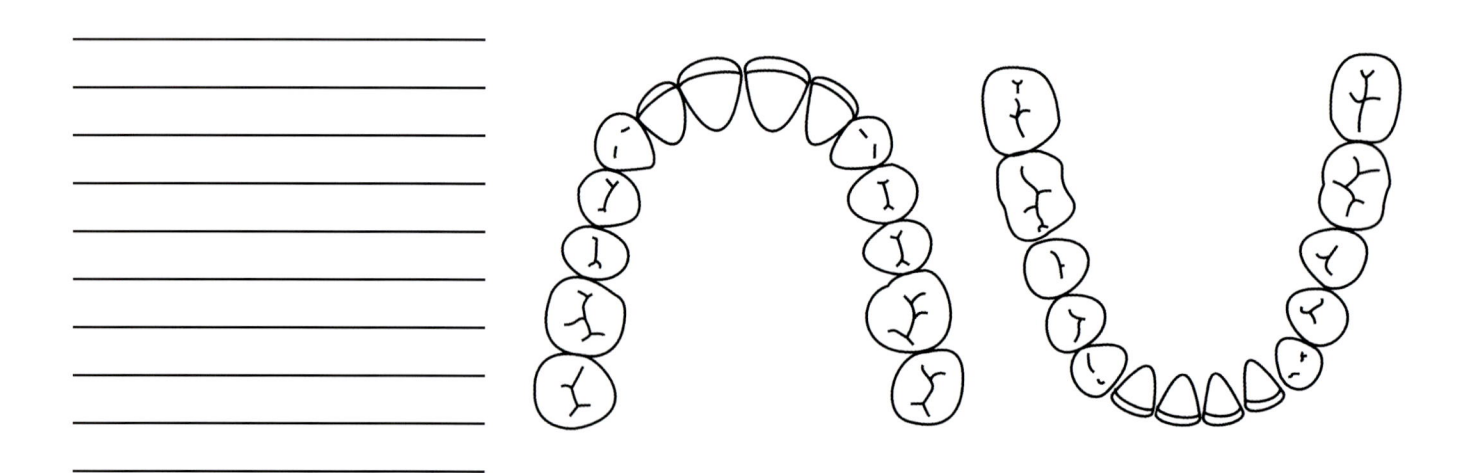

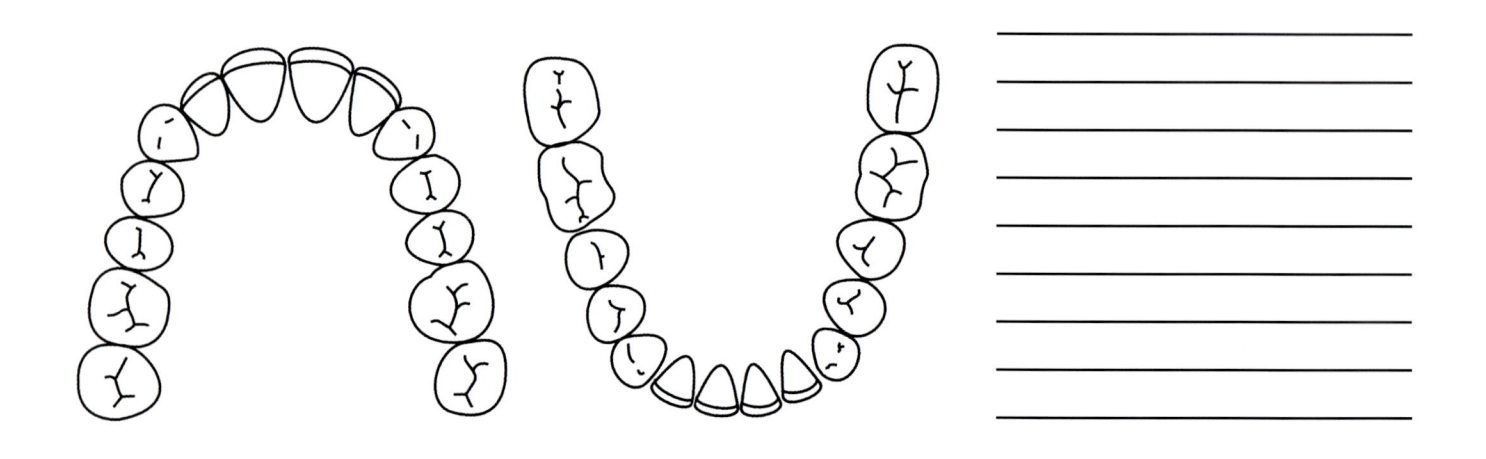

SPACE MAINTENANCE

2011 The Space Maintainer   U/L

Early loss of a primary molar often allows the adult first molar to tip and move mesially. The basic unilateral space maintainer is used for holding molar position.

Note - The forces during eating can cause this space maintainer to move gingivally at the loop. This can cause tissue irritation and will allow the banded molar to tip mesially. A better choice would be appliance #2012 or #2072.

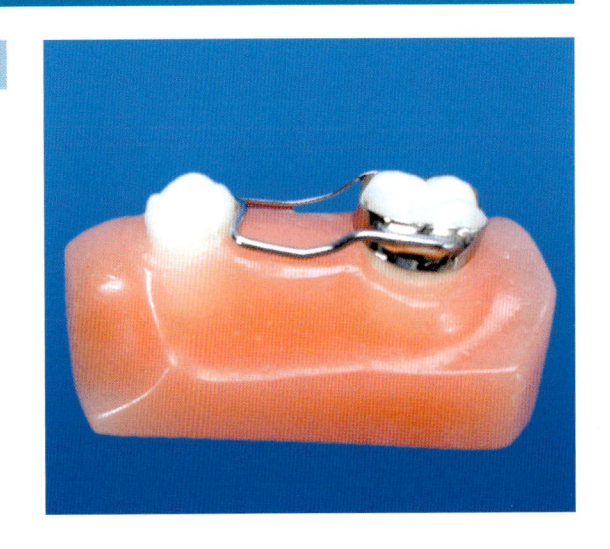

2012 Modified Space Maintainer   U/L

The early loss of a primary second molar often allows the adult first molar to tip and move mesially. This modified unilateral space maintainer features an occlusal rest on the adjacent tooth. The occlusal rest will prevent the forces of mastication from moving the loop gingivally.

Note - Sometimes it will be necessary to prepare a rest seat in the supporting tooth to keep the occlusion clear of any interference. Also, added retention can be gained by bonding the rest into position with composite resin.

2012B Bonded Spacer   U/L

When a tooth is not fully erupted, making a custom band for it is impossible and selecting a preformed band that is going to fit is almost as difficult. However, it still may be possible to place a space maintainer if a sufficient amount of tooth structure is exposed to place an all-bonded unilateral spacer like the one shown here.

This appliance is bonded to both the buccal and lingual surface of the partially erupted molar. When the other abutment tooth has a well-defined occlusal surface, a simple wire rest will suffice. Otherwise, bonding with a direct-bond pad as illustrated in the insert photo, is recommended.

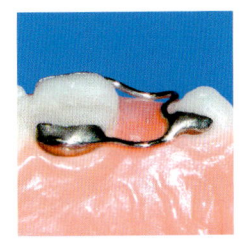

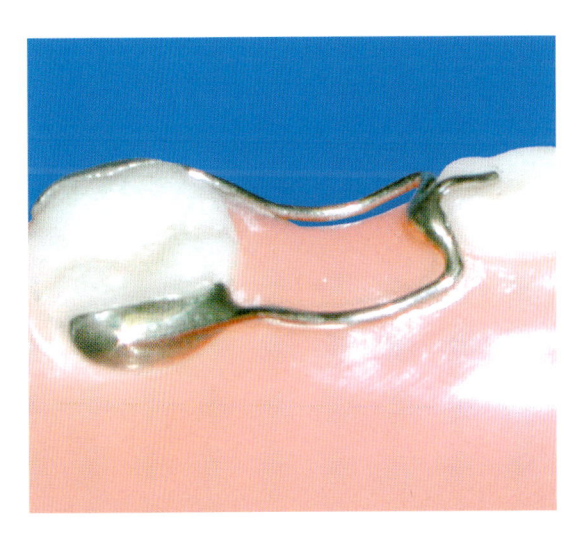

SPACE MAINTENANCE

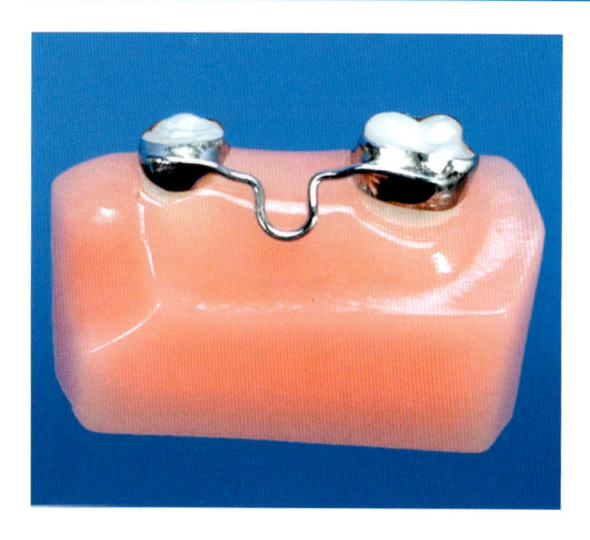

2013 Buccal Bar   U/L

Two bands and a buccal bar are used for maintaining space where a long span prohibits the use of a basic space maintainer. Slight adjustment of the loop makes this appliance useful when the path of insertion is not parallel between the abutment teeth. Adjustment of the loop after insertion will allow you to regain a small amount of lost space.

2014 Occlusal Bar   U/L

This two-band space maintainer with an occlusal bar is designed to prevent super-eruption of the opposing teeth. This cleansable design allows patients to easily maintain their oral hygiene. However, be sure the banded teeth have a parallel path of insertion before prescribing this appliance.

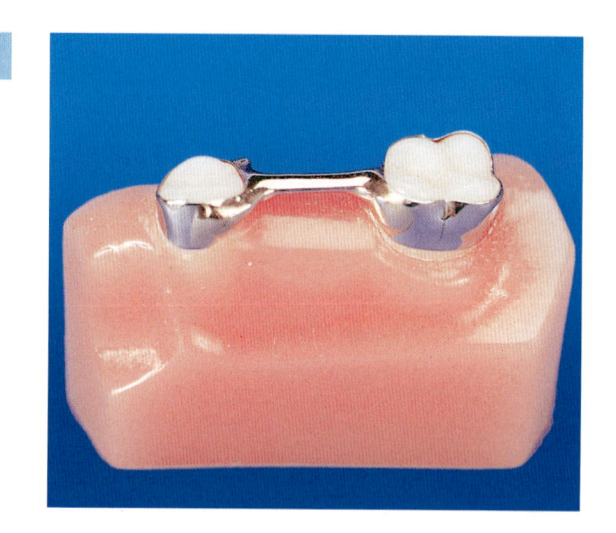

Note - To place the occlusal bar in the ideal position, the laboratory must be supplied with an opposing model and a bite relationship.

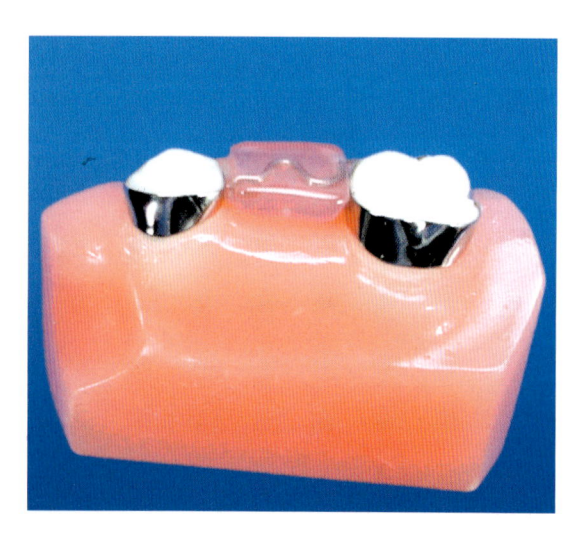

2023 Occlusal Pad   U/L

This two-band space maintainer has an acrylic pad over the edentulous region. It is designed with the occlusal surface of the pad in function with the opposing teeth and the tissue side cleared away to eliminate any interference with the normal eruption of the succedaneous teeth. Before choosing this design, be sure the teeth to be banded have a parallel path of insertion.

Note - This appliance can act as a food trap. This can be controlled easily with the use of an oral irrigator.

SPACE MAINTENANCE

2021 Crown and Loop   U/L

A crown may be used in conjunction with a space maintainer. Although a crown can be fitted to a model of the prepared tooth, it is always better to furnish the lab with a prepared crown of your choice. As with the other unilateral space maintainers, an occlusal rest on the adjacent tooth will prevent unwanted mesial tipping of the molar.

Note - When taking an impression for this appliance, it is best to take the impression with the crown in place. Then, pour the impression with the crown firmly seated in the impression.

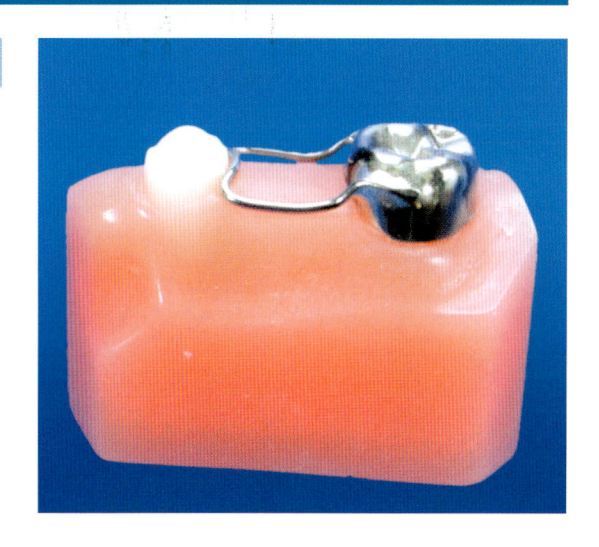

2021R Crown and Loop - with rest   U/L

When your treatment plan requires that a crown and loop space maintainer be used for an extended period of time, it is suggested that the appliance include a rest on the abutment tooth to prevent unwanted mesial movement and tipping. Sometimes it will be necessary to prepare a rest seat in the supporting tooth to keep the occlusion clear of any interference. Added retention can also be gained by bonding the rest into position with composite resin.

Note - When taking an impression for this appliance, it is best to take the impression with the crown in place. Then, pour the impression with the crown firmly seated in the impression.

2022 Distal Shoe   U/L

A single band with a distal extension that is placed through the tissue can be used to guide the eruption of the six-year molar when the primary second molar has been lost prematurely. To accomplish this, you must send an x-ray or mark the mesial edge of the six-year molar on the model for correct placement of the guide. Also, indicate the desired depth of the shoe that will extend beneath the tissue to contact the erupting tooth.

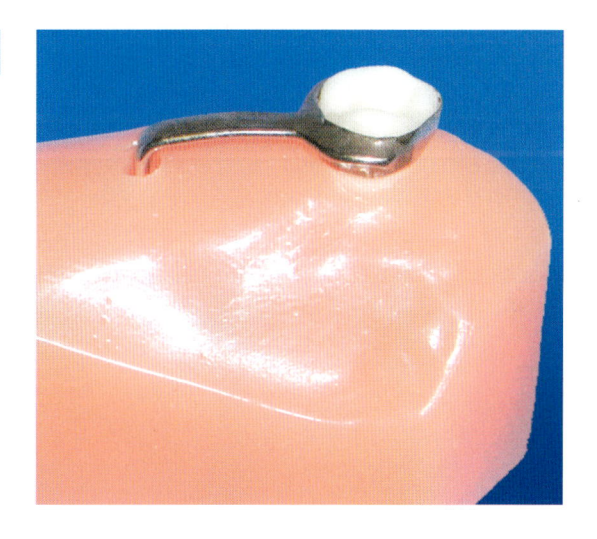

SPACE MAINTENANCE

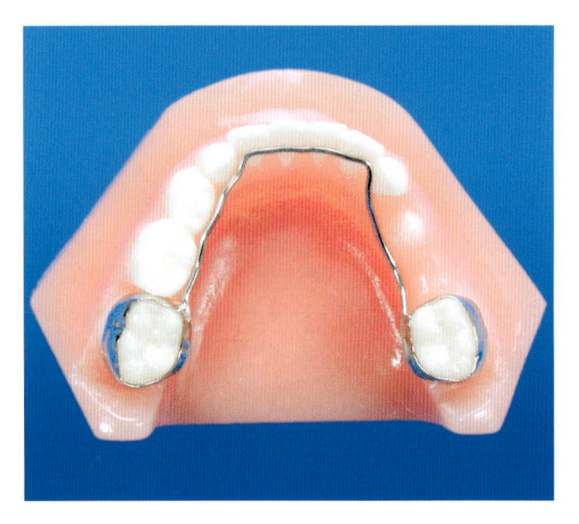

2072 Lingual Arch   U/L

The Lingual Arch is considered the "appliance of choice" to maintain arch length even when the space to be maintained is unilateral. This simple retainer prevents both mesial and lingual tipping of the molars while maintaining the arch length. The most common design is composed of an arch wire soldered to two bands. When prescribing this appliance, please indicate clearly if you have a wire placement preference on the lingual of the anterior teeth.

2016 Lingual Arch with Stops   U/L

When a primary cuspid is lost prematurely, the anteriors can shift into its position. This causes a loss of arch length in that area. This can be prevented with the use of a lingual arch wire with stops. In the design shown here, loops have also been added to the arch wire. These loops allow the doctor to adjust the length of the arch wire to gain a small amount of arch length.

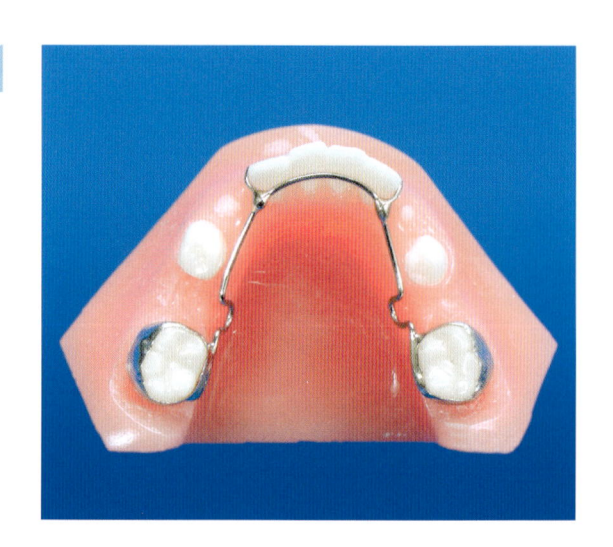

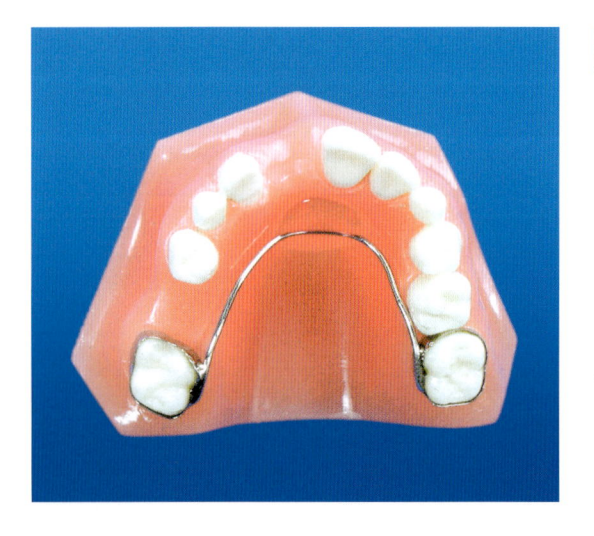

2025 The Nance   U

The Nance appliance is designed to prevent arch length loss by maintaining the position of the maxillary molars. To accomplish this, it uses an acrylic button in the pre-maxillary region of the palate to add stability. This design is also frequently used during full banding and bracketing to create an anchorage unit.

Note - This appliance must be monitored carefully as the acrylic pad can act as a food trap. Left unresolved, the pad could actually become embedded in the tissue. This can easily be controlled with the use of an oral irrigator.

SPACE MAINTENANCE

2026 Transpalatal   U

This appliance is used to hold the position of the maxillary molars, maintain the leeway space, and prevent molar extrusion when the patient is in the transitional stage of development. By using a wire that follows the vault of the palate, the possibility of a lingual arch wire interfering with the normal eruption of one of the bicuspids is eliminated. The appliance is comfortable and does not interfere with normal speech.

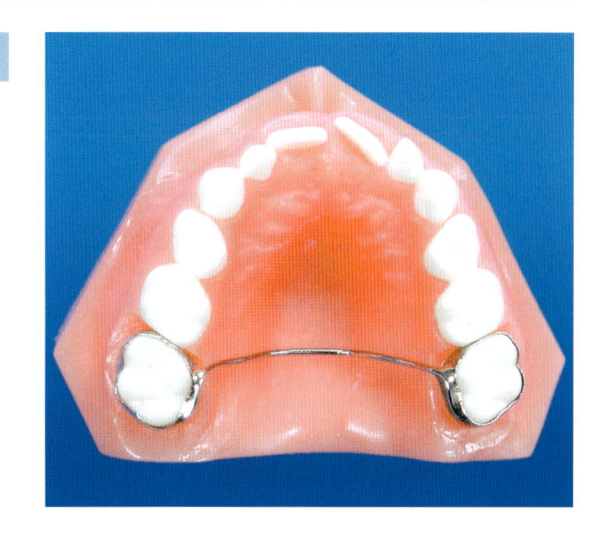

2026A Transpalatal with Omega Loop   U

By adding a mid-palatal Omega loop to the standard transpalatal design, this appliance not only acts as an anchor, but when carefully activated can be used to rotate, torque, distalize or intrude the molars. Adjustment techniques are available upon request.

2133 Removable Lingual   U/L

Special attachments to the bands permit the construction of a lingual arch wire that is removable for easy adjustment of the loops or for adding attachments. Pictured here is a horizontal attachment that allows the doctor to remove the wire in a mesial direction.

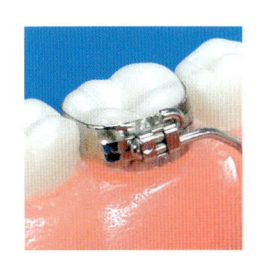

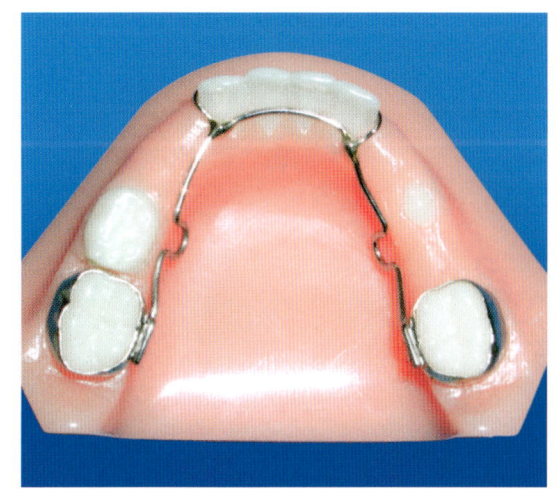

2.5

SPACE MAINTENANCE

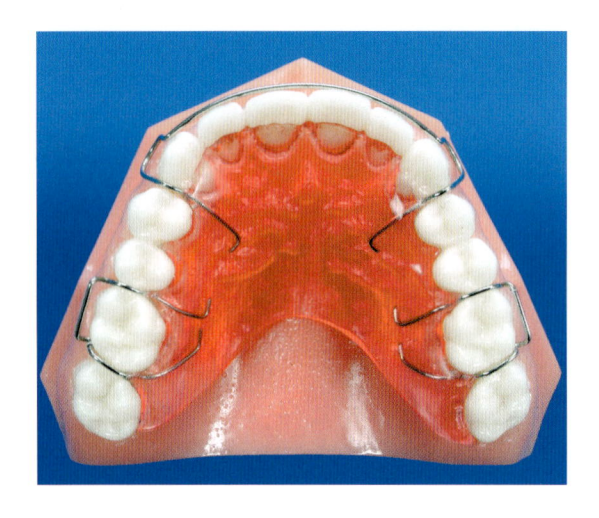

1161 Maxillary Final Retainer   U

When you have a cooperative patient, a removable retainer is an excellent way to maintain space. The basic Hawley retainer features Adams clasps on the first molars and a standard, tightly adapted Hawley type labial arch wire running from the distal of both cuspids. The acrylic should be well adapted to the palate and the lingual aspect of the teeth. Also, every effort should be made to keep it thin for comfort. Don't forget to let your patient choose a color or design. It's a great way to motivate your younger patients.

Note - Always send the lab both upper and lower casts along with a bite relationship for fabrication of this appliance.

1162 Simple Mandibular Retainer   L

Shown here is a simple mandibular removable retainer. This basic Hawley has the standard Hawley type labial arch wire. Adams clasps and rests are placed on the molars for posterior stability and to keep the appliance from over-seating into the tissue.

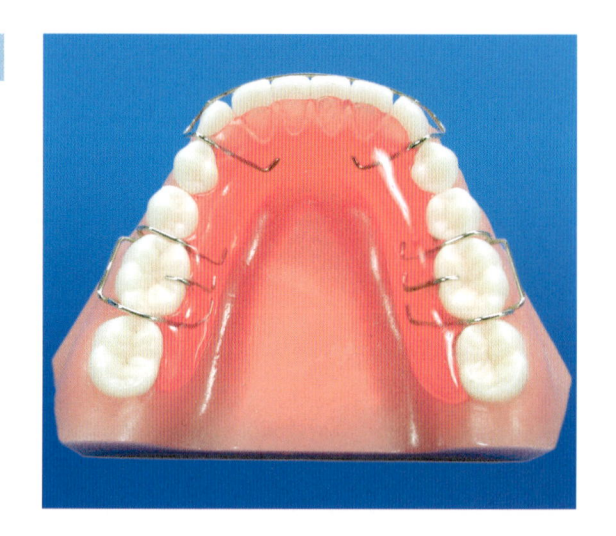

Note - Always send the lab both upper and lower casts along with a bite relationship for fabrication of this appliance.

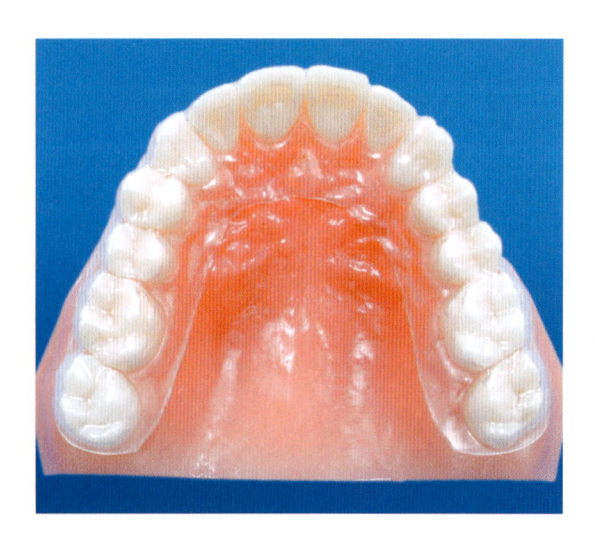

1116E - Essix   U/L

The Essix retainer is a popular retainer for the extremely appearance-conscious patient. It is fabricated by thermoforming a thin sheet of Essix material over the entire arch. Essix material is made of a clear acrylic that is tough, stain and abrasive resistant and has the light-reflecting properties to make the teeth appear brilliant when the retainer is in place. The appliance, as illustrated here, covers the buccal, labial, and lingual surfaces and extends onto the gingival tissue.

Note - Please provide a detailed description when ordering this appliance if you have a specific finish line in mind.

SPACE MAINTENANCE

2502 Wilson 3D® Lingual Arch   L

The Wilson 3D® system has special attachments to the bands that permit the lingual arch to be removed in a vertical direction. The 3D® Lingual Arch wire is a very versatile modular component. The adjustment loops in the wire (referred to as "activators") make this lingual arch much more than just an arch length space-maintaining device. The activator is a diamond-shaped loop that is easily adjusted with a flat-on-round light wire plier. Proper adjustment of the activator loops can provide a number of different movements such as: anterior-posterior arch length increase, buccal expansion, distal molar movement, molar torque or tip, and molar rotation. The adjustments, and the directional movements possible, are superbly described and illustrated in the Enhanced Orthodontics Mechanotherapy Manual available from RMO or Space Maintainers.

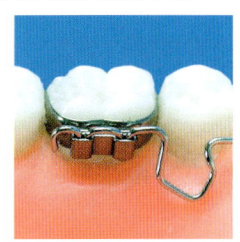

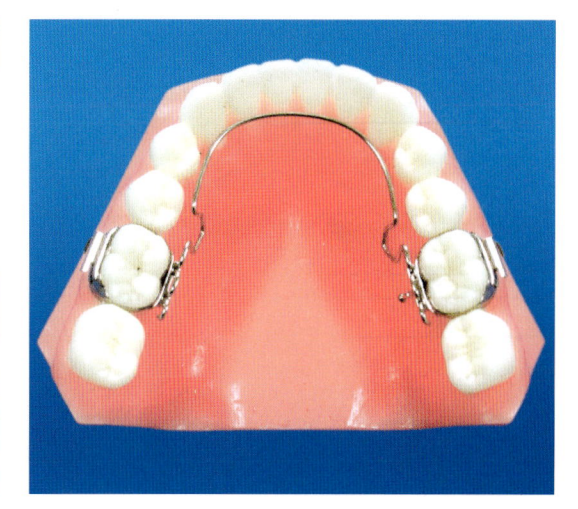

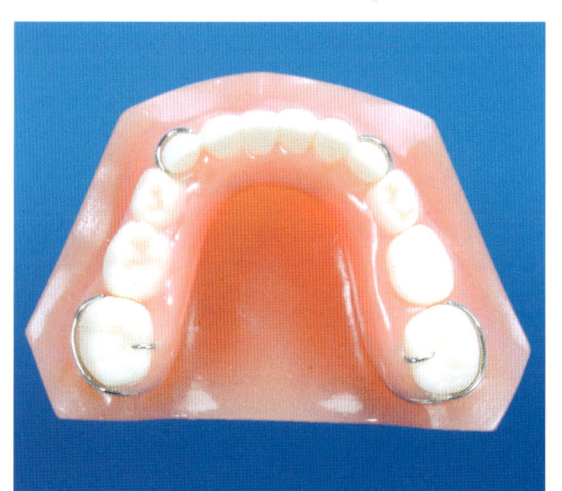

4173A Lower Pedo Partial   L

Four 'C' type clasps provide the retention for this removable partial. Any number of teeth may be replaced. However, as with all bridges and partials, an opposing model and bite registration are necessary for proper construction. As the permanent teeth erupt, an acrylic bur may be used to remove the acrylic pontics.

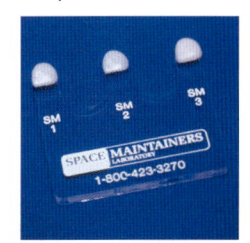

4173B Upper Pedo Partial   U

This removable appliance features replacement teeth for the four primary anteriors. It is often called a "flipper" because patients tend to play with it, flipping it in and out. This can easily be avoided by creating extra retention with a combination of additional clasps and/or direct bonded buttons as shown in the insert photo. However, patient cooperation is essential when using removable pedo partials. If cooperation is questionable, we recommend using a fixed approach.

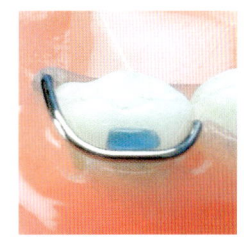

Note - As with all bridges and partials, opposing models and a bite registration are necessary for proper construction.

2.7

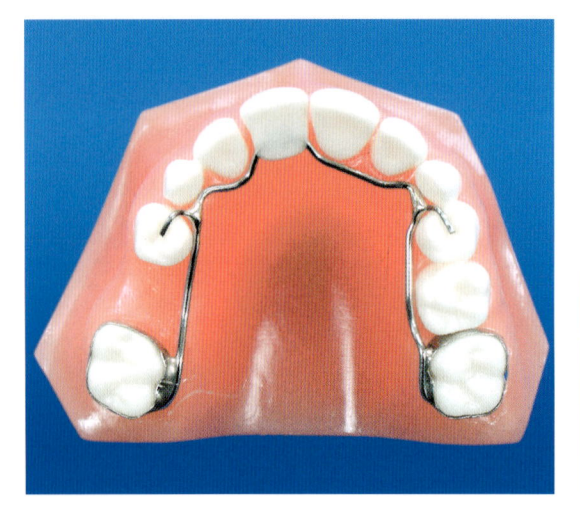

SPACE MAINTENANCE

4172 Fixed Banded Temporary Anterior Bridge U/L

By utilizing bands on the molars or premolars and a lingual arch wire, an esthetically pleasing temporary fixed anterior space maintainer may be constructed. Each anterior tooth (up to four) is fitted to a wire that has been soldered to the arch wire. Acrylic is then applied to bond them into a single unit. Primary or adult replacement teeth are available in the appropriate Bioform™ and Vita shades. This appliance can give the patient very pleasing esthetics, but requires extra care as it is vulnerable to distortion and breakage.

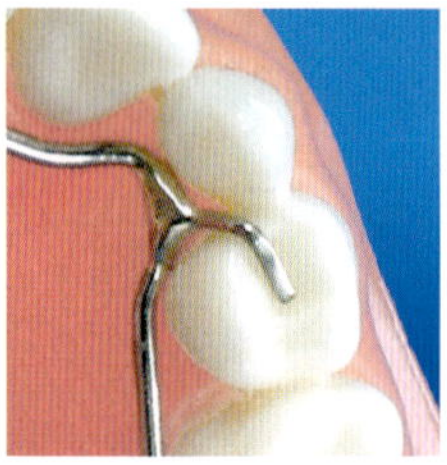

Note - We recommend that you always prepare rest seats in the supporting teeth. This will allow you to bond the occlusal rests into position, gaining extra retention while keeping the occlusion clear of any interference.

4210 Pedo Bridge   U/L

This patient-pleasing fixed appliance can accommodate up to four primary replacement teeth attached to a maxillary lingual arch. Each tooth is individually reinforced to prevent breakage, which can be a problem with this design. Placing rest seats and bonding rests into place will prevent the patient from bending or breaking the appliance.

Note - As with all bridges and partials, opposing models and a bite registration are necessary for proper construction.

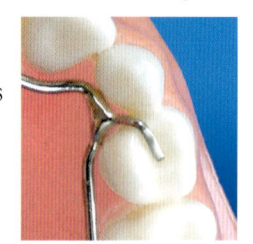

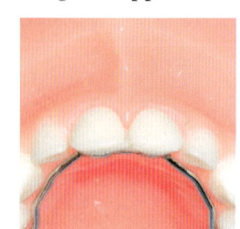

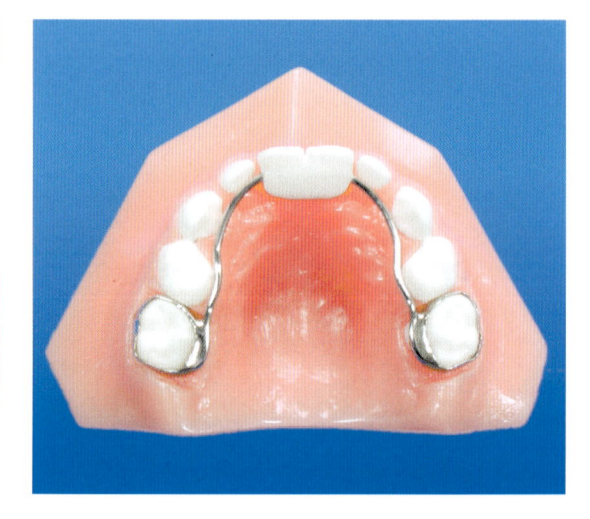

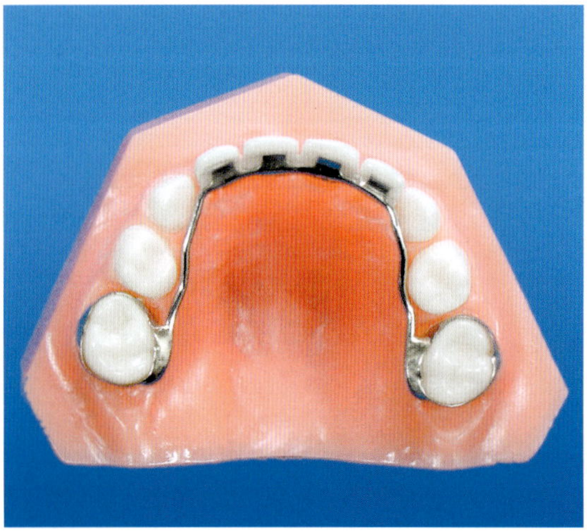

4310 Groper Fixed Anterior Bridge   U/L

Esthetics and strength are the key advantages to this popular design. The anterior bridge is made extra strong by attaching each tooth separately to a specially designed, stainless steel pad. Each unit is then welded and soldered to the arch wire. Placing rest seats and bonding rests into place will prevent the patient from bending or breaking the appliance.

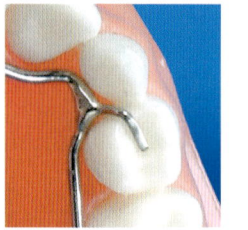

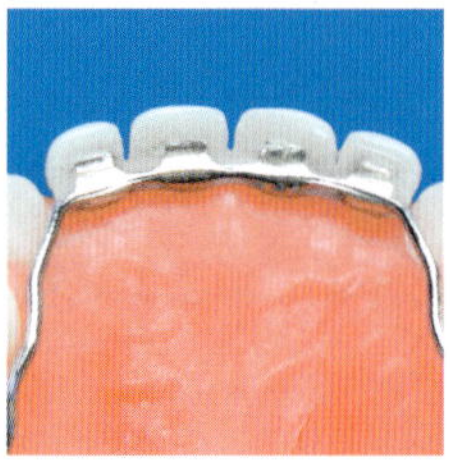

Note - As with all bridges and partials, opposing models and a bite registration are necessary for proper construction.

SPACE MAINTENANCE

4310C Groper Fixed Anterior Bridge - with crowns U/L

This appliance is the same as #2017 but utilizes stainless steel crowns in the place of bands on the molars. This design is often used when the abutment teeth are partially compromised, or when superior strength of the overall appliance is desired. Additional stability can be achieved by adding rests to the lingual wire and then bonding them to the lingual surface of the primary cuspids or first primary molars. This is particularly useful for patients who tend to be tough on their appliances.

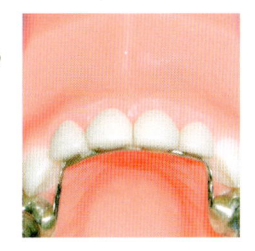

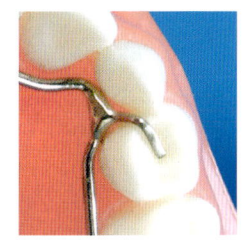

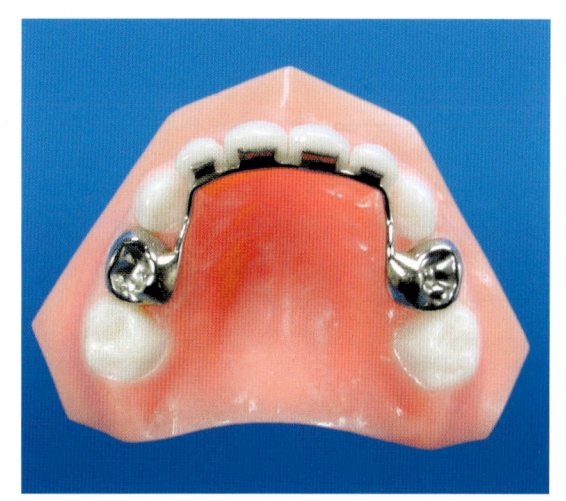

Important - When taking an impression for this appliance, it is best to take the impression with the crowns in place. Then, pour the impression with the crowns firmly seated in the impression and check the poured-up model for accuracy before sending to the lab.

Note - As with all bridges and partials, opposing models and a bite registration are necessary for proper construction.

Design Notes:

2.9

Design Notes

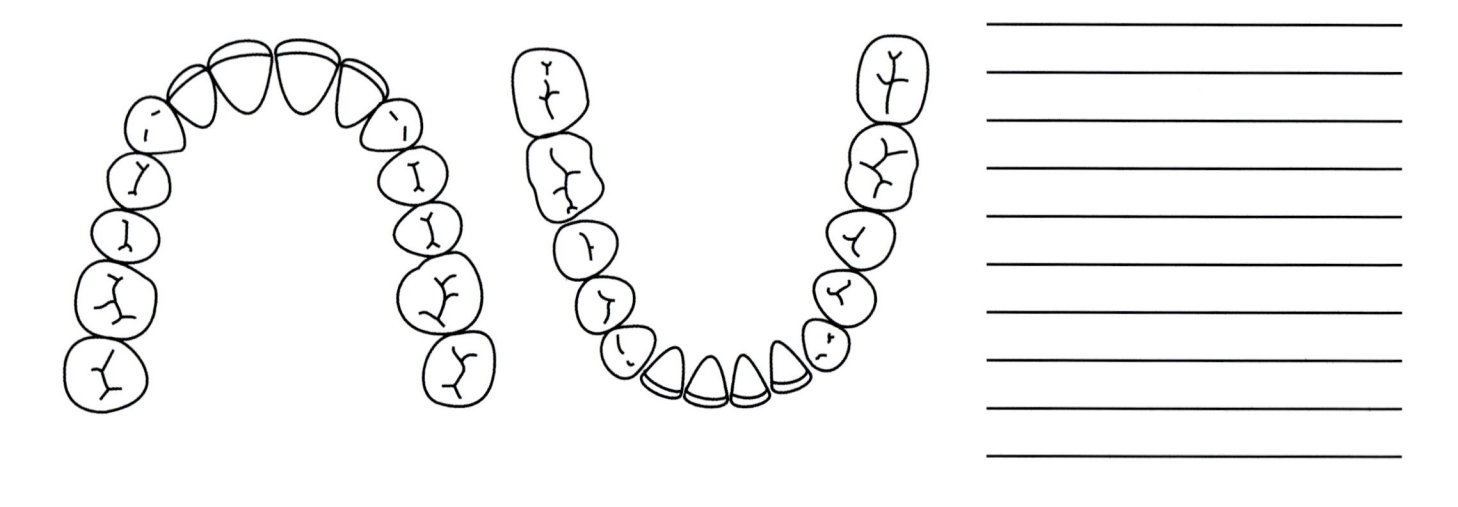

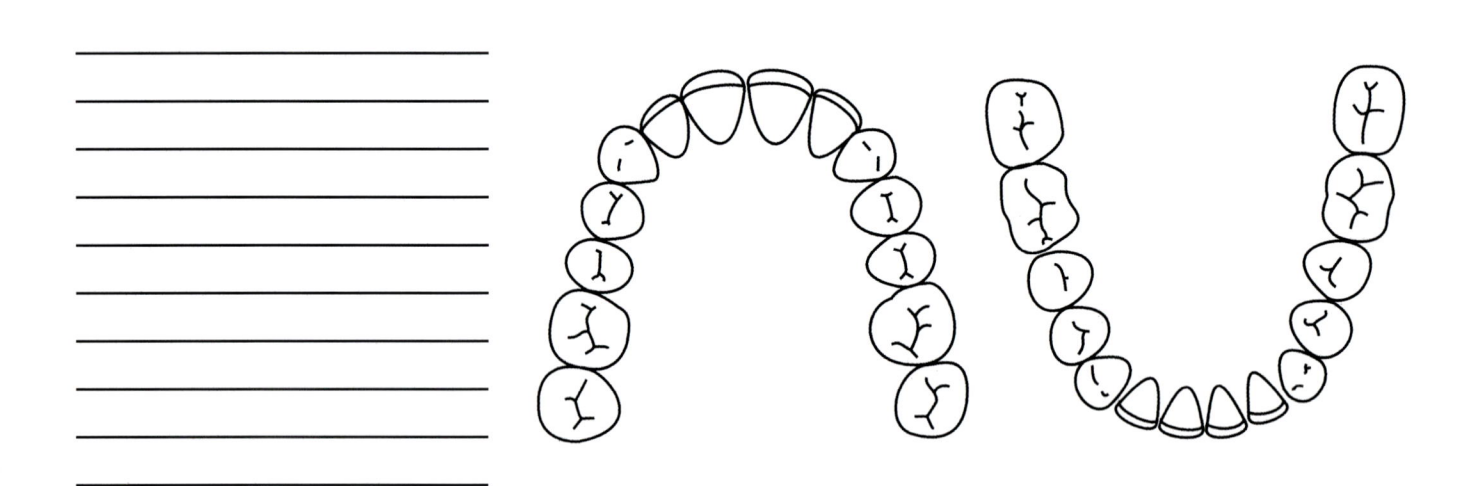

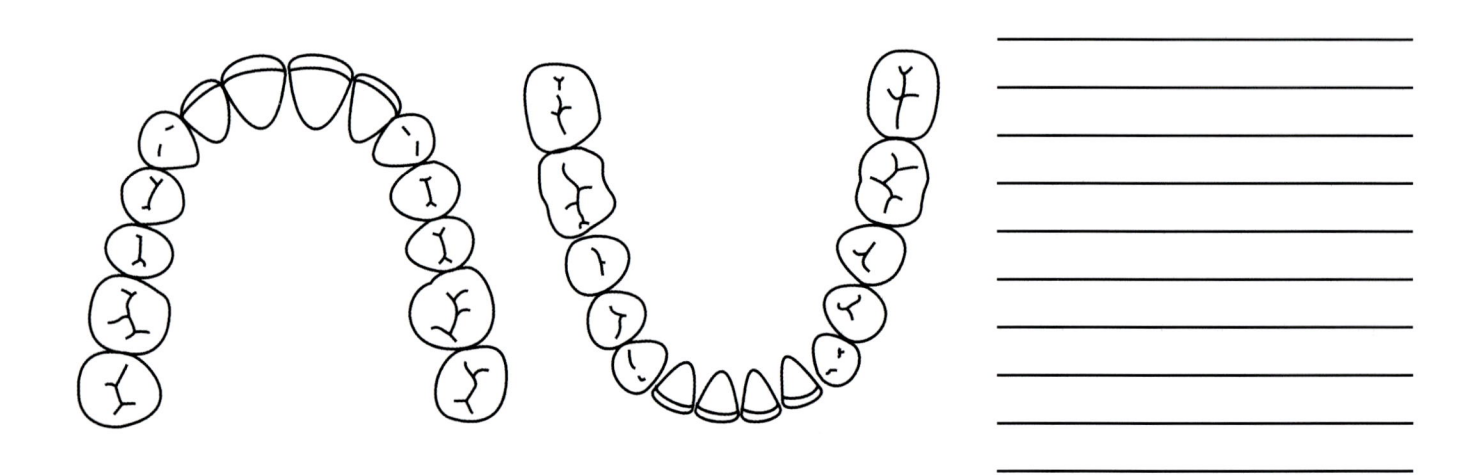

HABITS

an overview: HABITS

Chapter 3

Children

The existence of an oral habit should be noted during the clinical examination of a child. If this habit is creating an abnormal skeletal pattern or occlusal scheme, appliance intervention is usually indicated. However, the child must want to stop the habit. To achieve success, the child's cooperation and willingness to work with the dentist is essential.

Habits can be responsible for a number of orthopedic and orthodontic problems and should be addressed as soon as they are recognized. When treated immediately most of the problems caused by a habit can be reversed. However when no intervention occurs a serious malocclusion is inevitable.

For example, a thumb or finger habit can initially cause facial movement of the upper incisors and lingual movement of the lower incisors. Left untreated, it can lead to a canted maxilla and the creation of a skeletal anterior open bite, a constricted maxilla, a posterior crossbite and a skeletal Class II relationship.

Lip biting and lip sucking of the lower lip can cause the maxillary incisors to tip labially and the mandibular incisors to tip lingually. Over time this can lead to a significant increase in the amount of overjet. Biting or sucking the upper lip can actually inhibit the normal development of the pre-maxilla.

Although the etiology of a tongue thrust is often debated, the need to address the problem early is not. If a thrusting pattern remains past the age of 4 to 5, there is an increasing likelihood that this pattern will remain. An untreated tongue thrust can do great damage to the developing arches. The most common result of a tongue thrust is the creation of an anterior open bite with flared anteriors. A retruded mandible and posterior crossbite may also accompany this condition. Even the child's speech patterns can be negatively affected.

Nocturnal grinding or bruxism can occur in children. Grinding or bruxing is usually a sign of an existing malocclusion. Breaking the habit usually involves alleviating the cause. For example, a child with a narrow upper arch who hits abnormally in the cuspid region can usually be treated easily with a simple expansion appliance. Once the interference is removed, the grinding will usually stop. Bruxism can also be an indicator that a patient is suffering from an airway problem, as there is a clear correlation between children who grind their teeth and those who snore.

Rarely, with the exception of a physically or mentally challenged individual, is the problem severe enough to cause serious dental problems. If excessive wear becomes apparent, the use of a splint or an orthopedic appliance may be indicated. These appliances are covered in detail in following sections of this text.

an overview: HABITS

Chapter 3

Adults

Thrusting problems often remain throughout adulthood. In fact, it is not uncommon to see an anterior open bite recur even after orthodontic therapy has been completed. At bare minimum some form of long-term retention is often needed to prevent this recurrence from happening. For an excellent review of retention appliances, please look at the chapter in this book titled Finishing and Maintaining.

Another unusual habit that occurs in adults is cheek biting. This habit is difficult to control, but with the help of an appliance it is often possible to change this pattern or, at least, prevent further damage to the occlusion and tissue from occurring.

As our society becomes more complex, the incidence of the bruxism seems to be on the increase. A wide variety of treatment approaches and appliance designs are available for the treatment of these disorders. Regardless of the treatment technique, early intervention can prevent many of the severe problems associated with this problem. Although this topic is covered in depth in subsequent sections of this book a quick overview of bruxism splints is provided for you here.

Splints come in a variety of designs. Traditionally, they have been made from a hard acrylic material. Bruxism or disengaging splints induce relaxation of the masticatory muscles. This is accomplished, presumably by reducing, modifying, or more widely distributing the afferent neural input from the occluding teeth. Occlusion correcting splints temporarily eliminate chronic and acute malocclusion. Some techniques require a smooth bite plane, others call for having the occlusal facets ground into the completed splint, still others call for cuspid rise or anterior guidance inclines.

To provide you with the finest splint appliances possible, you need to provide the lab with:

• A properly taken wax construction bite. The bite must be taken at the correct vertical opening and anterior/posterior position desired for the completed appliance. This will enable the technician to articulate the models so that they can exactly duplicate the patient's actual occlusal relationship. The completed appliance should then fit with a minimum of chair time required for final adjustments.

• An accurate set of dental casts. For proper retention, ease of insertion and removal, the model for splint construction must be carefully surveyed and undercuts blocked out by the laboratory before the appliance is constructed.

Design Notes

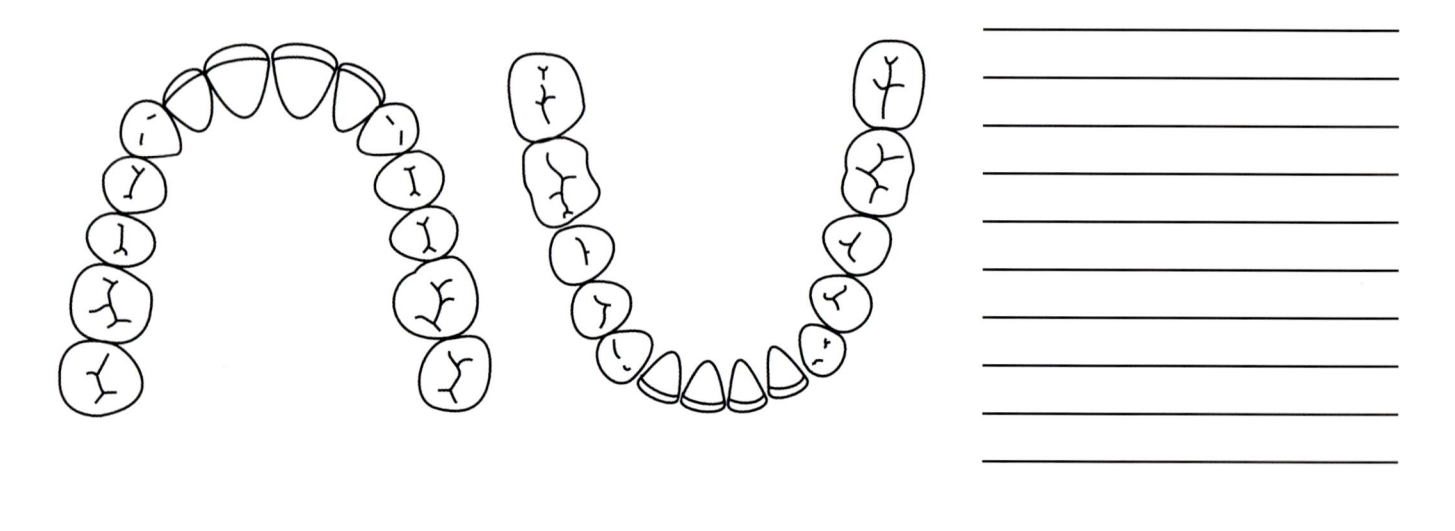

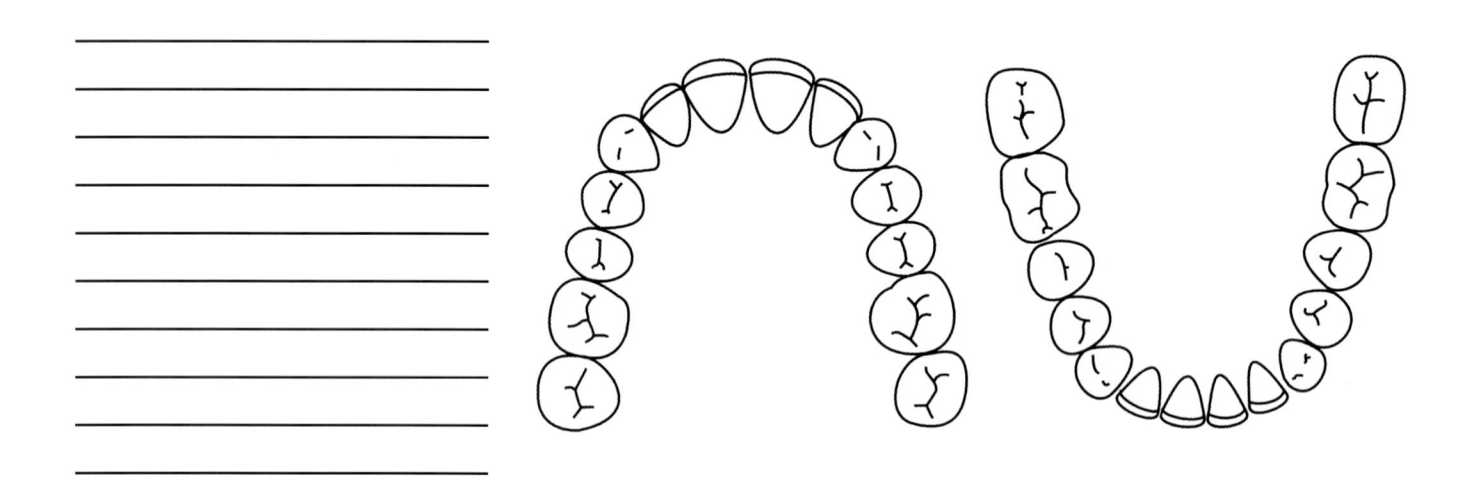

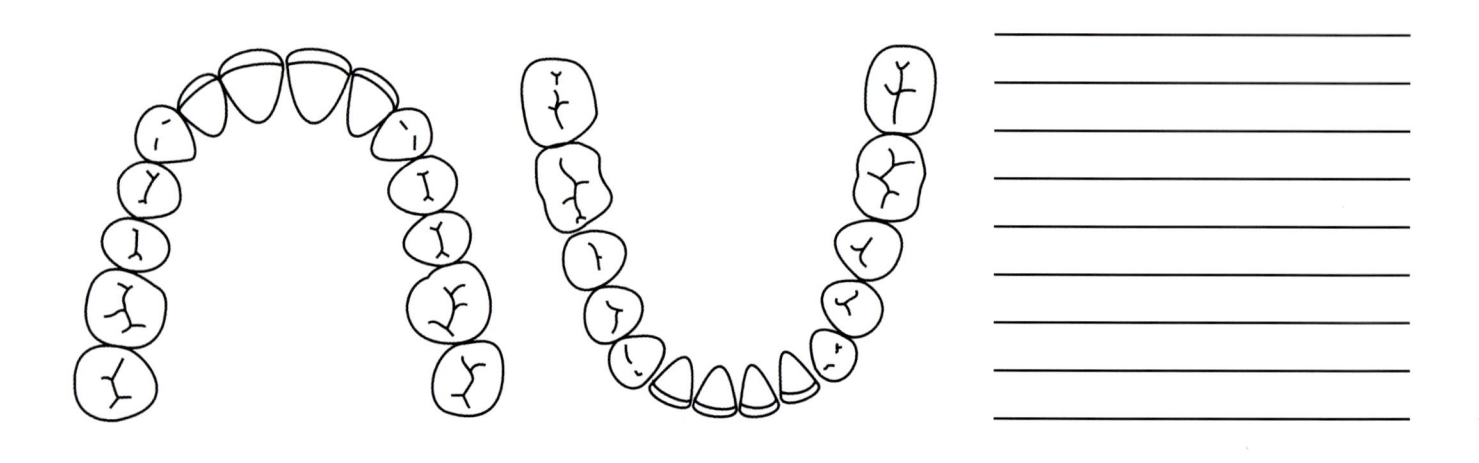

HABITS

2114 Upper Hay Rake   U

Discouraging thumb sucking, by making it as uncomfortable as possible, is the purpose of this appliance. This interference is often enough to allow the facial muscles to act upon the anteriors and return them to their normal position. Most clinicians consider this as the appliance of last resort.

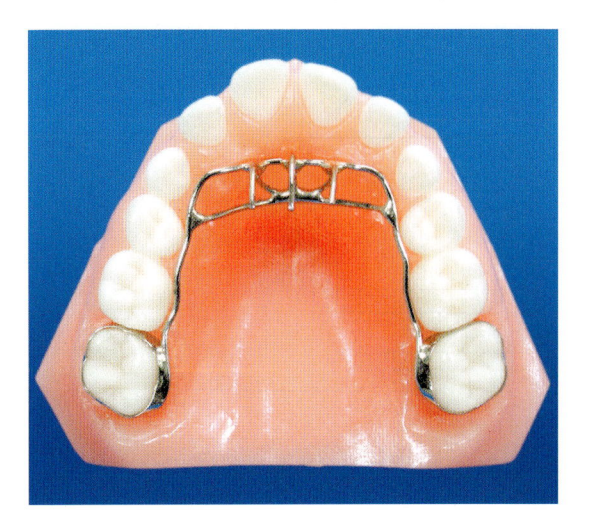

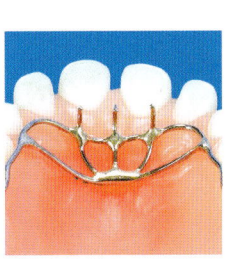

Note - With all habit appliances, an opposing model and bite relationship are required.

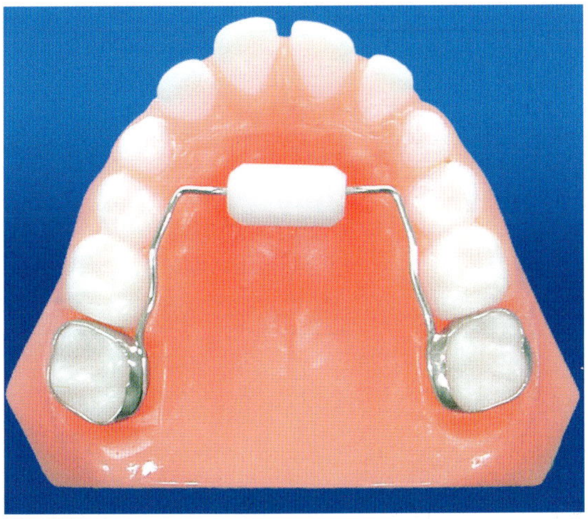

2113 Blue Grass Appliance   U

This device works through counter-conditioning. A teflon roller is placed in the most superior aspect of the palate. When patients try to thumb suck, the roller prevents them from experiencing the satisfaction of suckling. Instead, they use their tongue and spin the roller. This has proven to be a much more positive approach to controlling finger and thumb sucking habits as patients feel they have acquired a new toy. The Blue Grass appliance is particularly useful in the mixed dentition stage of development.

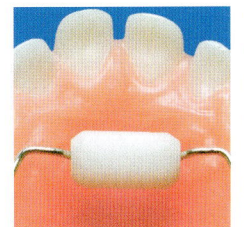

Note - With all habit appliances, an opposing model and bite relationship are required.

2111 Fixed Tongue Loops   U

Tongue loops may be used to control the effects of tongue thrusting or to prevent a patient from thumb sucking. This interference is often enough to allow the facial muscles to act upon the anteriors and return them to their normal position. By adding a spinner as shown in appliance #2110, myofunctional therapy can be initiated. If more aggressive treatment is needed, simply cut off the apex of the loops and straighten the wires. This will create a modified Hay Rake.

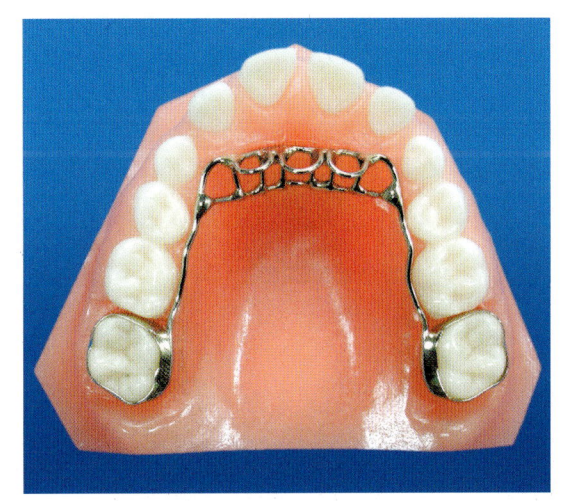

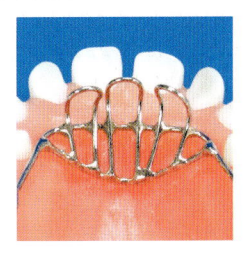

Note - With all habit appliances, an opposing model and bite relationship are required.

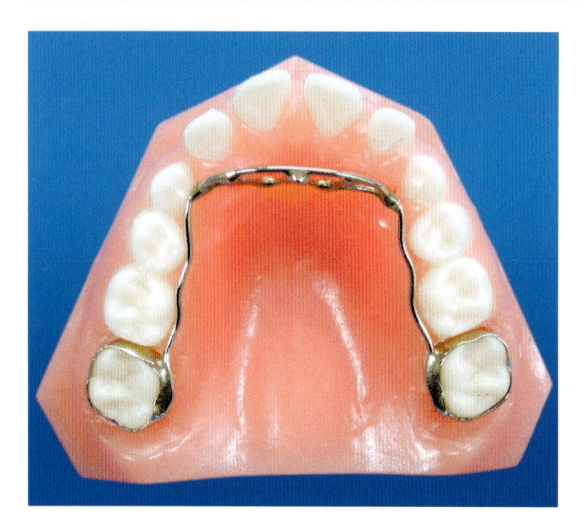

HABITS

2112 Tongue Fence   U

For extra strength, a double wire fence with inter-connecting supports may be used to control the effects of tongue thrusting or to prevent a patient from thumb sucking. As with appliance #2111, this interference is often enough to allow the facial muscles to act upon the anteriors and return them to their normal position. If the appliance is to be maintained for 6-8 months, bonding additional rests into position with composite resin will be helpful to stabilize the appliance. When doing so, it is best to prepare a rest seat in the supporting tooth to keep the bite clear of any occlusal interference.

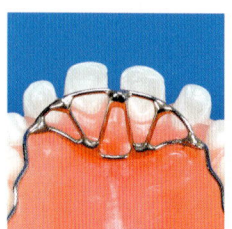

Note - With all habit appliances, an opposing model and bite relationship are required.

1113 Removable Tongue Loops   U

Habit loops can be added to a removable Hawley retainer to control the effects of tongue thrusting or to prevent thumb sucking in a cooperative patient. As with its fixed counterpart, the loops offer enough interference to allow the facial muscles to act upon the anteriors and return them to their normal position. However, this appliance is also designed to allow you to actively move flared anteriors lingually. Simply relieve the acrylic from the lingual aspect of the anteriors and tighten the labial bow.

Note - With all habit appliances, an opposing model and bite relationship are required.

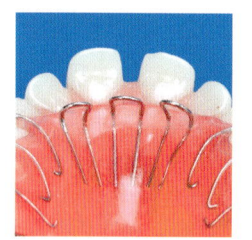

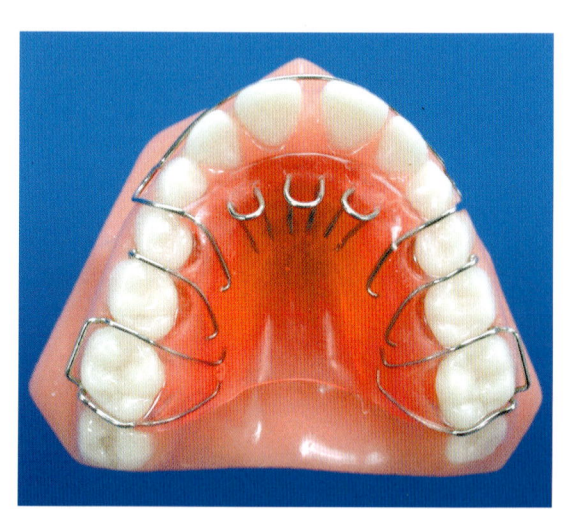

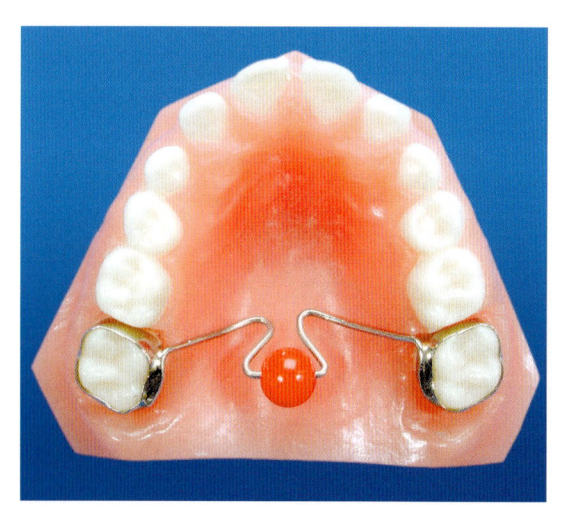

2110 Spinning Bead Tongue Retrainer   U

This myofunctional device is used to retrain proper tongue position. Patient cooperation is generally not required as the appliance evokes a spontaneous reaction to play with the spinner and position the dorsum of the tongue against the soft palate. This appliance is commonly used in conjunction with tongue loops (appliance #2111).

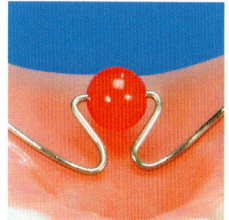

Note - Many practitioners incorporate this type of myofunctional therapy into their fixed orthodontic treatment. When this is the case, lingual sheaths are often used to maintain this appliance so that the bands do not need to be replaced when tongue therapy is complete.

HABITS

2115 Lower Tongue Thrust Inhibitor   L

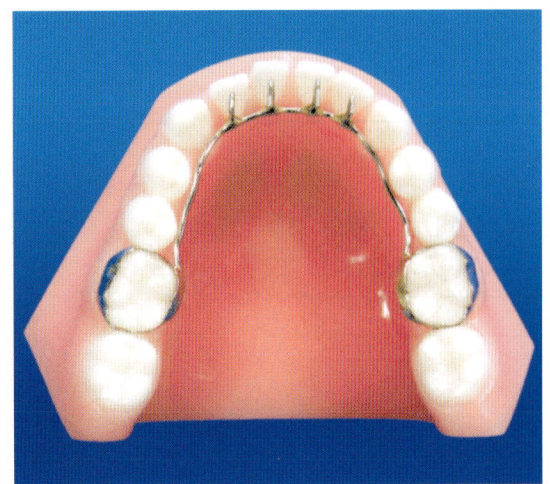

This tongue-thrusting appliance is used to prevent the tongue from placing a labial force against the lower anteriors. It can be attached to bands on the primary or permanent molars and is often used in conjunction with anterior bracketing when closing anterior open bites. When the bite is closed, the prongs can be reduced in length but should be kept in until lip seal has been established. In severe open bite cases, it may be necessary to place prongs like these on a banded bicuspid-to-bicuspid lingual retainer.

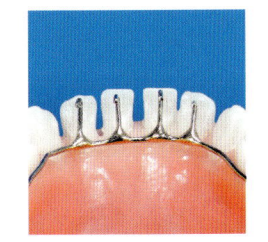

Note - With all habit appliances, an opposing model and bite relationship are required.

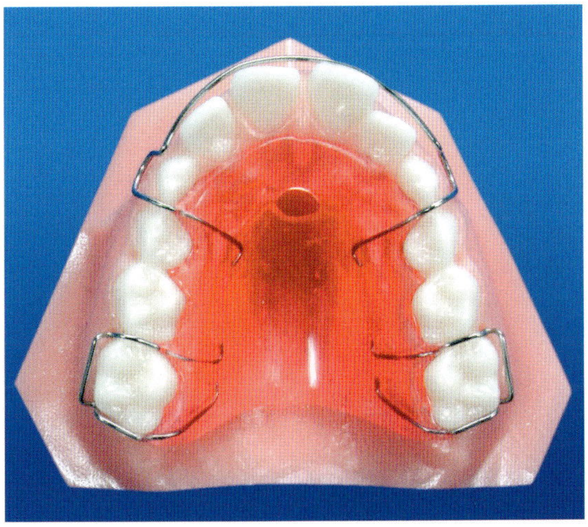

1114 Removable Tongue Positioner   U

In patients with an aberrant swallowing pattern, the tongue often comes forward with tremendous force against the anteriors causing them to move labially. One method to correct this pattern is to use the tongue-positioning appliance described here. It consists of a Hawley retainer constructed with a 5mm hole in the acrylic in the center of the palate, lingual to the anteriors. The patient is instructed to position the tip of the tongue in this hole during swallowing and to practice this new pattern as much as possible.

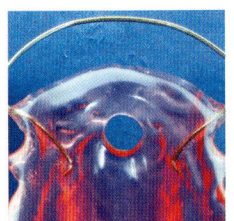

Note - With all habit appliances, an opposing model and bite relationship are required.

1119 Lateral Tongue Thrust Inhibitor   U

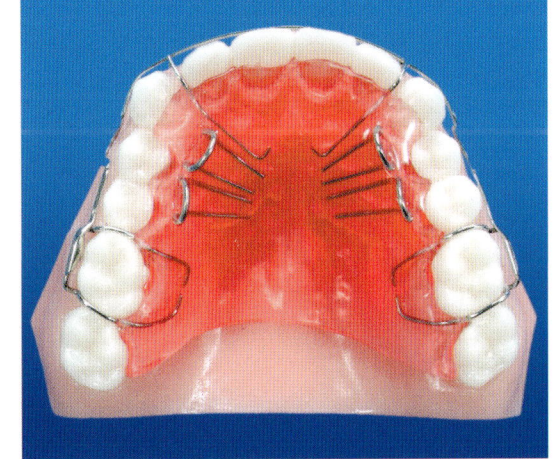

Sometimes patients develop a lateral tongue thrust. When this happens, it can inhibit the eruption of the bicuspids, cuspids, and cause an arch asymmetry to occur. To break this pattern, tongue loops are placed lingual to the premolars and cuspids in a Hawley retainer, and the labial bow is carried all the way back to the molars. Wearing the appliance prevents the tongue from being displaced laterally during swallowing and helps to keep the patient's cheek away as well. This permits the posterior teeth to erupt into occlusion. Bonded buttons and inter-arch elastics are often used to encourage eruption.

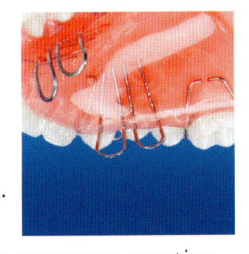

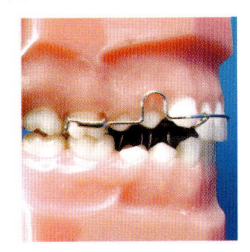

Note - An opposing model and bite relationship are required.

HABITS

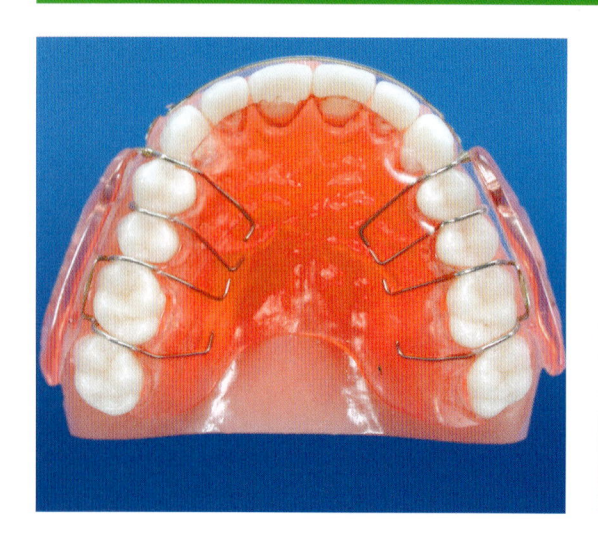

1117 Cheek Biting Inhibitor   U

Cheek biting can be habitual or due to an improper occlusal relationship. Buccal shields can be used to prevent the habit of sucking or chewing of the cheeks. While it may not address the underlying cause of the problem, the appliance is useful in controlling the habit and allowing the tissues to heal.

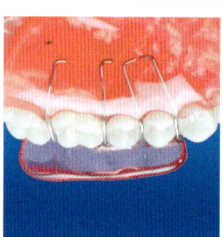

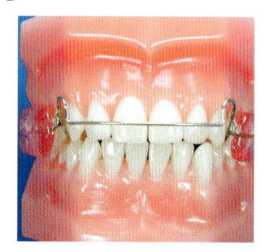

Note - It is essential to take impressions that reach into the vestibule to properly design and place the buccal shields.

2118 Lip Biting Inhibitor   L

A common habit in both children and adults is lip sucking or biting. One method used to break this habit is to place a labial shield. A lip shield can also be incorporated into a removable appliance. Be careful when using this appliance as the facial muscles used during swallowing are strong enough to distal drive the molars if left unattended.

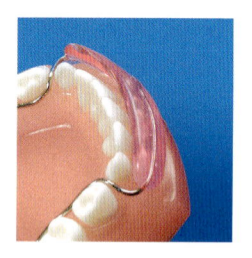

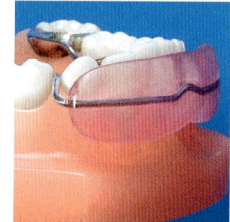

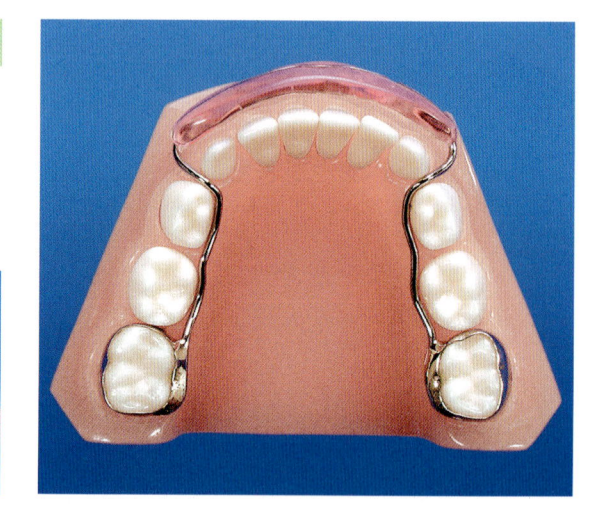

2150H Dillingham Habit/Expansion Appliance   U

Over time, a tongue thrust will cause the patient to have a narrow, underdeveloped maxilla. When this occurs, an appliance is needed that will not only discourage the harmful habit but will also function as an expansion appliance. This hygienically designed appliance accomplishes both goals and requires minimal patient cooperation to maximize your results.

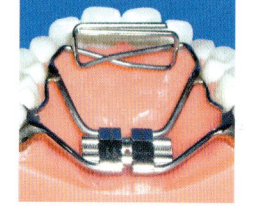

HABITS

3012 Bionator™

This Bionator, commonly referred to as the Bionator II, is designed to correct anterior open bites in Class I and Class II malocclusions.

The posterior teeth are covered with acrylic to prevent their eruption while the acrylic is kept away from the incisors to permit closure of the open bite. The mid-line expansion screw can be used for arch development when it is indicated. Adding a "Balters Type" labial wire will also enhance lateral arch width development.

Note: If desired, the lower incisors can be capped with acrylic if you wish to prevent their eruption. If so, please be sure to include this on your lab prescription.

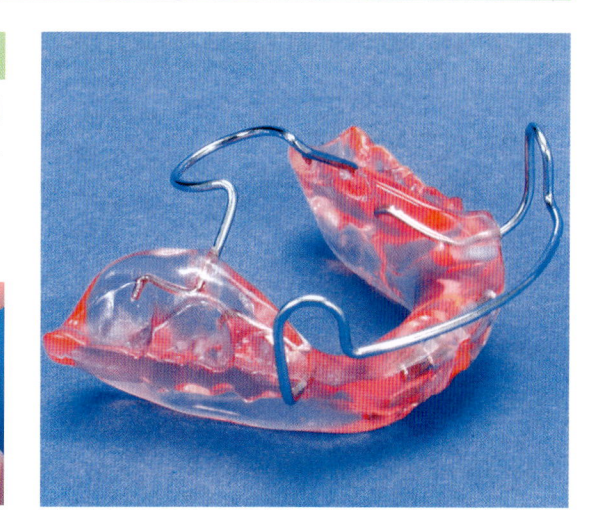

Design Notes:

Design Notes

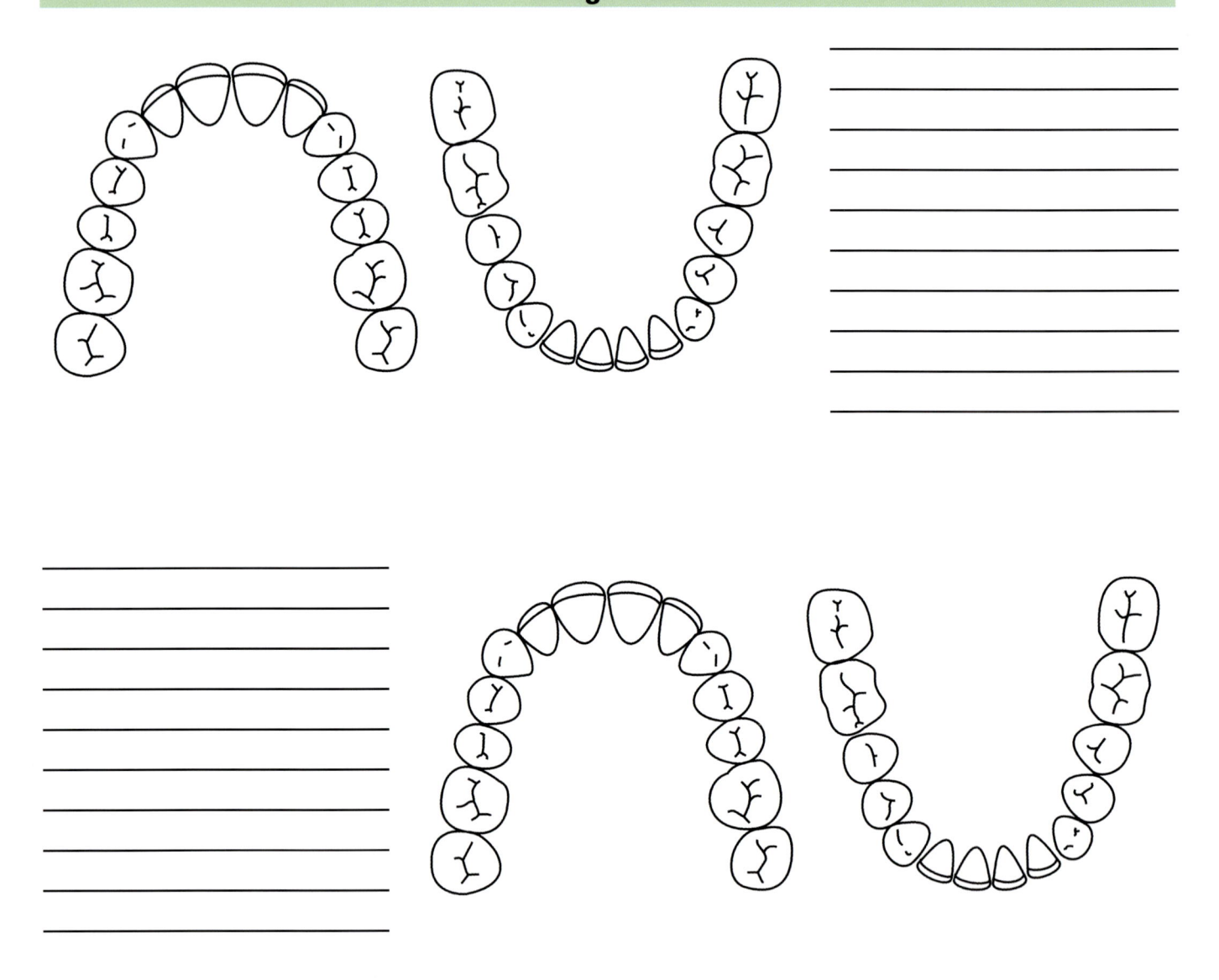

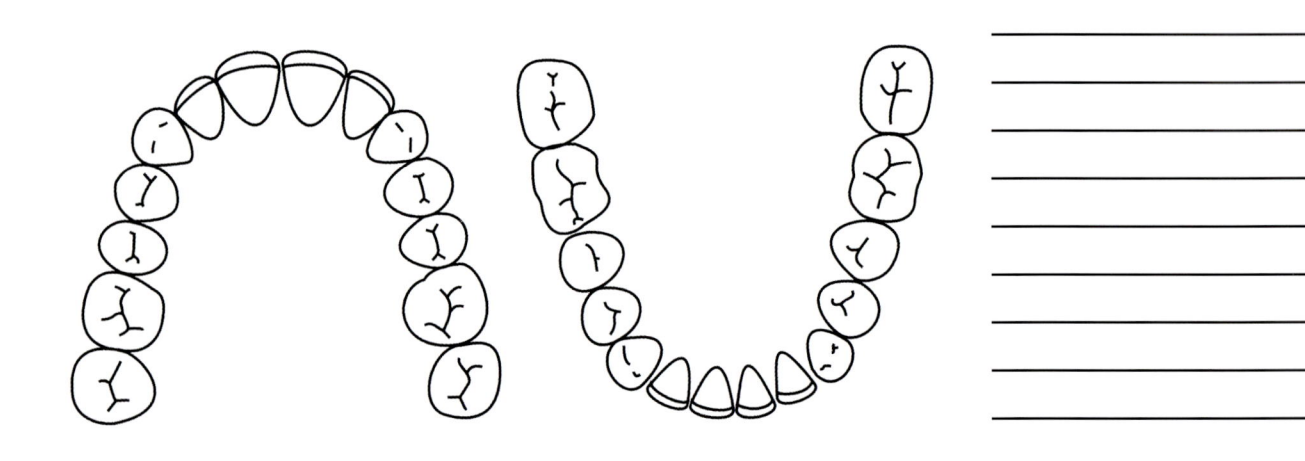

REGAINING SPACE

an overview: REGAINING LOST SPACE

Chapter 4

Children

When dental development occurs normally at every stage and these stages occur in the proper sequence, there is a good chance a normal, healthy, permanent dentition and occlusion will be established. Unfortunately, many factors can adversely affect normal occlusal development. Some of the more common problems seen are:

- **The Early Extraction of the Second Primary Molar** - because of the high prevalence of caries found in second primary molars, it is not unusual to lose this tooth. Normally the eruption of the first permanent molar is guided by the distal surface of the second primary molar. When premature loss occurs and the primary molar space is not well maintained, the first molar often moves mesially before the second bicuspid can erupt.

- **The Early Loss of a Primary Cuspid** - normally the location and arrangement of the permanent incisors are guided by the mesial surface of the primary canine. When this tooth is prematurely lost, arch length can be reduced by both mesial drift of the posterior teeth and distal drifting of the incisors. The midline can also shift and cause the development of an arch asymmetry.

- **An Abnormal Eruption Sequence** - normally the greater mesio-distal width of the primary molars provides enough space for the easy eruption of the bicuspids and cuspids. Should the arch length become shortened due to an unfavorable sequence of eruption, the cuspid may have insufficient space for its final positioning and can be forced to erupt in labioversion with a decided mesial inclination. If the adult second molar erupts prior to the second bicuspid, its strong mesial driving force may move the first molar and cause it to block out the eruption of the second bicuspid.

When space from the premature loss of a primary tooth has not been maintained, an appliance to regain lost space is necessary to prevent crowding and malocclusion. The following section offers a wide variety of appliances for most of these situations. While it may not completely eliminate the need for comprehensive orthodontic treatment, space regaining done at an early stage of development can often prevent a serious orthodontic problem from occurring.

Adults

Once a patient has a full complement of adult teeth, regaining lost space becomes much more difficult. For example, a first molar that has drifted mesially due to a premature loss of a primary second molar is much harder to move distally once the adult second molar has erupted. To regain the space for the bicuspid, you will have to move both teeth. This is very difficult to do at one time and usually involves multiple steps to accomplish.

In an adult, a basic treatment goal is to create enough space so that all the adult dentition can be aligned in the arch form. This is usually accomplished through a combination of techniques ranging from distalizing molars, to lateral arch development, to air rotor slenderizing. Some of the basic designs used to accomplish this tooth movement are seen here. However, a variety of adult space regaining techniques are covered in the sections on arch development, restorative enhancement, partials/bridges and periodontal appliances as well.

REGAINING LOST SPACE

2031 Looped Coil Space Regainer   U/L

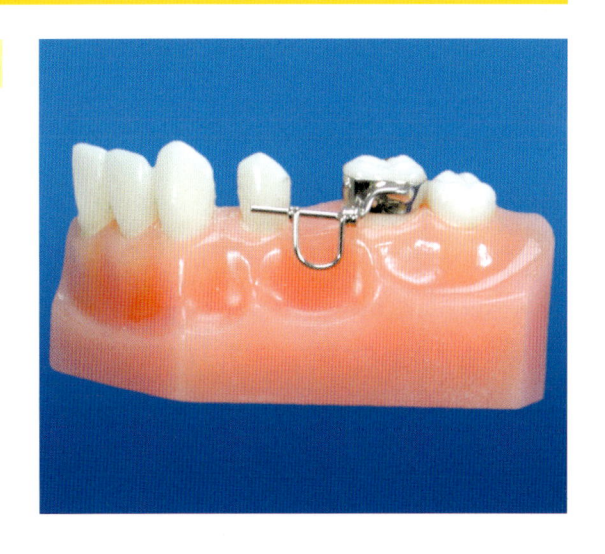

The need to gain space for an un-erupted bicuspid is a common problem. When first and second molars are present, a bicuspid can be moved mesially with this simple appliance. It consists of a band on the molar with a wrap-around looped finger spring to apply mesial pressure to the bicuspid. Once cemented into place, the appliance is adjusted in the mouth by flattening the loop with a 139-bird beak plier. This appliance is not recommended for moving more than one tooth or for moving a molar distally.

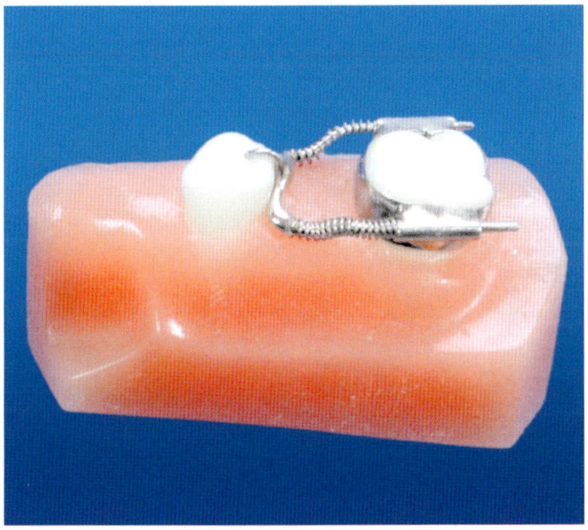

2032 Sliding Loop Space Regainer   U/L

Regaining space may be accomplished by using a band and loop unilateral space maintainer with sliding molar tubes and coil springs. This setup applies constant tension and may be used to move a premolar mesially with some reciprocal distal movement of the permanent molar. To adjust the appliance, simply stretch the coil springs prior to the initial seating of the appliance. No further adjustment is usually necessary.

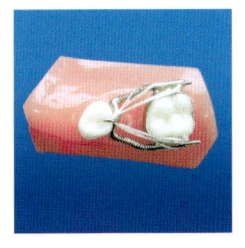

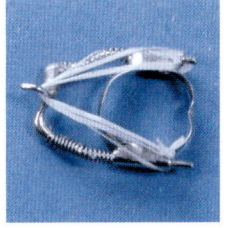

Note - To aid in easy insertion of this appliance it is recommended to first pre-assemble the activated appliance on the working model. Then use dental floss as illustrated to hold the activated loop passive during cementation.

2033 Sliding Distal Shoe   U/L

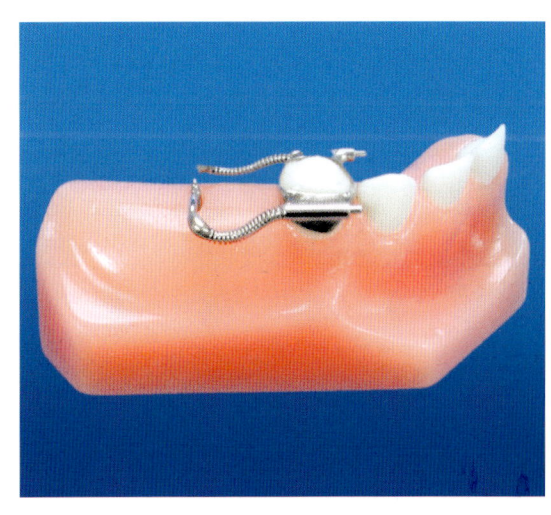

This expanding distal shoe engages a mesially erupting six-year molar and guides it distally when the primary second molar has been lost prematurely. Light coil springs over the loop wire provide the needed pressure for distalization. To accomplish this, you must send an X-ray or mark the mesial edge of the six-year molar on the model for correct placement of the guide. Also, indicate the desired depth of the shoe that will extend beneath the tissue to contact the erupting tooth.

Note - The banded tooth must be in contact with the adjacent tooth and should have an intact root for proper anchorage.

REGAINING LOST SPACE

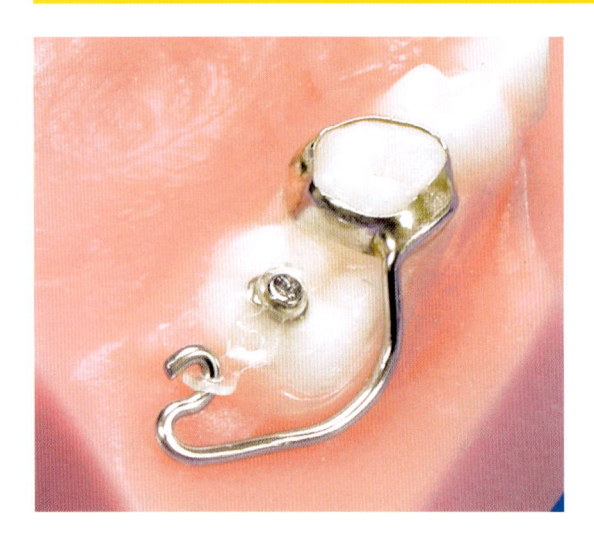

2027 Elastic Halterman Appliance   U/L

This design is indicated when the erupting six-year molar is caught under the distal edge of a primary second molar. A mushroom-shaped button is bonded to the occlusal surface of the erupting molar. A band with a hook that extends distal to the molar is cemented to the primary second molar. Chain elastic is used between the hook and the button to provide the distal force needed to move the six-year molar. (For adult applications, see the Restorative Enhancements section.)

Note - Always send an opposing cast to evaluate if there is sufficient occlusal clearance for this appliance.

2028 Ectopic Spring Distalizer   U/L

Designed in principle to function the same as the Elastic Halterman, this appliance features a recurved wire spring to achieve the distal movement of the six-year molar that is caught under the primary second molar. Placement of the occlusal button is usually on the distal aspect of the erupting molar.

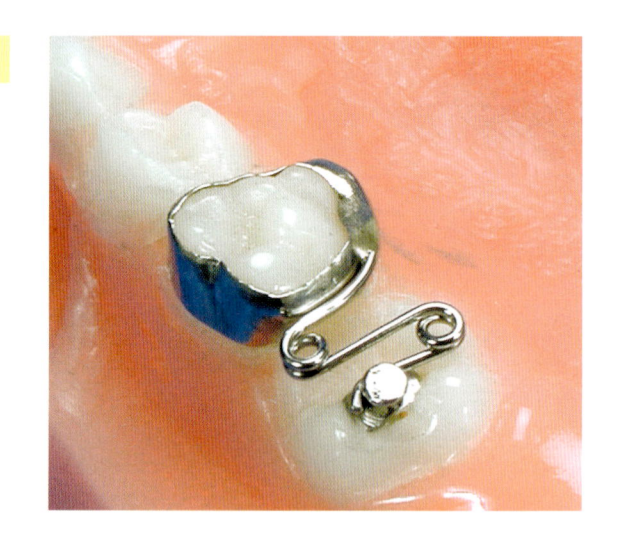

Note - Always send an opposing cast to evaluate if there is sufficient occlusal clearance for this appliance.

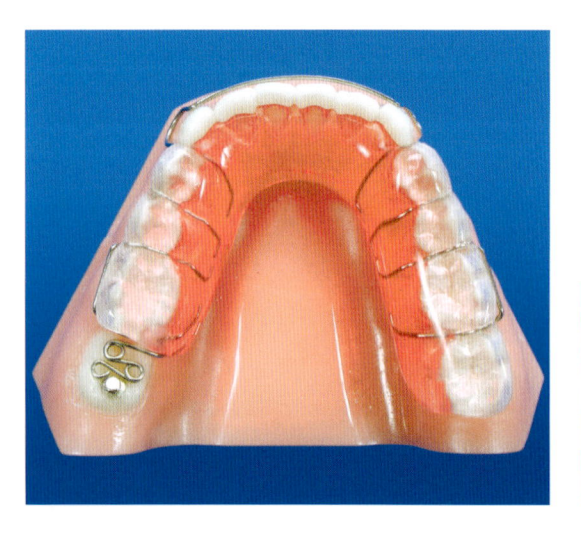

1044 Removable Ectopic Distalizer   U/L

This appliance is quite effective in distalizing an ectopically erupting molar when there is insufficient vertical clearance to use the fixed Ectopic Spring Distalizer #2028. In this case, vertical clearance is achieved by adding occlusal coverage to the removable appliance.

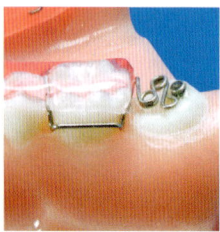

Activating the finger spring soldered to the molar clasp places a positive distal driving force against the button that is bonded to the occlusal of the second molar. Typically, this appliance needs to be worn for a relatively short period of time.

REGAINING LOST SPACE

2035 Jackscrew Appliance   U/L

Two nuts, placed on a threaded arch wire, provide the force for this device. It is designed to regain space without tipping or rotating the teeth. Reciprocal movement of the molar distally and the bicuspid mesially will be effected by the proximity of the adjacent teeth.

In order to restrict the movement of one of the abutment teeth, it is necessary to add additional anchorage as illustrated on appliance #2041. Activating the jackscrew is accomplished with a small, open-end type wrench (available from your laboratory).

The nut against the buccal tube is adjusted first to provide the needed force. The second nut is then tightened against the first nut to act as a lock.

Note - A popular option to this design is appliance #2038

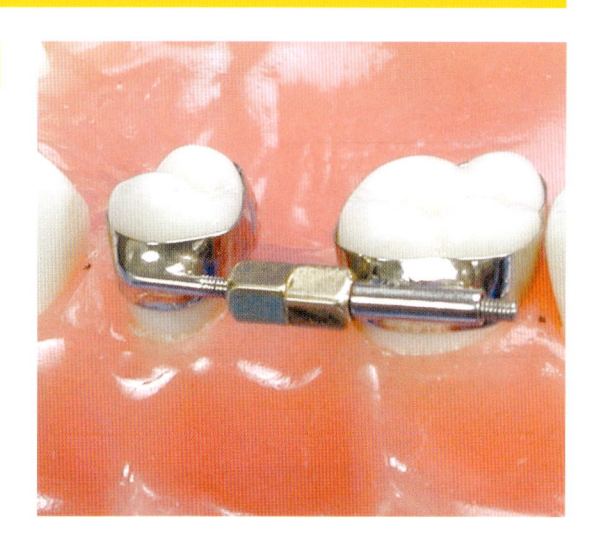

2038 Unilateral Gurin Lock   U/L

This appliance uses nickel titanium coil spring activated by an adjustable Gurin lock to regain space without tipping or rotating the teeth. The amount of reciprocal movement of the molar distally and the bicuspid mesially will be effected by the proximity of the adjacent teeth.

In order to restrict the movement of one of the abutment teeth, it is necessary to add additional anchorage as illustrated on appliance #2041. Activating the Gurin lock is easily accomplished with a special box wrench (available from your laboratory).

2041 Jackscrew Distalizer   U/L

When regaining space, sometimes all the movement needs to be in one direction. Using a jackscrew, as in appliance #2035, with labial/lingual arch wires, will give you the added anchorage you need to accomplish this uni-directional force.

Hint - A small dab of premixed cold-cure acrylic may also be applied to the threads behind the second nut to further ensure that the screw maintains its force and does not back up.

Note - A popular option to the jackscrew is the use of nickel titanium coil spring activated by an adjustable Gurin lock as illustrated in appliance #2041G.

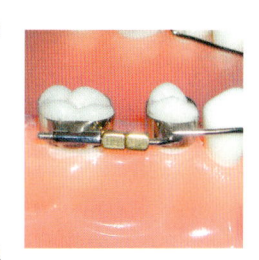

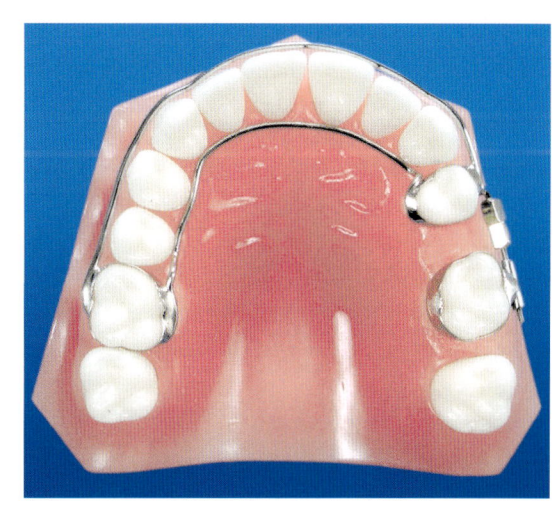

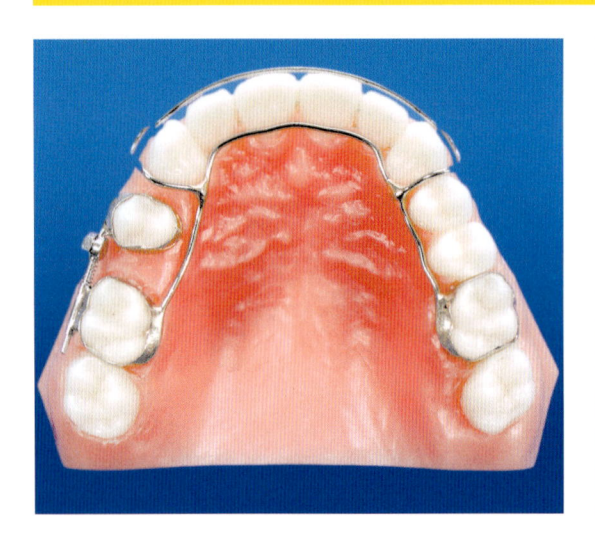

REGAINING LOST SPACE

2041G Gurin Lock Regainer   U/L

This appliance illustrates the typical anchorage system used when you wish to unilaterally move a bicuspid mesially while preventing reciprocal movement of the other teeth. This appliance uses nickel titanium coil spring and an adjustable Gurin lock. Activating the Gurin lock is easily accomplished with a special box wrench (available from your laboratory).

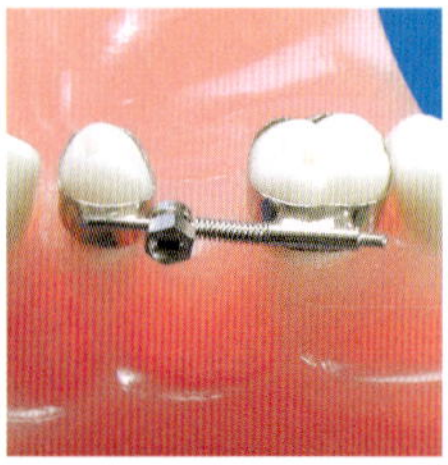

2037 Fixed Sectional Distalizer   U/L

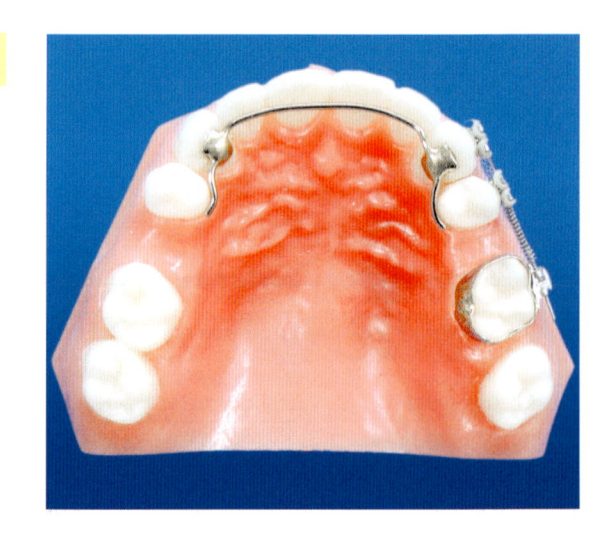

Whether you need to distalize a molar to allow room for the eruption of an impacted bicuspid, or you simply need to recapture the ideal space for a pontic, the fixed sectional distalizer is often the appliance of choice.

This appliance will bodily move a molar that has drifted mesially. Patients readily accept this design because the facial surfaces of the anteriors do not need to be bracketed. Instead, adequate anchorage is accomplished by placement of a lingual-bonded retainer that includes the first bicuspids. Brackets are placed on the cuspid and first bicuspid to support a sectional wire that runs through the buccal tube of the molar band. Nickel titanium coil spring is compressed on the sectional wire prior to ligating it to the brackets on the bicuspid and cuspid.

If desired, a Gurin lock can be placed on the sectional wire distal to the bicuspid for subsequent adjustments; however, this is typically not necessary unless a significant amount of distalization is required.

4.4

REGAINING LOST SPACE

2045 CD Distalizer U/L

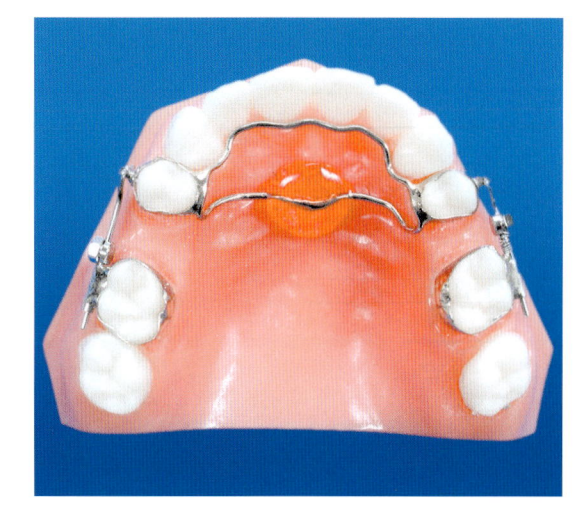

This photo illustrates the original design of this popular molar distalizing appliance. It, of course, can be used on either arch and can be used in a unilateral or bilateral configuration.

The anterior portion of this appliance typically attaches to the first bicuspid bands with a Nance button and often an additional lingual wire to act as anchorage. Vertical tubes on the buccal aspect of these bicuspid bands accept the .032 guide wires that run back through the horizontal tubes on the molar bands. Gurin locks and open coil springs are placed, as illustrated, to provide the necessary distalizing force to the molars.

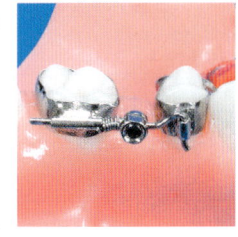

Adjustments are made approximately every 3-4 weeks. The vertical tubes on this appliance allow it to be placed segmentally, by first cementing the anterior segment, and then by placing the molar bands with the .032 guide wires inserted in the tubes as individual units. The appliance shown here illustrates the force module necessary to distalize #14 and the use of the Gurin lock to maintain the already distalized #3.

Note - When selecting this appliance, please provide the lab with detailed instructions.

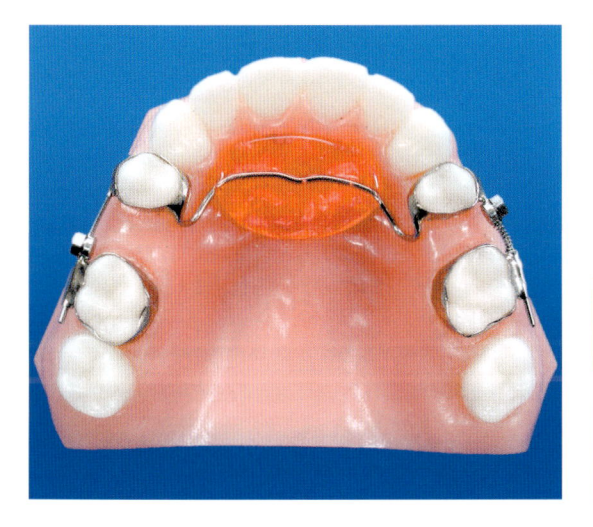

2045M Modified CD Distalizer U/L

This appliance works the same way as the CD Distalizer (appliance #2045). However, the design has been modified so that the guide wires are soldered to the first bicuspids rather than using the vertical tube assembly to attach them to the bicuspids. The advantages of this design are superior strength and added comfort to the patient, as the attachments to the bicuspids are smooth and reduced in overall bulk. Although this design requires all four bands to be seated at once, this is typically not a problem. The appliance shown here illustrates the force module necessary to distalize #14 and the use of the Gurin lock to maintain the already distalized #3.

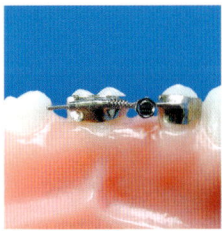

Note - Gurin locks and open coil spring provide the necessary distalizing force to the molars.

4.5

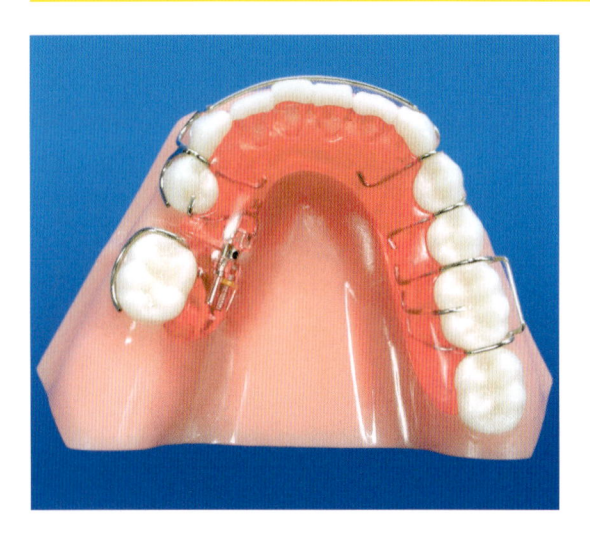

REGAINING SPACE

1042 Removable Space Regainer   U/L

Early loss of primary teeth can allow a first molar to drift mesially and block the eruption of the bicuspids. This removable appliance uses an expansion screw to distal drive the molar, regaining the space needed for the eruption of the bicuspid. Adjustments are made 1/4 turn once each week with the wrench provided.

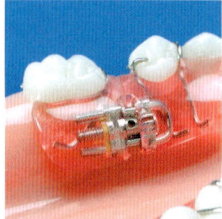

As illustrated in this photo, there is no occlusal rest on the first permanent molar. This will allow the molar to upright as it moves distally.

Note - When distalizing a first molar, it is important to take an x-ray of the second molar to make sure distalization will not cause its impaction.

Hint - When using "C" clasps as illustrated here, consider the use of bonded composite ledges on the buccal of the clasped molars if retention is a concern.

1042D Removable Molar Distalizer   U/L

To move two adjacent molars distally with a removable appliance, maximum anchorage must be utilized while each molar is moved individually. This can be accomplished with one appliance that has two screws aligned next to each other by sequentially turning the screws.

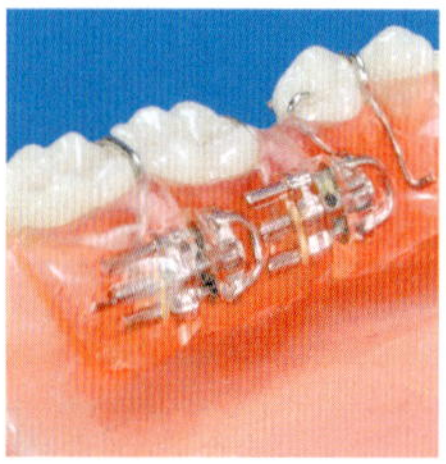

First, move the second molar by adjusting the distal-most screw. Once you have achieved the desired distalization of the second molar, you may begin adjusting the mesial screw to distalize the first molar. It is important to remember that as the mesial screw is opened one turn, the distal screw needs to be closed one turn. This will keep the second molar in its new position as the first molar is distalized to meet it.

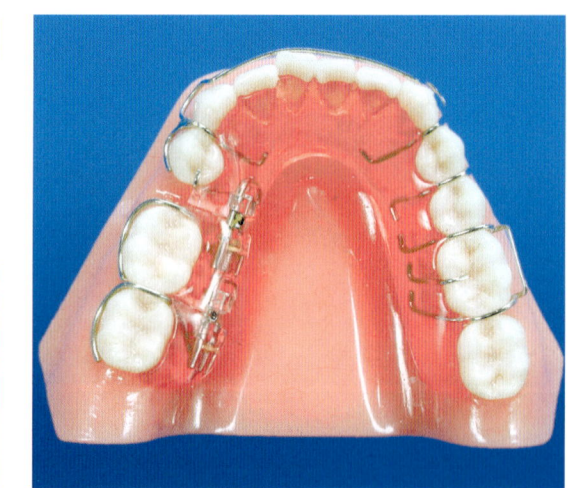

Note - When distalizing both first and second molars, it is important to properly instruct the patient about the precise adjustment technique and sequence.

REGAINING SPACE

1043 Split Acrylic Space Regainer   U/L

When only two to three millimeters of lost space needs to be regained, and the edentulous area is at least 8mm, using the split-saddle appliance is a good choice. Opening the wire loops prior to insertion easily activates this device. Periodic adjustment is usually required to help keep the appliance active.

Note - The edentulous region must be at least 8mm in length in order to accommodate the acrylic and wire loops that make up the split saddle.

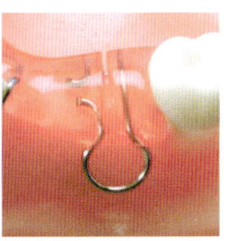

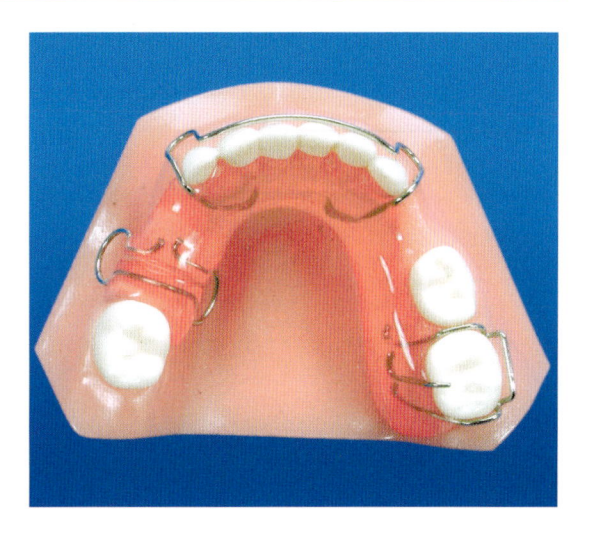

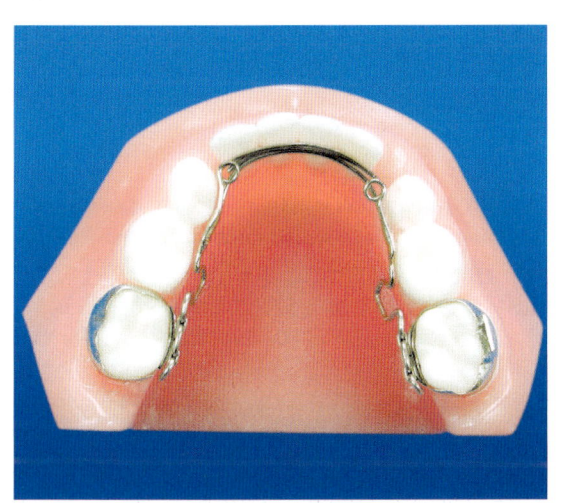

2502M Adjustable Lingual   U/L

This lingual arch features lingual lap springs to align the incisors and adjustment loops to move them labially to regain lost cuspid space. The lingual arch wire is attached to the bands with Wilson vertical attachments. This allows you to remove the arch wire and easily adjust the lap springs and adjustment loops out of the patient's mouth. Regular adjustments of the loops will continue to move the anteriors labially.

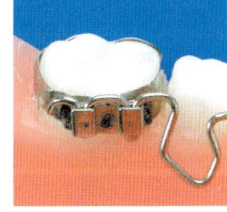

Note - Make sure to protect the attachments from cement by placing wax in them prior to cementation.

4.7

REGAINING SPACE

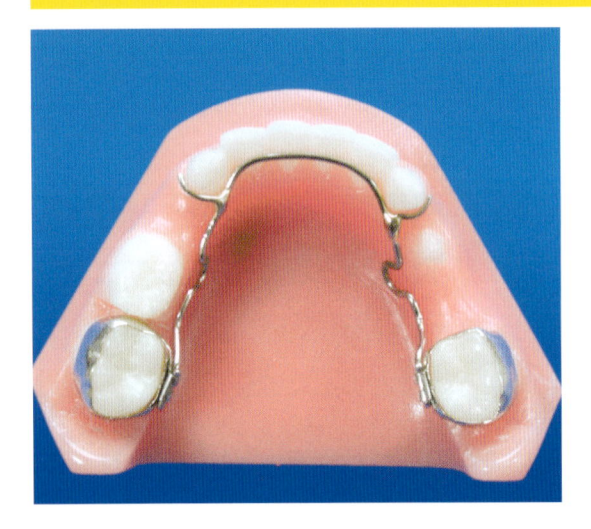

2133 Horizontal Removable   U/L

Early loss of the primary cuspids along with the loss of primary molars can cause a decrease in arch length by molars drifting forward and anteriors moving distally off of the mid-line.

In this example, primary molars have been lost early, leading to a loss in arch length. The appliance shown here is ideal for regaining a small amount of arch length while preventing the anteriors from shifting into the edentulous space.

Horizontal lingual sheaths allow you to remove the arch wire in a mesial or distal direction without disturbing the molar bands. This will allow you to remove the arch wire and make the necessary adjustments out of the patient's mouth to increase arch length.

Note - Make sure to protect the attachments from cement by placing wax in them prior to cementation.

2044 Adjustable Loop Lingual   U/L

The Adjustable Loop Lingual appliance is a fixed anterior sagittal that allows you to regain lost anterior space and align lower anterior crowding. Using a standard lingual arch wire as a base, this appliance features a second, lighter gauge wire with adjustable loops to apply pressure against the anterior teeth. As the loops are flattened, the wire is free to slide along the fixed lingual wire in a labial direction.

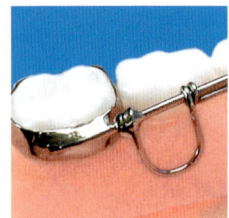

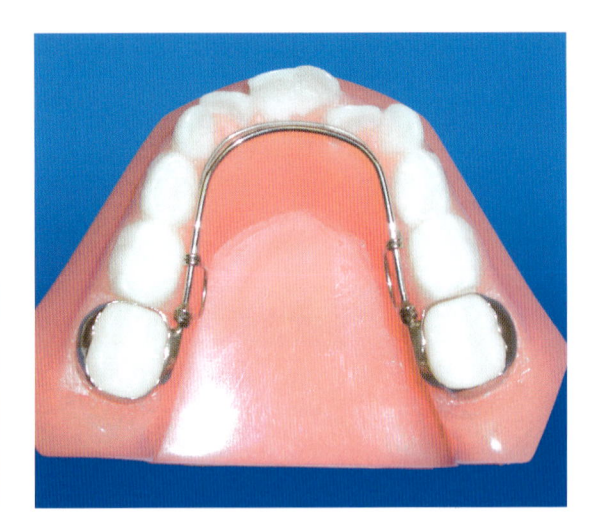

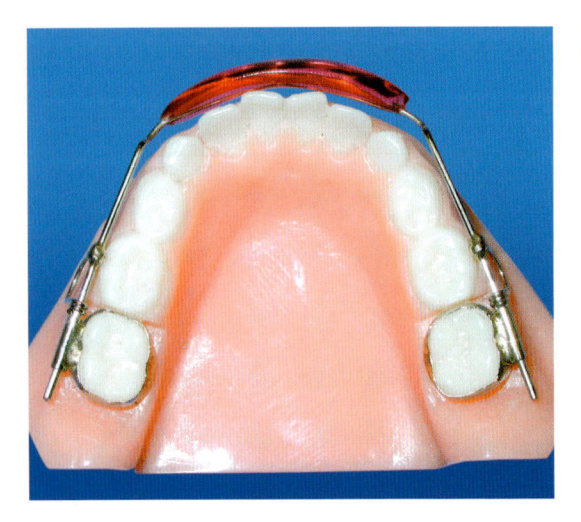

2142 Muscle Anchorage Appliance   L

This mandibular space regainer utilizes a labial lip bumper that inserts through buccal tubes on the molar bands. Lip pressure creates a distal force that moves the molars posteriorly. To adjust the position of the lip bumper, simply open or close the loops that are soldered to the labial wire. The appliance also alters the equilibrium of forces acting upon the incisors. Removing the resistance of the lip against these teeth allows the tongue to move the incisors forward.

REGAINING SPACE

1073 Moving Anteriors Labially   U

In the case of a Pseudo Class III or end-to-end bite relationship caused by an underdeveloped pre-maxilla, this anterior sagittal is often used to move the maxillary anteriors labially.

By using an expansion screw in an anterior-posterior direction the anterior acrylic section moves the pre-maxilla forward. The labial arch wire moves with this section and provides additional stability. Finger springs can be added for individual tooth movement and, when appropriate, T-springs can be used to provide lingual movement of the cuspids.

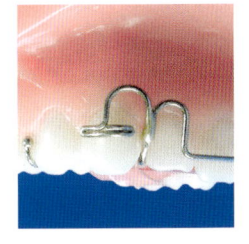

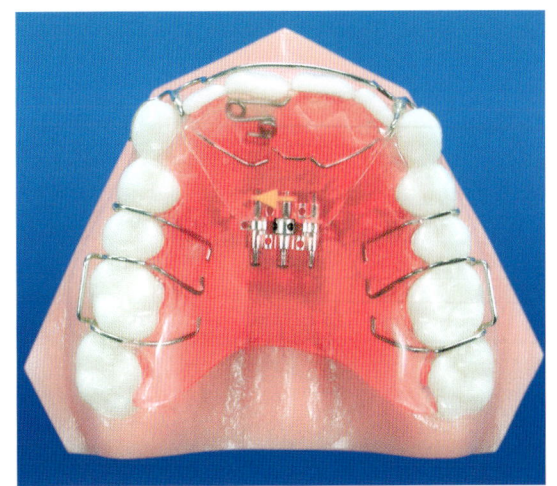

Note - In this appliance it is important to understand that cuspid movement cannot occur until space is available.

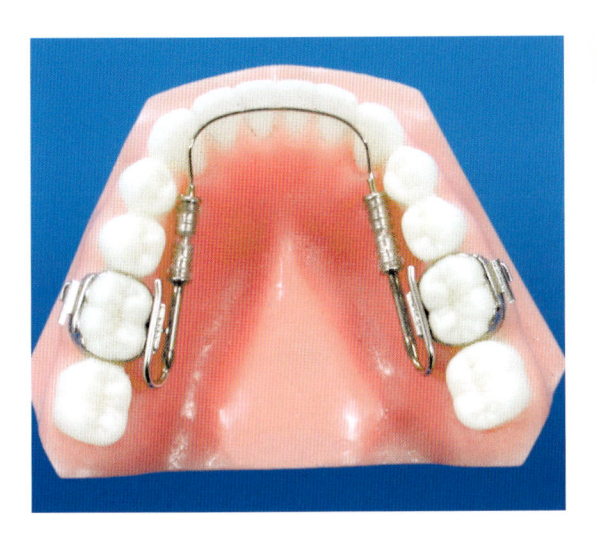

2511 Clark Trombone   U/L

The principal goal of this appliance is to manage a loss in arch length by using a pre-activated system. The original design of this appliance used coil springs to provide the necessary force, and chain elastic attached to mesial and distal hooks to control the force. In the new design shown here, the AP force is provided through a unique Compression Tube Activator that is comprised of fine bore silicone tubing. Replacing the springs and hooks with this new material has improved the stability and safety of the appliance.

The advantages of this appliance are that it is removable from the bands giving the doctor complete control, it is virtually invisible, and it can be used in conjunction with any conventional fixed appliance technique.

Design Notes:

_____
_____
_____
_____
_____
_____
_____
_____
_____

4.9

Design Notes

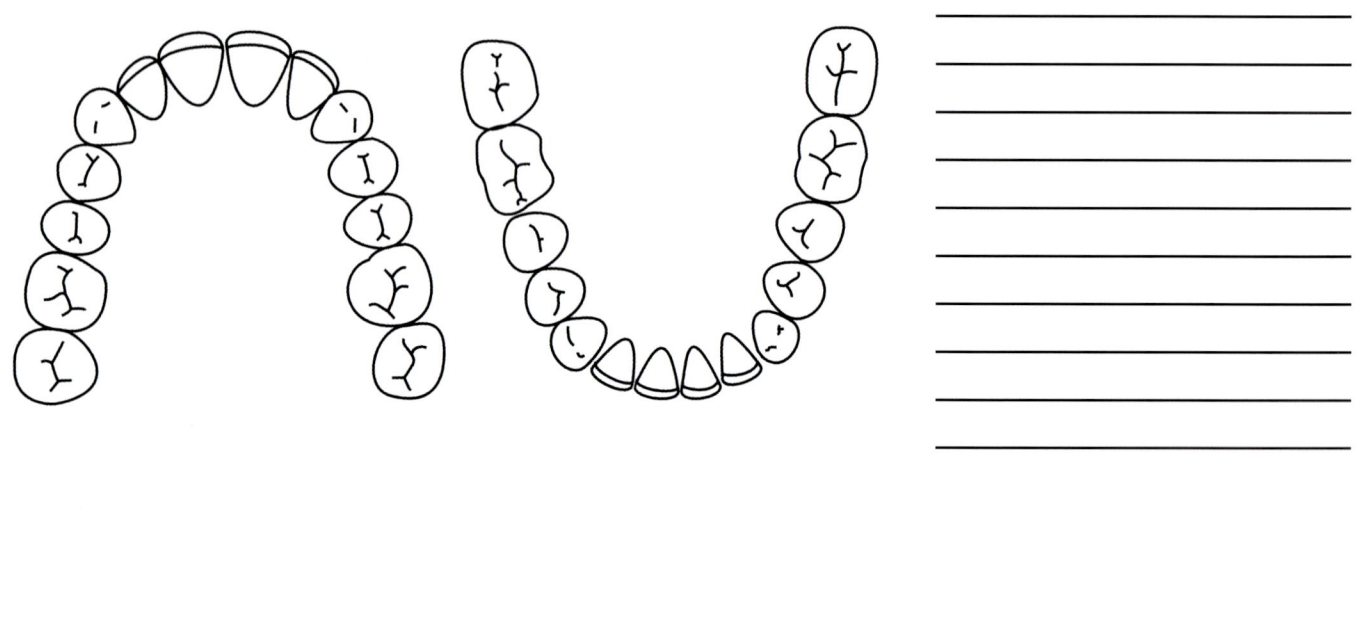

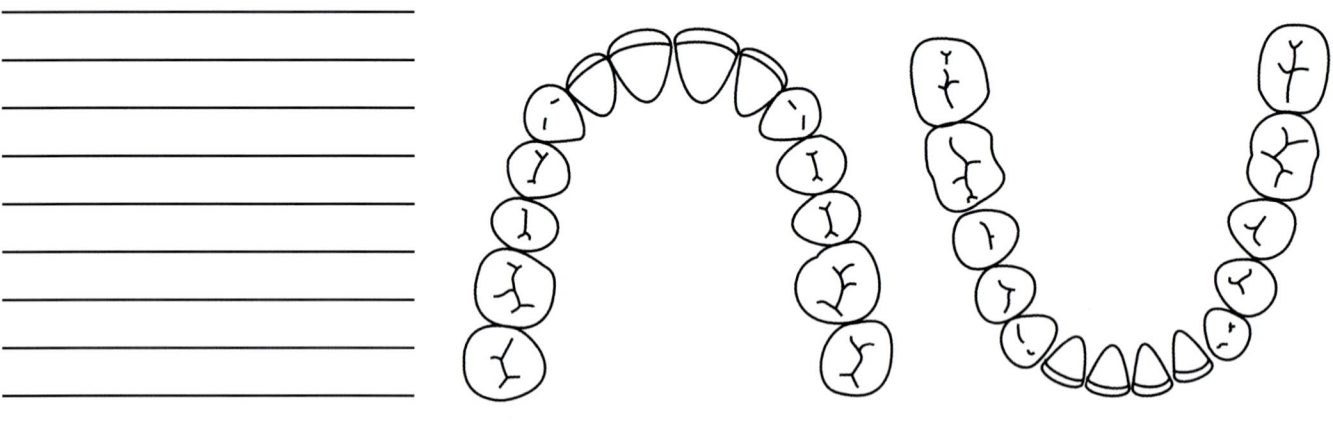

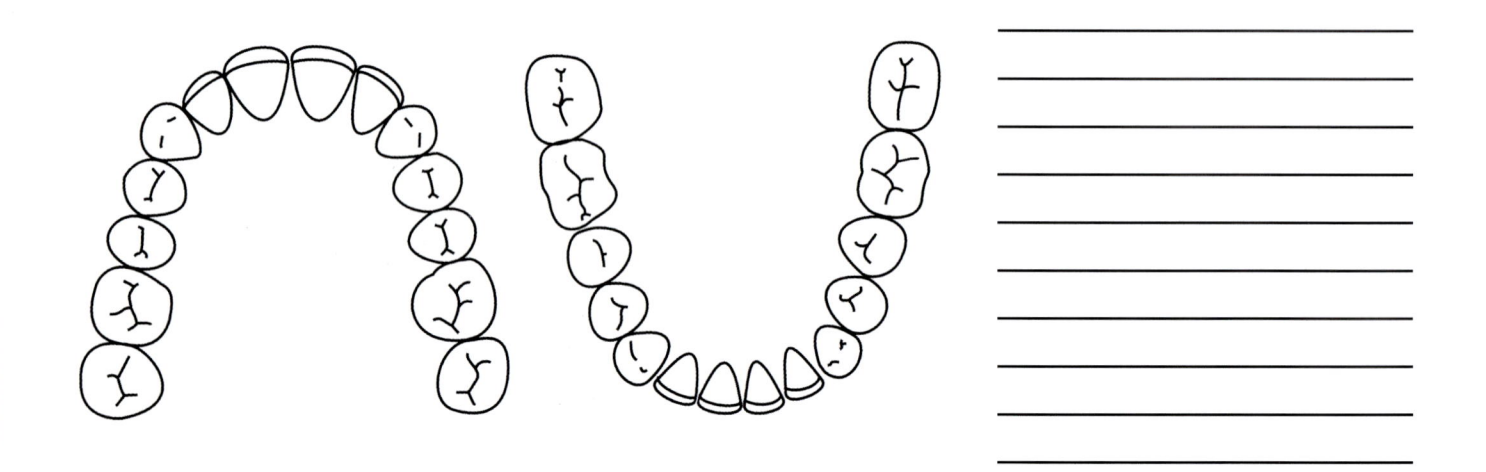

CLOSING SPACE

an overview: CLOSING SPACE

Chapter 5

Children and Adults

Tongue thrusting, tooth size discrepancy, periodontal disease and posterior bite collapse are just a few of the factors that can cause a patient to have excessive space. Only when you identify the cause of the problem can you properly select an appliance that will close the space and allow you to keep it closed.

The most common result of a tongue thrust is the creation of an anterior open bite with flared anteriors. Although the etiology of a tongue thrust is often debated, the need to address the problem early is not. If a thrusting pattern remains past the age of 4 to 5, there is an increasing likelihood that this pattern will remain. When an appliance is used to close excess space caused by a tongue thrust, it is best to choose a design that also addresses the thrusting problem. If this is not done, tongue forces will just cause the problem to re-occur.

Nocturnal grinding or bruxism can breakdown the protective mechanisms provided by the posterior occlusion. When this occurs, undo forces are placed on the anteriors causing them to flair. Many of the appliances shown in this section can be used to gather the anteriors. However these appliances should only be used after the loss in vertical dimension has been corrected. This is usually accomplished through a combination of orthodontics and restorative therapy.

Periodontal disease can also be a factor causing anterior flaring and the creation of excessive space. An anterior retraction appliance should be used after periodontal therapy is completed. In these cases, it may be necessary to splint the teeth together after retraction and space closure is completed.

Managing space problems caused by a tooth size discrepancy are usually handled by combining a small amount of tooth movement with some form of cosmetic restorative therapy. The key to success here is not to impinge upon the space needed for the tongue. Therefore one must exercise caution when using any form of retraction mechanics to close the excess space.

When choosing an appliance it is important to remember that fixed appliances are capable of moving the teeth bodily while removable appliances tend to tip teeth. As with most appliance designs found in this book, many combinations of different components are possible to accomplish a given objective.

CLOSING SPACE

2051 Diastema Controller   U/L

The simplest appliance to bodily move two teeth and close a diastema is the Diastema Controller. It is composed of two brackets and a segmental guide wire that is tied to the brackets with metal ligature ties. An elastic is then carried from the distal of each bracket to provide an equal force on both teeth in a mesial direction. The guide wire assures bodily movement and prevents unwanted rotations or changes in the axial inclination. Elastics of the appropriate size are provided with each appliance. The patient should be instructed to change them daily for the best results.

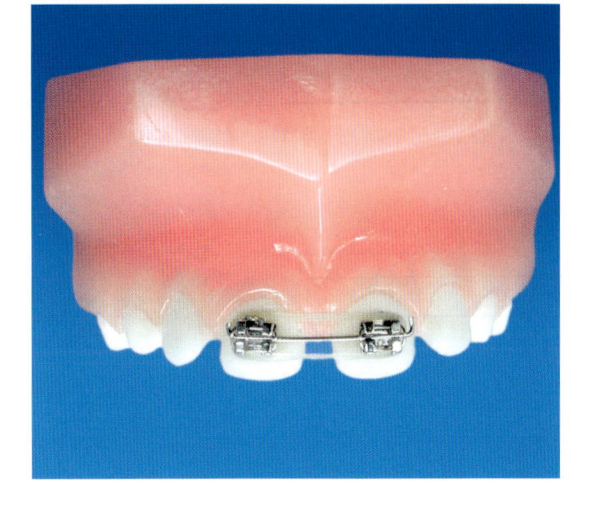

Note - The metal ligature ties should be tightened just enough to maintain the guide wire in place. Over-tightening these ties will create excess friction and slow down the closure process.

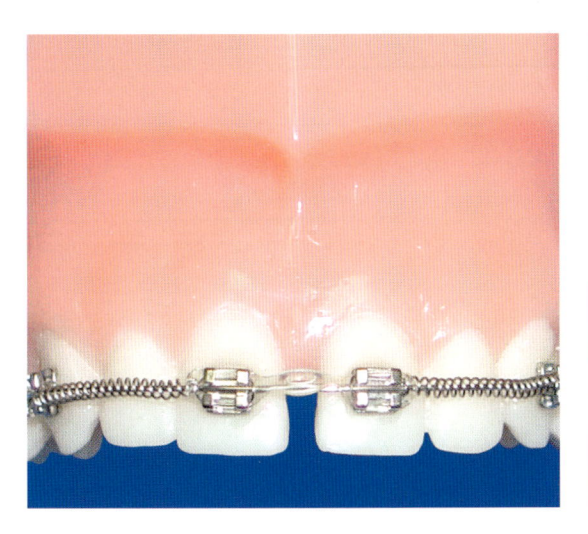

2053 Diastema Closing   U/L

When closing a diastema, differential amounts of mesial movement of the centrals are often needed. Here, force is applied from both chain elastics and coil springs.

An arch wire has been placed from cuspid to cuspid to act as a guide and keep the centrals from tipping. The initial length of coil spring placed distal to the central is equal to the distance between the brackets plus the width of the central bracket. This amount will typically move the tooth 1.5mm.

Increasing the amount of coil spring distal to one central can move it faster than the other. However, the teeth should not be moved faster than approximately 1mm per month to prevent root resorption. Because this is such an active appliance, the patient should be seen every two weeks.

Note - To prevent unwanted movement of the cuspids, a lingual bonded 3-to-3 retainer can be placed to create an anchorage unit, holding the cuspids in place.

Design Notes:

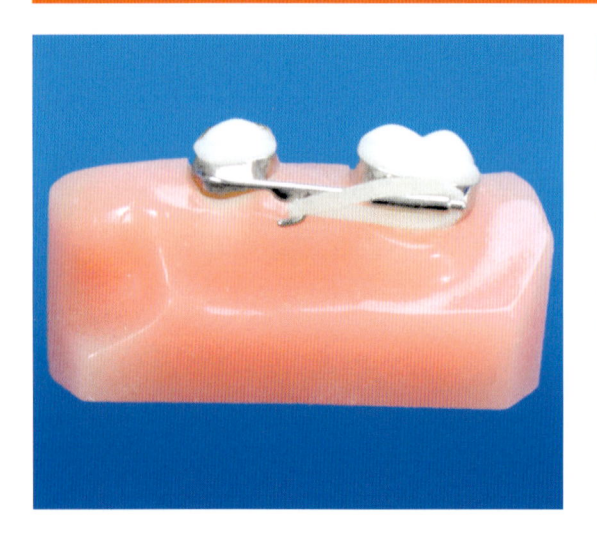

CLOSING SPACE

2052 Sliding Buccal Bar U/L

This appliance allows for reciprocal movement of both teeth to close the space between them. Elastics provide the force, while the bar, extending through the tube soldered to the molar band, keeps the teeth from tipping as movement occurs. Elastics, of the appropriate size, are provided with each appliance and the patient should be instructed to change them daily. When you wish to eliminate the movement of one of the abutment teeth, employ the anchorage concepts as illustrated on appliances #2041 or #2041G in Chapter 4.

1076 Removable with Anterior Finger Springs U/L

When space exists between teeth because the teeth are tipped, finger springs can be used to tip the crowns back over the roots and close the space. Here, the finger springs are designed to close up excess space between the centrals by tipping them mesially. Closing the diastema will create the space needed to align the laterals. The labial arch wire, Adams clasps, and ball clasps provide the needed retention for this active appliance.

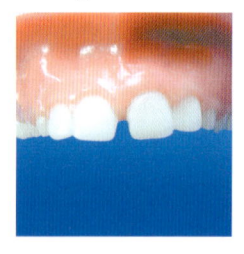

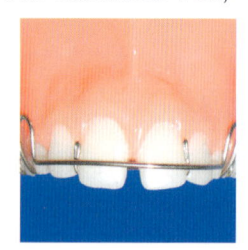

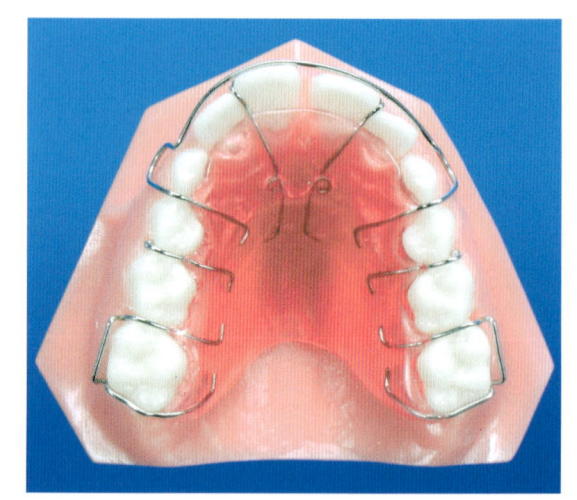

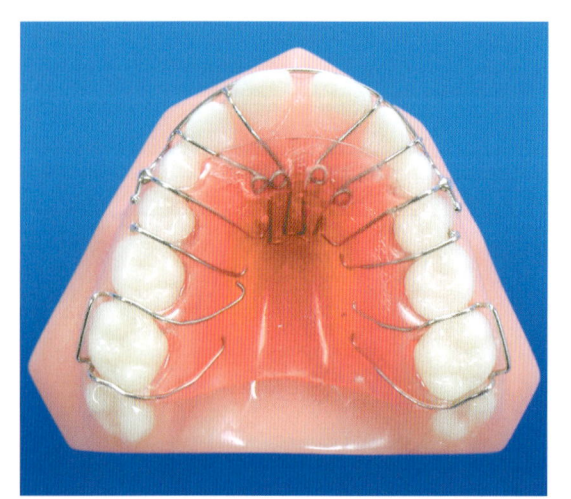

1121 Mesial and Lingual Anterior Movement   U/L

Sometimes anteriors need to be moved both mesially and lingually to close up excessive space. This removable Hawley type appliance features finger springs for mesial movement of the centrals and laterals and an elastic force over the labial surface of the anteriors to move them lingually. Adjustments are easily accomplished by using finger pressure to activate the spring wires and by changing the elastic every day. Once the desired tooth movement has been accomplished, the labial bow can be adjusted to allow the appliance to be worn as a final retainer.

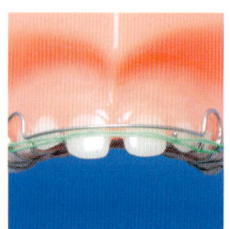

Note - Make sure to relieve the acrylic away from the lingual aspect of the anteriors before attempting to move them lingually.

CLOSING SPACE

1122 Apron Spring Appliance   U/L

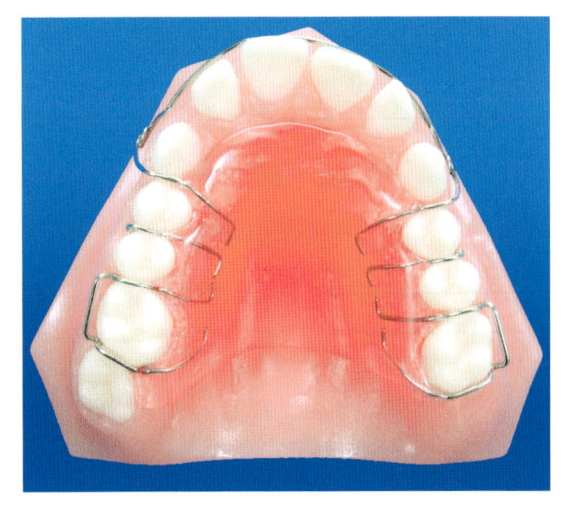

An alternative to retracting flared anteriors with an elastic force is the Apron Spring Appliance. This removable appliance uses light spring pressure to gently guide the centrals and laterals lingually. When this protrusive position is associated with a habit, tongue or thumb, control loops can readily be incorporated into the palatal area to provide habit control. Minimal adjustment is required to keep the appliance active.

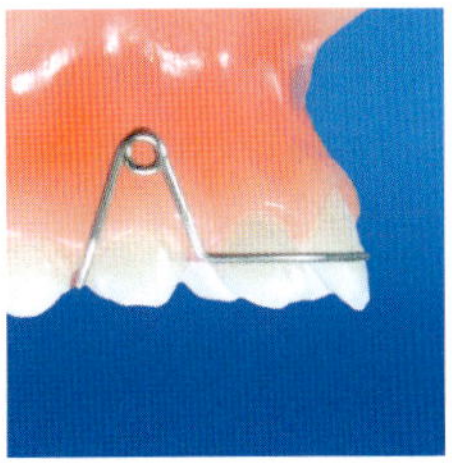

Note - Make sure to relieve the acrylic away from the lingual aspect of the anteriors before attempting to move them lingually.

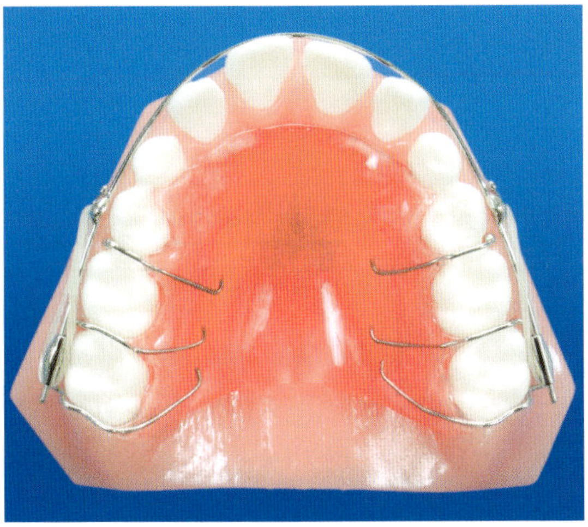

1123 Sliding Labial Appliance   U/L

When the anteriors are not severely proclined, a Sliding Labial Appliance can provide a constant, light lingual pressure sufficient to retract the anteriors and close up a small amount of excess space. The amount of force is controlled by the size of the elastic stretched between the hooks on the labial wire and the tube soldered to the Adams clasps through which it slides.

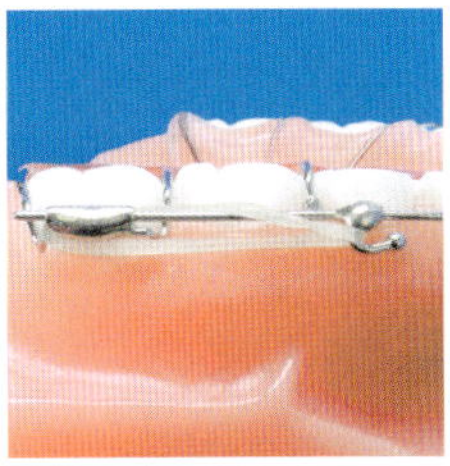

Note - Make sure to relieve the acrylic away from the lingual aspect of the anteriors before attempting to move them lingually.

1124 Retraction Expansion Screws   U/L

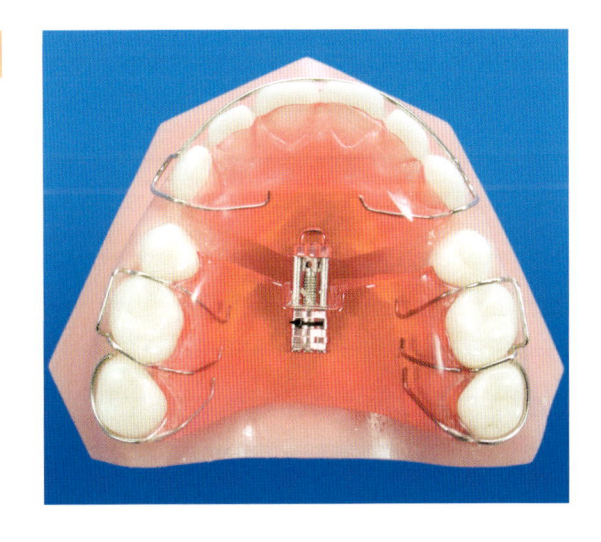

The most common area of relapse after finishing a bicuspid extraction case is in the area distal to the cuspids. This space can be closed and maintained by placing an expansion screw in the open position, between two sections of an acrylic appliance, and drawing the sections together. Extra retention is provided by using both "C" and Adams clasps bilaterally.

Note - This space-closing technique is only to be used after a thorough evaluation of the patient's vertical dimension and upper and lower anterior relationship have been completed. Care must be taken not to deepen the bite or lock the mandible into a retruded position.

CLOSING SPACE

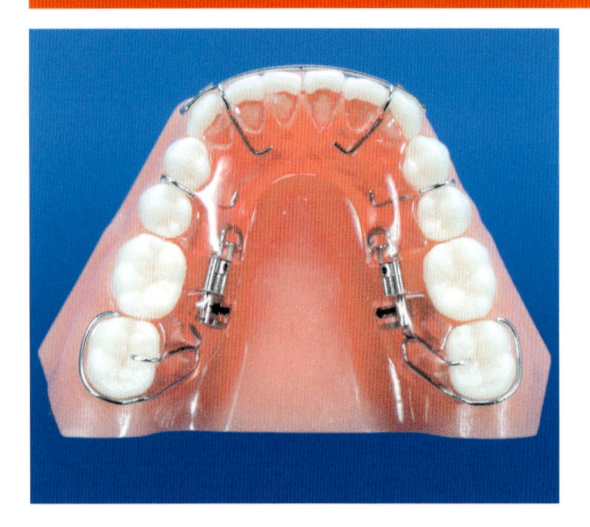

1125 Posterior Space Closure   U/L

Abnormal occlusal forces, periodontal disease, and poor restorative work can cause interproximal spacing to occur in the posterior segments. This often leads to food impaction that is not only annoying but can also contribute to a worsening of the periodontal condition. This excess space can be easily reversed with an appliance like the one shown here.

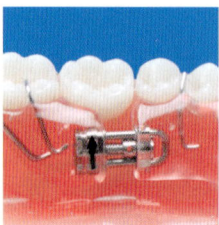

Anchorage is the key to successfully closing this space. The appliance typically requires anterior retention using a combination of bilateral clasping and a labial bow. Then, stainless "retraction" screws are placed bilaterally as needed to close the interproximal spaces through mesial movement of the molars.

Typically, heavy "C" clasps are placed around the distal of the last molars and the acrylic is removed from the interproximal areas around the teeth needing mesial movement.

Design Notes:

INDIVIDUAL TOOTH MOVEMENT

an overview: INDIVIDUAL TOOTH MOVEMENT

Chapter 6

Children

When treating children, it is important to regularly monitor their growth and development. The clinician should constantly check to see if any interceptive orthodontics will be necessary. Even in cases where the arches are nicely developed and the skeletal relationship is well balanced, there is often the need for some minor tooth movement. This is the case because the sequence of eruption seems to be slightly different for every patient.

For example, it is not uncommon for a primary central to exfoliate late and cause an adult central to erupt lingually. When this is the case, a simple appliance can be used to help guide this central back into its normal position.

Another common situation where minor tooth movement is appropriate is when the cuspids are forced to erupt in a mesial-buccal position because the first bicuspids erupted before them. When the arch length is sufficient, the cuspids can easily be brought back into the arch by first moving the bicuspids distally prior to retracting the cuspids.

When an appliance is properly designed, it can be used to accomplish multiple tooth movements. For example, by using numerous springs, one appliance can be used to close the space between the centrals, to create room for blocked out laterals and then guide the laterals into place. To accomplish these movements, the springs must be adjusted sequentially. Do not attempt to activate all the springs at once.

Adults

Today, more than ever, cosmetic dentistry is an integral part of an active practice. You shouldn't call yourself a cosmetic dentist if you are unable recognize when orthodontic therapy would enhance your ability to create a superior esthetic result. Minor tooth movement, in conjunction with your restorative care, can be used in many ways to enhance a patient's appearance. For example, when an anterior is labially placed, a small amount of tooth movement will often allow you to use a less invasive procedure and minimize the amount of tooth reduction needed. This minor tooth movement procedure will allow you to place a veneer instead of a crown, which usually gives the patient a better esthetic result.

INDIVIDUAL TOOTH MOVEMENT

1071 Micro-Screw   U/L

Individual teeth can easily be moved labially with a removable appliance. Here, a micro-screw is being used. This special screw has a spring-loaded piston within its housing. By adjusting the screw one-half turn weekly, a constant pressure can be maintained on the tooth to be moved. A special screwdriver is available from your laboratory.

Micro-screws work well when direct labial or buccal movement is needed and if the tooth is sufficiently erupted (at least 4mm of the lingual surface needs to be well exposed). If a tooth needs to be rotated as it is moved labially, it would be best to use a recurved finger spring or bonded brackets.

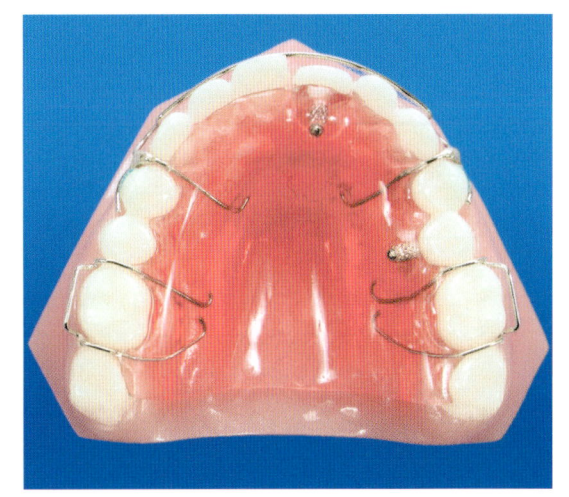

Caution - Do not over-adjust the micro-screw as this can damage the spring-loaded piston.

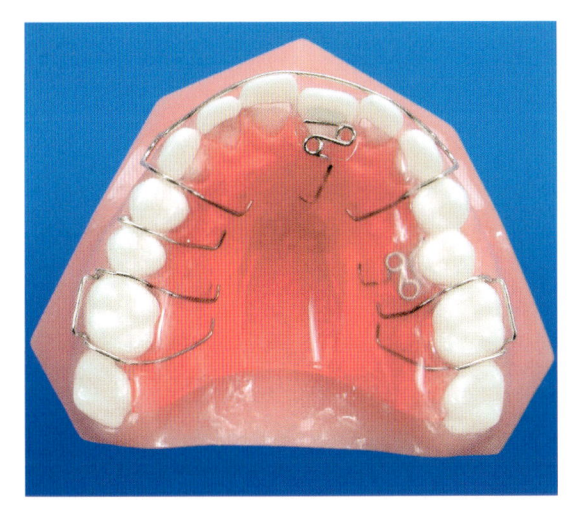

1072 Recurved Finger Spring   U/L

An alternative to a micro-screw for moving a tooth labially is the recurved spring. With proper positioning and adjustment, this spring can also be used to correct minor rotations. To activate these springs, simply pull forward on the spring's arm with a 139 bird-beak plier.

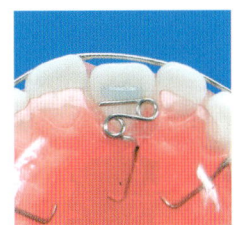

Typically, if the lingual surface of the tooth to be moved is quite vertical, the acrylic is left over the top of the finger spring.

However, if the lingual incline is rather shallow, it is suggested that a composite ledge be placed on the lingual of the tooth (illustrated in blue).

A composite ledge will prevent the activated finger spring from riding up the lingual incline of the central, greatly improving its effectiveness. When this is the case, it is recommended that the acrylic be cleared away from the top of the spring as shown. This makes it easier for the dentist to adjust the spring and for the patient to properly insert the activated appliance. Upon insertion, the patient needs to be certain that the spring arm "snaps" gingival to the composite ledge.

Note - It may necessary to open the bite with an anterior or posterior bite plane if any of the teeth are locked in lingual crossbite.

6.1

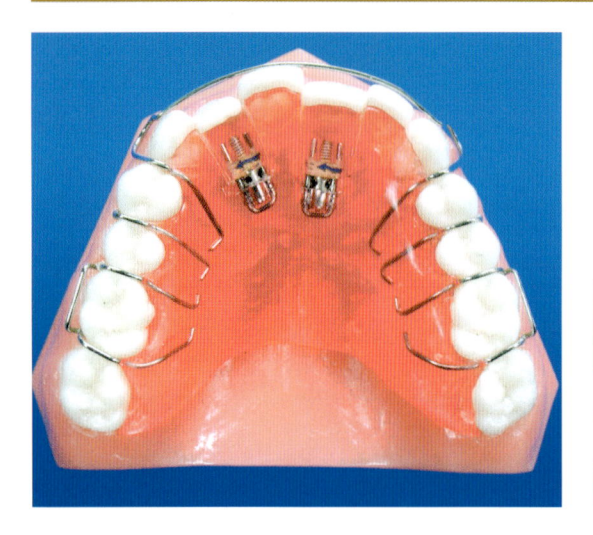

INDIVIDUAL TOOTH MOVEMENT

1091 Mini-Screw Appliance   U

In cases where you need to move a tooth labially and you choose not to use a recurved finger spring or a micro-screw, the use of a mini-screw is an excellent alternative. Because they are easy for the patient to adjust, some doctors use them in situations when the patient cannot readily return to their office on the recommended bi-weekly basis.

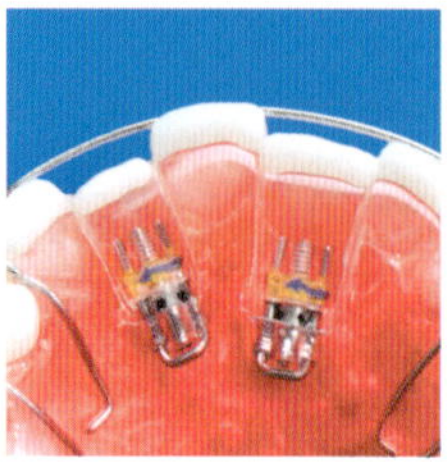

These screws add a modest amount of bulk to the anterior portion of the appliance creating an anterior bite plane. This typically is not a problem; however, the use of this design is contraindicated in a patient who already has an open bite and is a vertical grower.

1072B   Recurved Extrusion Spring   U/L

When a primary molar has been overly retained, it can inhibit the eruption of a succedaneous bicuspid in relation to the rest of the arch.

This unique appliance uses a recurved finger spring to aid in the eruption of a single bicuspid. A direct bond straight wire bracket is placed on the bicuspid to create an undercut for the helical recurved spring. The patient then simply inserts the activated appliance and "snaps" the activated spring under the gingival tie wings of the bracket. This not only expedites the eruption of the tooth, but also aids in appliance retention.

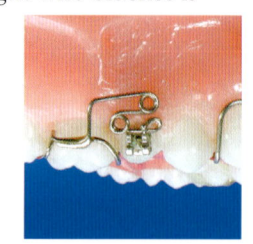

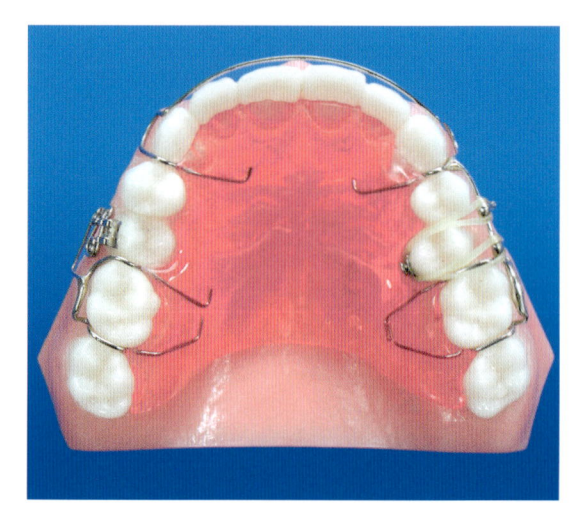

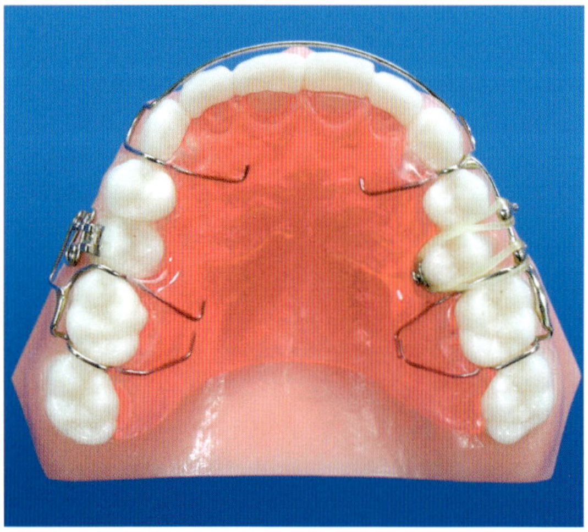

1072E   Fixed/Removable Buccal Sling-shot   U/L

Another method to move a bicuspid buccally, other than a finger spring, mini-screw, or micro-screw, is the use of a "sling-shot" elastic.

By bonding a button onto the lingual surface of the bicuspid, an elastic can be carried from hooks on the labial bow to this button to move the bicuspid buccally. This method is sometimes preferred to a finger spring or a micro-screw, especially when timely office visits are difficult for your patient.

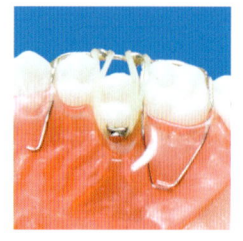

6.2

INDIVIDUAL TOOTH MOVEMENT

1076B Multi-spring Appliance   U/L

A properly designed removable appliance can be used to accomplish multiple tooth movements. In this example, our objective is to close the space between the centrals, create room in the arch form for the blocked out laterals, and guide the laterals into place. This design shows the use of two different mesial kicker springs to move the centrals, a re-curved spring to move one of the laterals labially, and a T-spring to move the other lateral lingually. To accomplish the numerous movements, they must be done sequentially. Do not attempt to activate all the springs at once.

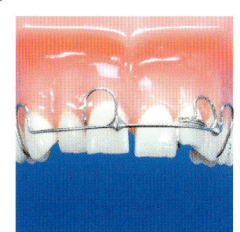

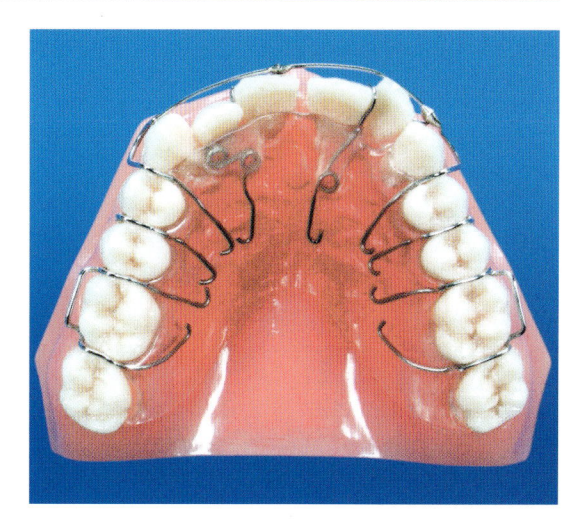

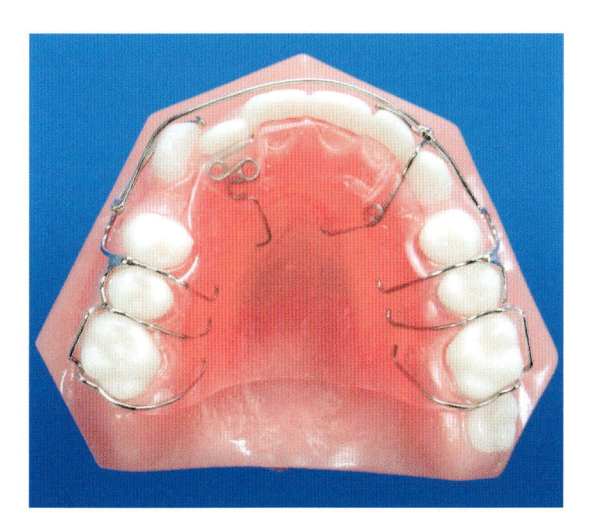

1076C Multi-spring Cuspid Retraction Appliance U/L

This is another design using finger springs to accomplish a variety of objectives. It is important to provide extra retention, in the form of "C" clasps soldered to the labial wire, when moving anterior teeth. To increase retention, a small composite button can be placed on the buccal just occlusal to the "C" clasp to create a retentive undercut. In situations where the mesial of the cuspid is not well exposed, the use of a bonded button or bracket will provide a positive contact point for the spring.

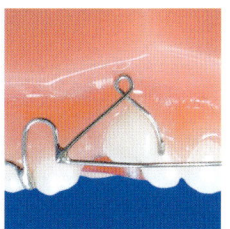

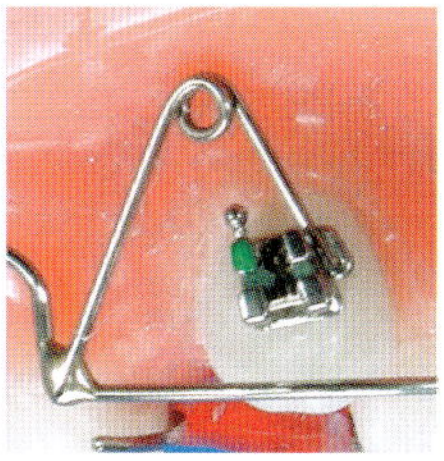

Maximum stability is necessary to keep the appliance fully seated when activating the finger springs. Remember, it is recommended to activate no more than two springs at any one time. Activating more than this tends to compromise overall appliance retention, slowing down treatment time.

6.3

INDIVIDUAL TOOTH MOVEMENT

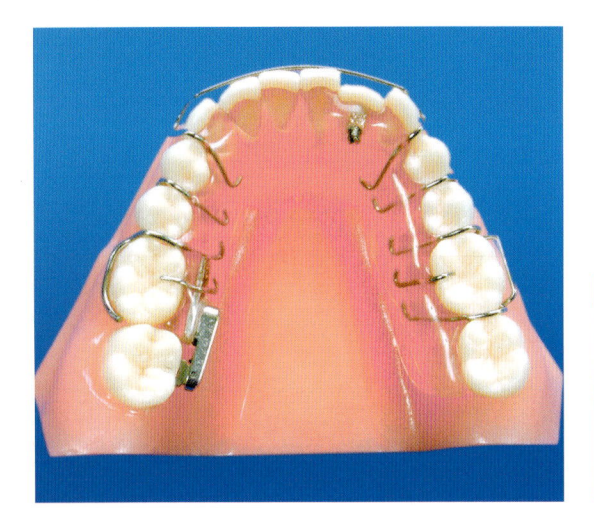

1334 Single Tooth Molar Uprighter   L

When the distal-most molar on the lower arch erupts in lingual version, this special expansion screw can upright it very efficiently, provided that no more than approximately 3mm of movement is needed. It affords a precisely controlled tipping of the crown without bodily movement. A key is provided with the appliance for the weekly adjustments.

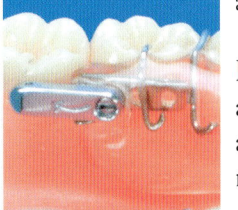

If the molar is in a locked lingual crossbite, it is advisable to request that a posterior bite plane be added to the appliance to facilitate this movement.

Note - This appliance also shows a micro-screw. This screw is a very effective way of moving a single tooth labially in both arches.

1076D Multi-spring Posterior Space Regainer U/L

Abnormal exfoliation and eruption patterns can cause erupting teeth to be blocked out of the arch form. When the overall arch length is sufficient, an appliance like the one shown here is ideal to move the bicuspids, allowing the submerged teeth to erupt.

This example also illustrates the proper use and placement of the retention components needed for this active appliance. Note that the labial arch wire used here is of the "Reverse Hawley" design. This affords cuspid support without having cross-over wires distal to the cuspids.

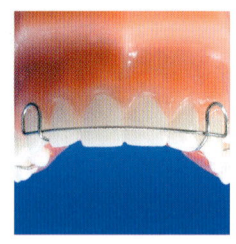

As a result, the right bicuspid can be moved into complete contact with the cuspid. Likewise, a "C" clasp (possibly used in conjunction with a composite ledge) is used on the left first molar to permit complete distalization of the left second bicuspid. These are all critical design considerations in this treatment scenario.

Design Notes:

INDIVIDUAL TOOTH MOVEMENT

1076E Multi-spring Molar Uprighter   U/L

This appliance illustrates the use of two very effective uprighting springs: the mushroom spring and the distal recurve. These springs are easy to adjust and can very effectively tip molars upright, usually with only two or three adjustments. Placing a rest on the molar being uprighted by the distal recurve, aids in controlling super-eruption when an opposing tooth is missing.

Note - When using a "C" clasp, consider the use of a composite ledge for superior retention.

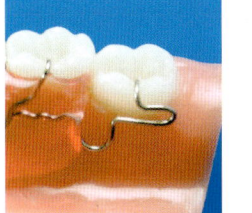

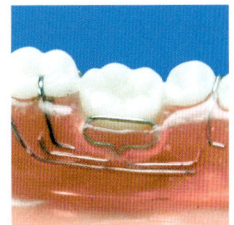

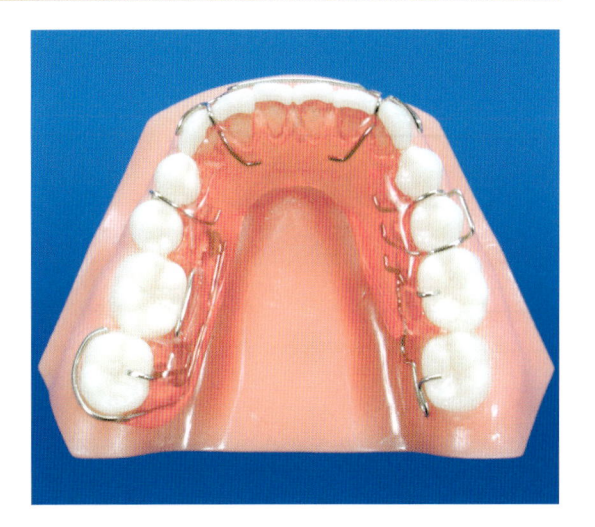

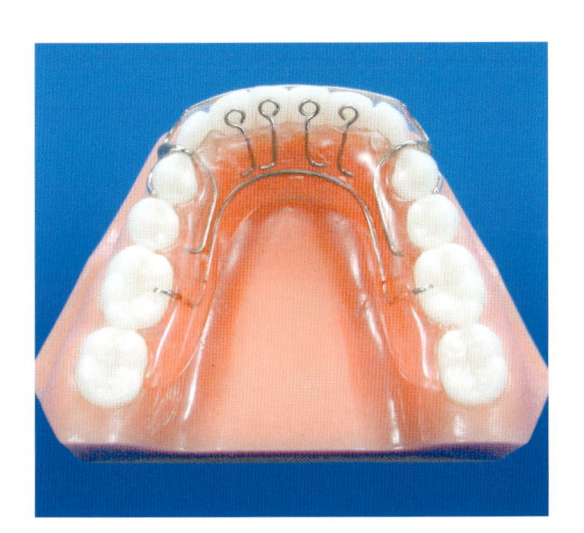

1076F Bloore Aligner   U/L

Patients who have a small amount of crowding in their upper or lower incisors often prefer to try to correct this problem without having to wear braces. The Bloore Aligner was designed specifically for that purpose. Springs, called eyelet arms, are placed lingual to each incisor and are individually activated to move the teeth into alignment. As needed, interproximal reductions and incisal re-contouring are utilized to gain room and provide an esthetic result.

Note - When used on the lower arch, it is important to make sure that the incisors are not coupling with the lingual of the uppers prior to initiating treatment, as vertical and AP clearance are required to successfully correct the lower anteriors.

Design Notes:

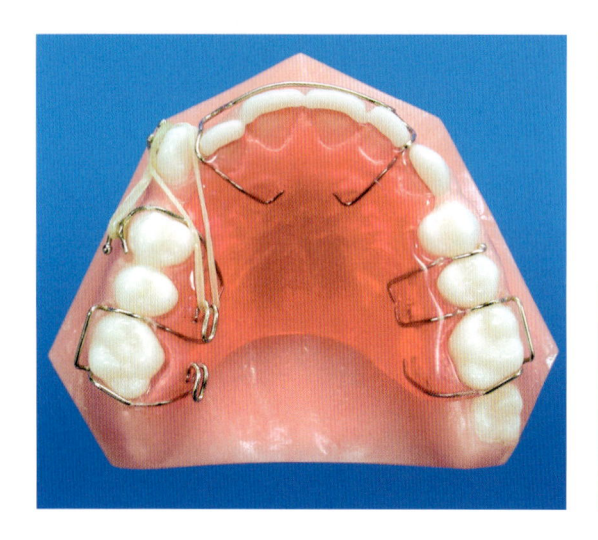

INDIVIDUAL TOOTH MOVEMENT

1054 Direct Bond Cuspid Retraction   U/L

Combining the versatility of a removable appliance with the positive control of a fixed attachment, we can even effectively retract a cuspid. In the appliance shown here, the attachments (buccal and lingual hooks and the bracket) can be strategically placed to move the cuspid distally as shown, lingually, or even to help it erupt.

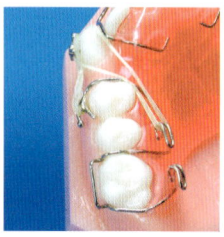

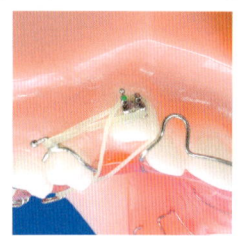

The appliance comes complete with the direct bond brackets ready for cementation and a supply of the appropriate size elastics. Little adjustment is necessary other than to change the elastics daily and keep the retentive clasps tight so the removable section remains stable.

1054B Direct Bond/Spring Cuspid Retraction   U/L

Occasionally an erupting cuspid may need to be tipped distally and lingually while the remainder of the arch needs little, if any, additional treatment. In this situation, you may consider the use of a combination removable appliance with a cuspid retraction spring and a direct bond straight wire bracket. The bracket not only provides a positive contact point for the activated spring, it also allows for the use of an elastic, if desired, to enhance the movement.

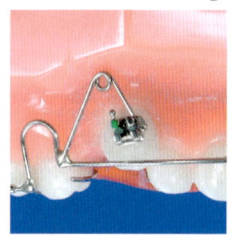

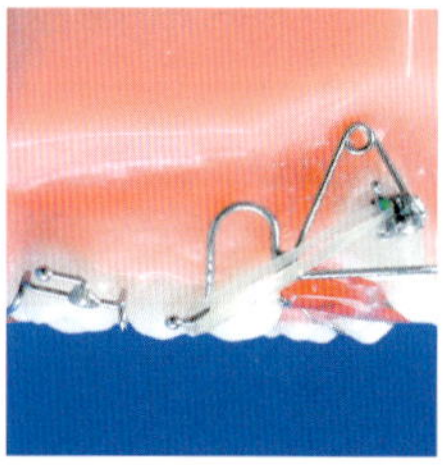

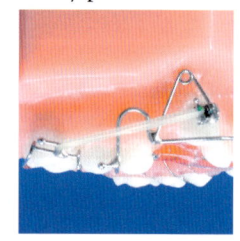

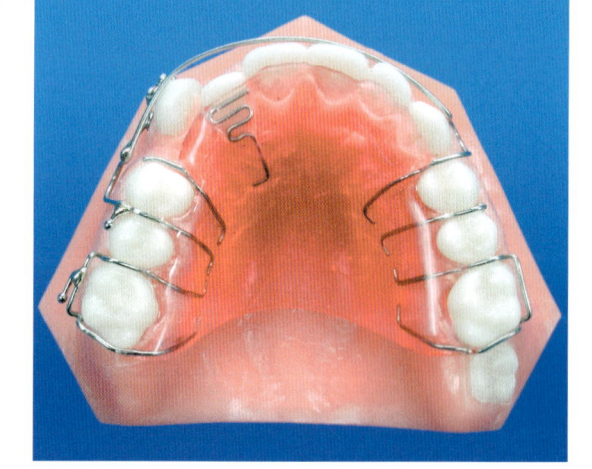

INDIVIDUAL TOOTH MOVEMENT

1063 Combination Fixed/Removable Appliance   U/L

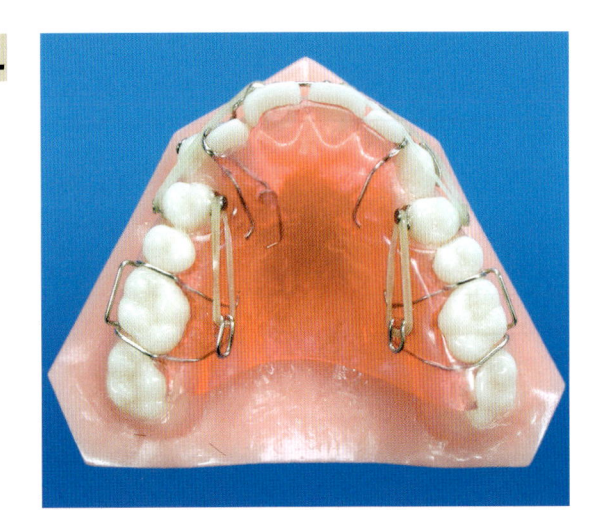

It was once very difficult to effect rotation of a molar or bicuspid using a removable device. This combination fixed-removable appliance has solved the problem.

As shown here, direct bond buttons can be placed on just those teeth needing rotation, with hooks for elastics placed wherever they are needed on the removable appliance. Using a mirror, the patient can be easily taught to hook up the elastics.

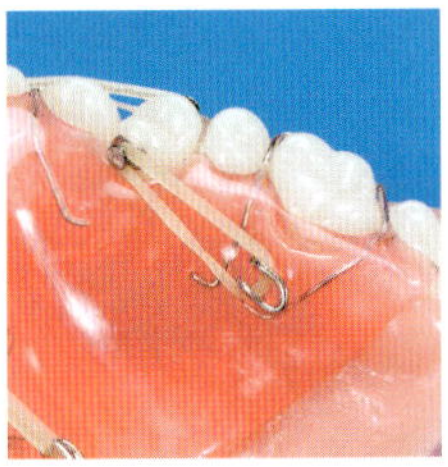

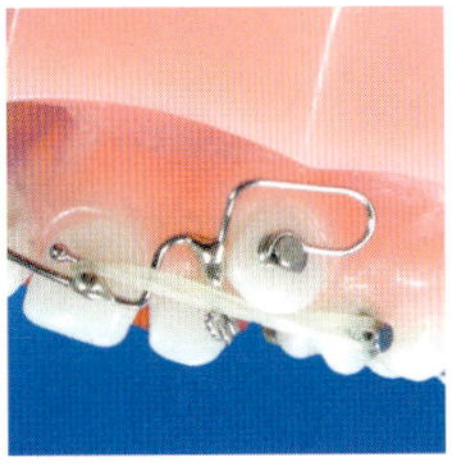

In addition, well-designed finger springs can also be added to afford other needed corrections. In this case, a combination finger spring/direct bond button is used on the right cuspid to aid in its eruption and distal positioning as the first bicuspid is rotated.

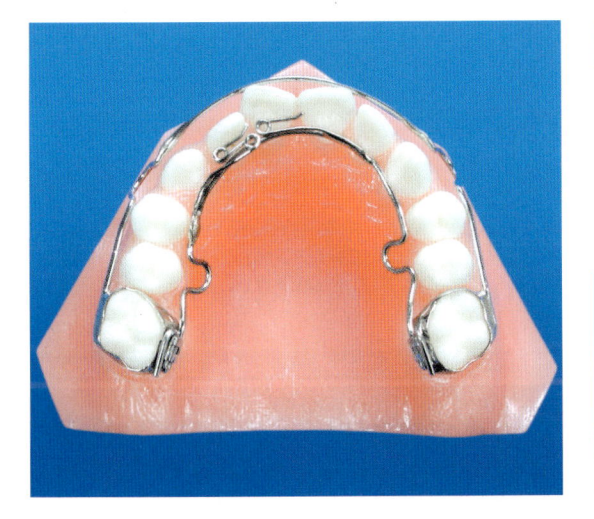

2061 Labial-Lingual Appliance   U/L

Almost anything that you can accomplish with a removable appliance can be done with a fixed appliance. This is very important when treating younger, less cooperative patients.

This fixed appliance includes two finger springs, one to rotate the central and the other to move the lateral labially into position. The labial arch has direct pressure arms in contact with the mesial edge of the centrals and adjustment loops opposite the cuspids. These loops may be closed as movement is accomplished to retain the results. The lingual arch is easily removed so that adjustments can be made out of the patient's mouth. Replacing it is just as easy.

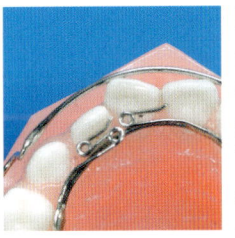

Note - To get an overview of all the components that can be added to a fixed appliance simply review Chapter One of this publication.

6.7

Design Notes

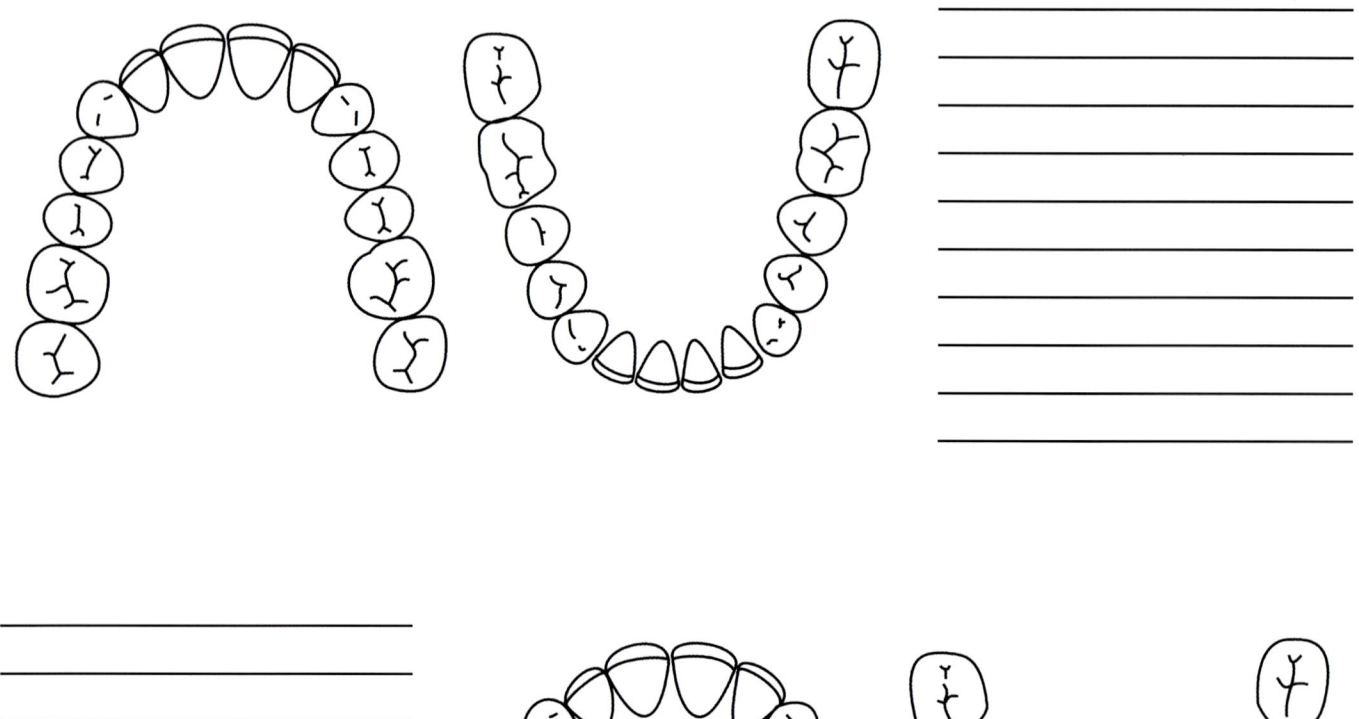

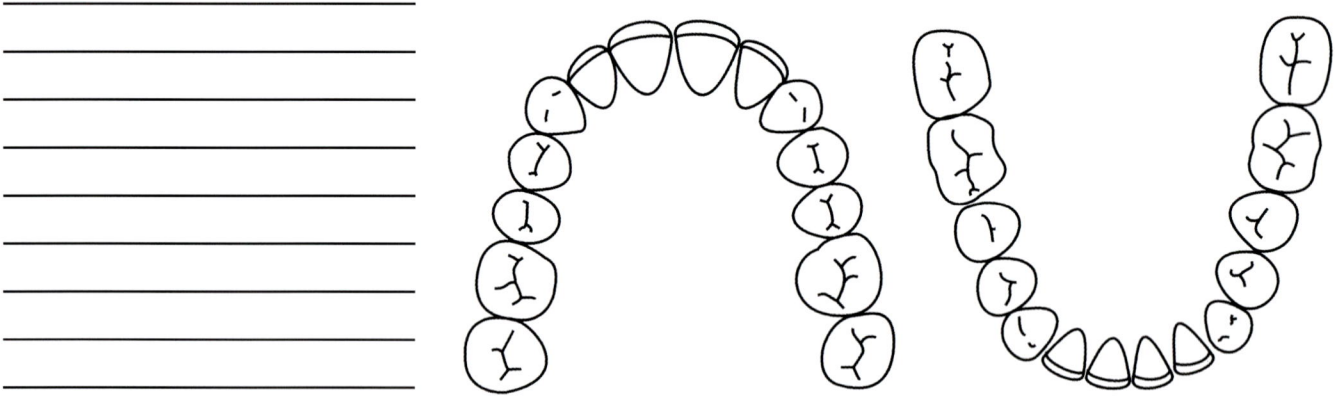

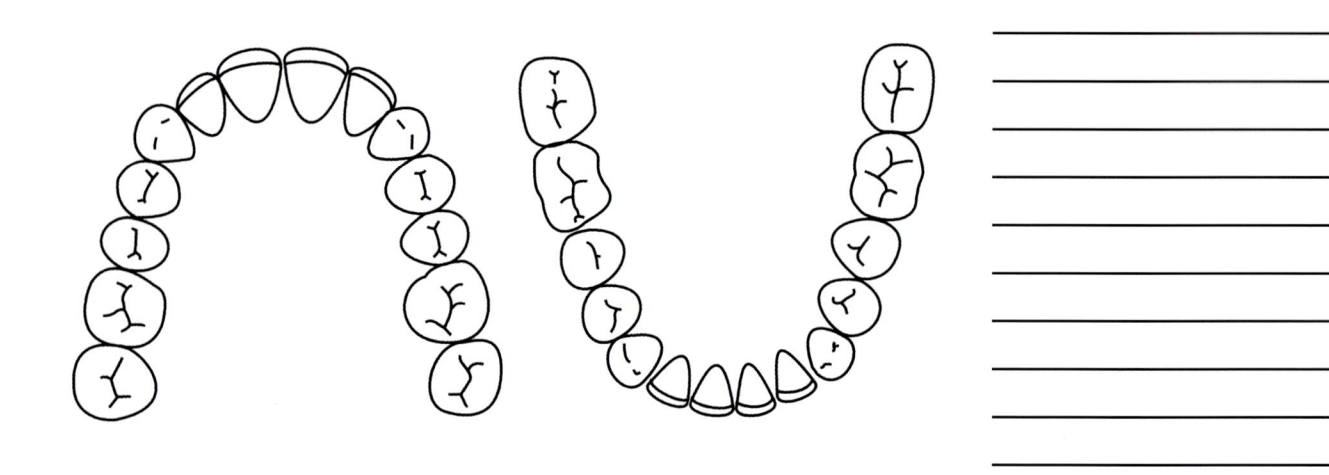

CROSSBITES

an overview: CROSSBITES

Chapter 7

Crossbites are one of the most common orthodontic problems that we see in growing children. They usually occur in the primary and mixed dentition as a result of disharmony in either the skeletal, functional, or dental components of the orthognathic system of the child.

Crossbites should be treated in the primary and mixed dentition. Allowing the malocclusion to continue into the permanent dentition without correction will result in a reduction of treatment options and provide a less than ideal environment for growth to proceed in an orderly fashion.

Specifically, an untreated crossbite can lead to gingival inflammation and recession of the investing tissues surrounding the mal-opposed teeth; occlusal trauma, enamel abrasion or fractures; the development of abnormal chewing and swallowing problems; abnormal growth of the maxilla and the mandible; the development of a permanent Class III dentofacial abnormality; asymmetric growth of the mandible and temporomandibular joint dysfunction.

Anterior Crossbites

There are three types of anterior crossbites found in children. They are the simple dental crossbite, the functional or pseudo crossbite, and the skeletal crossbite.

An anterior crossbite is defined as simple when it involves only one or two teeth and the mandible has a smooth arc of closure into an Angle Class I molar and cuspid relationship.

Patients who have a functional anterior crossbite, exhibit a forward shift of the mandible. This is usually caused by an early occlusal interference during closing. As the mandible shifts forward into centric occlusion, the incisors are placed into crossbite and the molars into a Class III relationship. Over time the maxillary incisors will become retroclined and the mandibular incisors will become proclined.

A true skeletal Class III, or mesiocclusion, is caused by a skeletal dysplasia involving mandibular hypertrophy, a marked shortening of the cranial base or maxilla, or a combination of both. The main characteristics they exhibit are that they will maintain a Class III molar relationship and an anterior crossbite in centric occlusion and centric relation while their arc of mandibular closure remains smooth without any occlusal interferences.

Posterior Crossbites

There are four types of posterior crossbites. They are a bilateral posterior crossbite, a laterocclusal unilateral posterior crossbite and a laterognathic unilateral posterior crossbite and a true unilateral posterior crossbite. Each category is unique and has specific diagnostic criteria.

When both posterior segments are in crossbite and the patient's skeletal midlines are aligned regardless of whether the mandible is at postural rest or in habitual occlusion, the patient has a bilateral crossbite. The cause of this crossbite is usually a narrow maxillary alveolar arch. Treatment usually consists of using a removable lateral expansion appliance with occlusal coverage, or in severe cases, a Rapid Palatal Expander may be indicated.

an overview: CROSSBITES

Chapter 7

A laterocclusal crossbite exists when, at mandibular postural rest, the posterior segments appear to be either in an end-to-end bite or in a bilateral crossbite, and the skeletal midlines are coincident and well centered. Then as soon as the teeth are brought into occlusion, a shift of the mandible laterally occurs leading to one side going into crossbite while the other appears to occlude normally. This lateroclusion is due to a functional adjustment of the mandible caused by a tooth interference. Although it is often hard to find the interference point, the shifting of the skeletal mid-lines is usually quite visible.

Because a laterocclusal crossbite is really a bilateral crossbite that appears to be unilateral, treatment is the same and is often done by merely widening the narrow maxillary arch with any uniform bilateral expansion appliance.

A functional shift left untreated for a prolonged period of time during the growth period can lead to asymmetric jaw development. This is called laterognathism. A laterognathic crossbite exists when the midline shift is present in both the occlusal and postural rest positions. This is a true facial skeletal asymmetry and quite difficult to treat. Transcranial x-rays, or tomograms, of TMJ must be taken and analyzed before treatment is initiated.

A true unilateral posterior crossbite exists when one posterior segment is in crossbite and the patient's skeletal midlines are aligned regardless of whether the mandible is at postural rest or in habitual occlusion. Correction of minor unilateral crossbites of this nature can be treated carefully with appliances designed to move only one quadrant buccally.

Design Notes

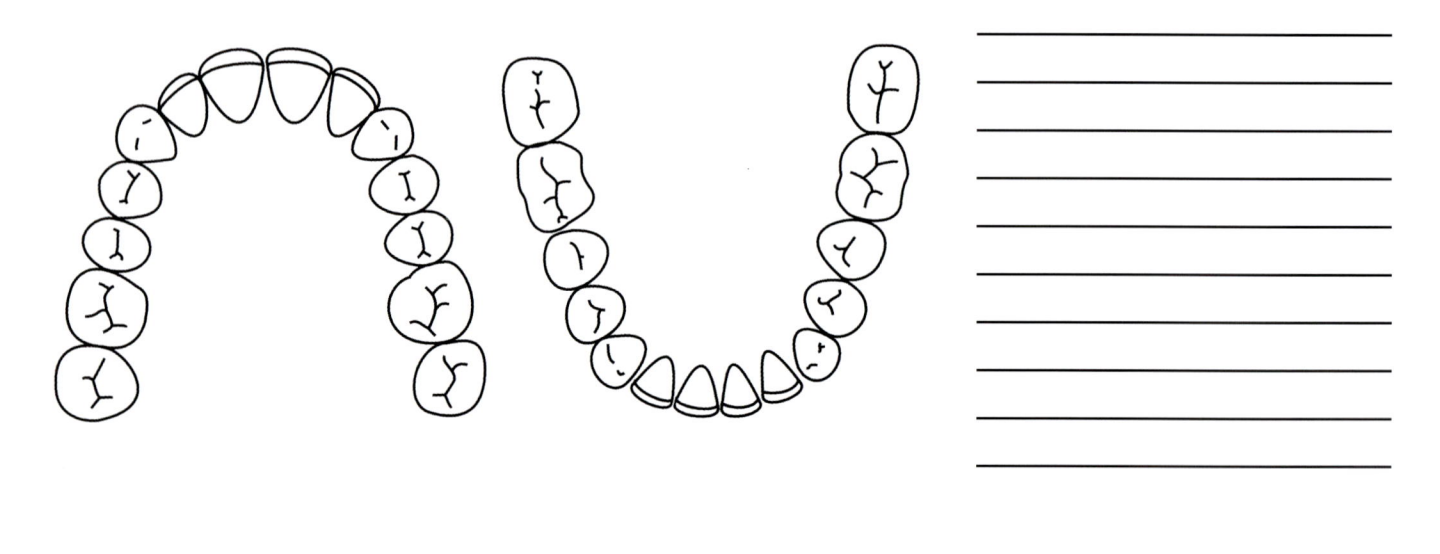

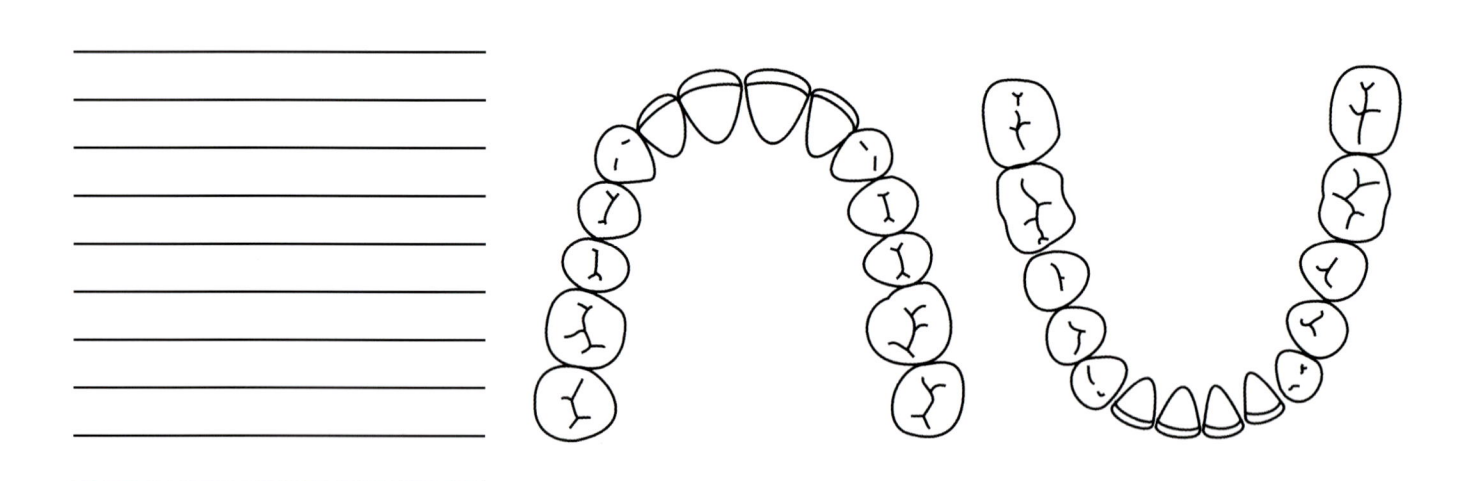

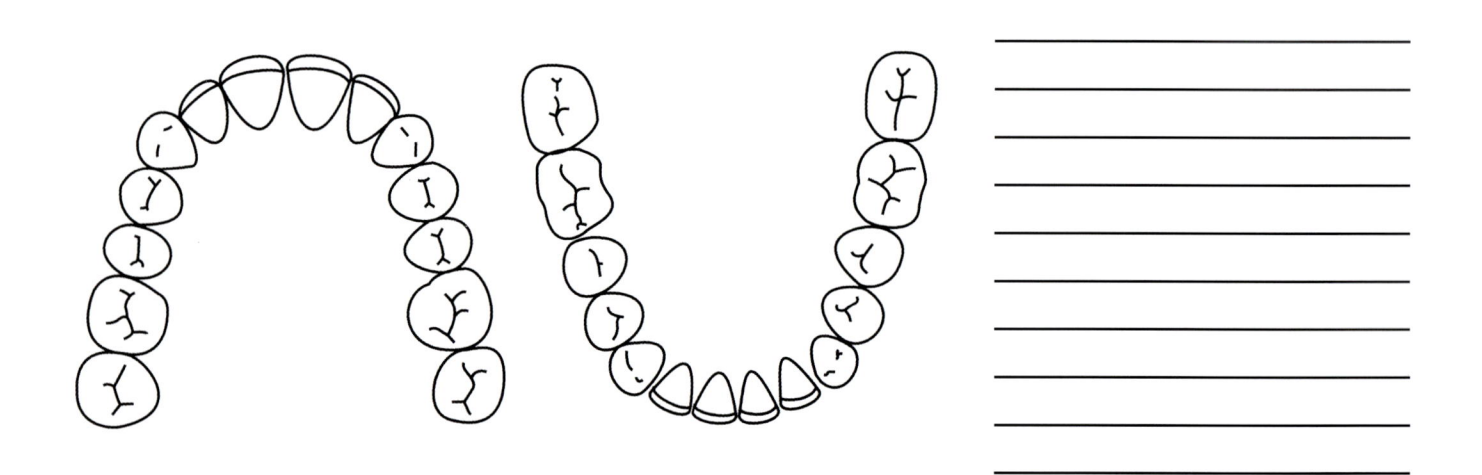

CROSSBITES

2081 Molar Crossbite Correction with Bands

It is not unusual for molars to erupt into crossbite. When this is a true single tooth crossbite (i.e. the midlines are concomitant and there is no visible shift of the mandible), it can easily be corrected with this simple appliance.

Here, maxillary and mandibular bands are made for the two molars. Hooks are placed on the buccal of the maxillary band and on the lingual of the mandibular band, so an elastic force can be used to correct the crossbite. This applies a reciprocal force moving both molars. If the patient is already in the adult dentition stage, slight occlusal adjustment of the molars, or the use of a bite plane, is often needed as the crossbite is treated.

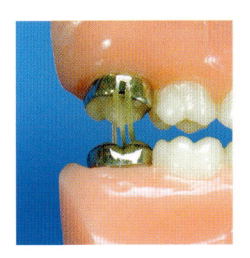

Once the condition is corrected, normal intercuspation is usually sufficient to maintain the results. Bands, as opposed to direct bond hooks alone, are recommended when significant occlusal interferences are present that may cause a direct bond bracket to be sheared off the tooth.

Note - If only one tooth needs to be moved, the other must be tied to an anchor unit or this approach will not work.

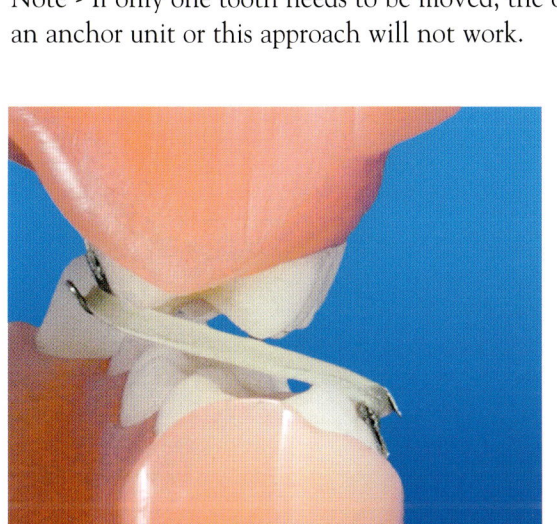

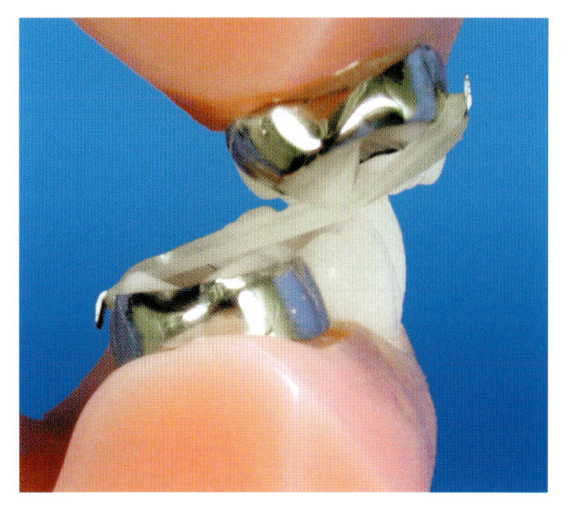

2082 Molar Crossbite Correction with Bonded Hooks

Many practitioners have found it easier to use bonded hooks instead of bands when they need to jump a molar crossbite. Here, direct bond hooks are placed on the buccal surface of the maxillary molar and on the lingual surface of the mandibular molar. Inter-arch elastics are then used to correct the crossbite. This applies a reciprocal force moving both molars.

If only one tooth needs to be moved, the other must be tied to an anchor unit or this approach will not work. Buttons can be used in place of hooks if desired; however, hooks retain the elastic better.

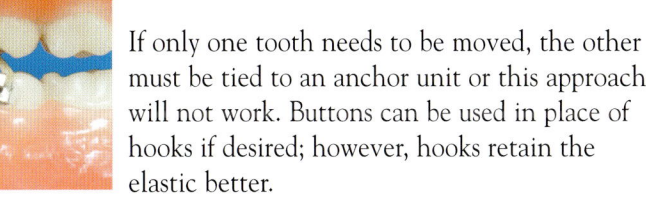

Note - If the patient is already in the adult dentition stage, slight occlusal adjustment of the molars or the use of a bite plane is often needed as the crossbite is treated. This can be accomplished by using a Hawley with an anterior bite plane or a bruxism splint. Once the condition is corrected, normal intercuspation is usually sufficient to maintain the results.

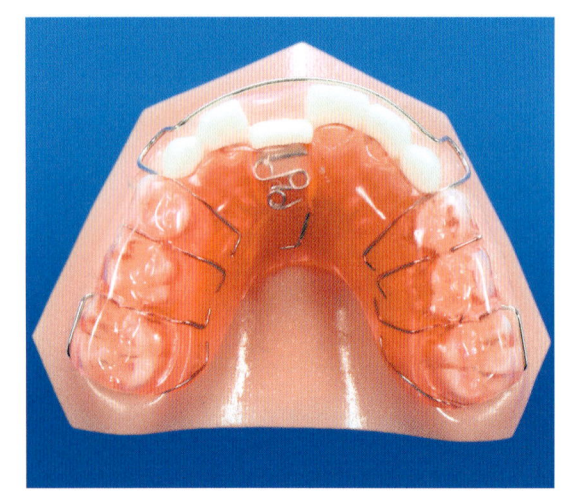

CROSSBITES

1075 Single Tooth Anterior Crossbite with Bite Plane U

Abnormal eruption patterns such as a retained primary can often cause one or two anteriors to erupt into crossbite. Choosing the best appliance to correct this problem is dependent upon the depth of the bite, the space available, and whether or not an occlusal interference is involved.

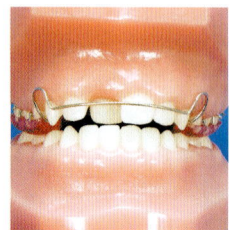

In this example, there is plenty of space in the arch to move the central forward, there are no occlusal interferences causing a mandibular shift, and the depth of the patient's bite is ideal.

To correct this crossbite, a simple Hawley with a posterior occlusal bite plane and a recurved spring is used. The occlusal bite plane clears the occlusion sufficiently to let the recurved spring move the anterior forward while preventing any unwanted change in the patient's ideal vertical dimension. It also aids in retention of the appliance. Once the crossbite is corrected, the bite plane can be removed and the appliance can serve as a retainer.

Note - If the spring is riding up the lingual incline of the central instead of pushing it forward, we recommend that you clear the acrylic away from the spring and add a small composite ledge on the lingual surface of the tooth to act as a positive stop for the spring. This can be seen in Chapter 6, appliance #1072. Removing the acrylic will also make it easier to adjust the spring with a 139 bird-beak plier.

1091 Mini-Screw Appliance   U

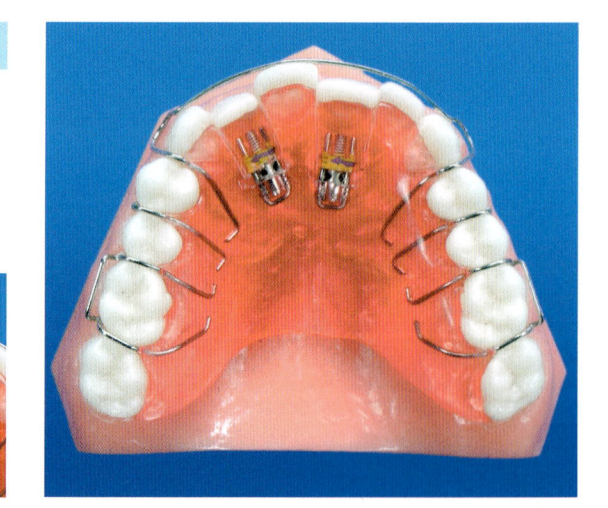

In cases where you need to move a tooth labially and you choose not to use a recurved finger spring or a micro-screw, the use of a mini-screw is an excellent alternative. Because they are easy for the patient to adjust, some doctors use them in situations when the patient cannot readily return to their office on the recommended bi-weekly basis.

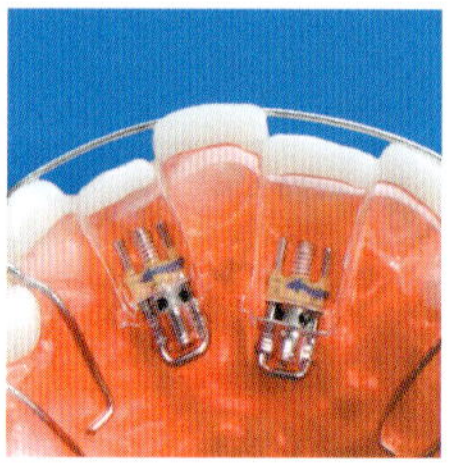

These screws add a modest amount of bulk to the anterior portion of the appliance creating an anterior bite plane. This usually supplies enough occlusal clearance to jump the crossbite.

Once the crossbite is jumped, it will be necessary to switch to a final retainer to stabilize the correction while the occlusion settles into place.

Note - If the patient has a skeletal open bite tendency, adding posterior coverage to this design would be appropriate to prevent any unwanted vertical changes from occurring.

CROSSBITES

1084 Single Tooth Posterior Crossbite U

Abnormal eruption patterns can cause a single molar to end up in crossbite. Choosing the best appliance to correct this problem is dependent upon the depth of the bite and whether or not there is adequate space in the arch to move the tooth back into position.

In this typical example, there is plenty of space to move the molar back into the arch. However, if your clinical and model examination indicates a significantly deep bite and the tooth is locked lingually, a small anterior bite plane should be added to the appliance.

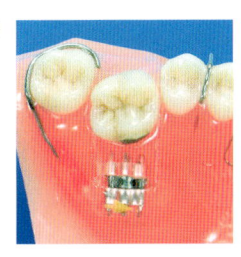

In this photo, a single expansion screw is used to exert pressure on the molar. With this expansion screw, you should expect to get both tipping and some bodily movement of this molar.

Note - All expansion screws of this type are adjusted once a week, one-quarter turn. Remember, as with all crossbite cases, always supply the lab with upper and lower models and a wax bite so we can check for any occlusal interference and assist you in selecting the right design.

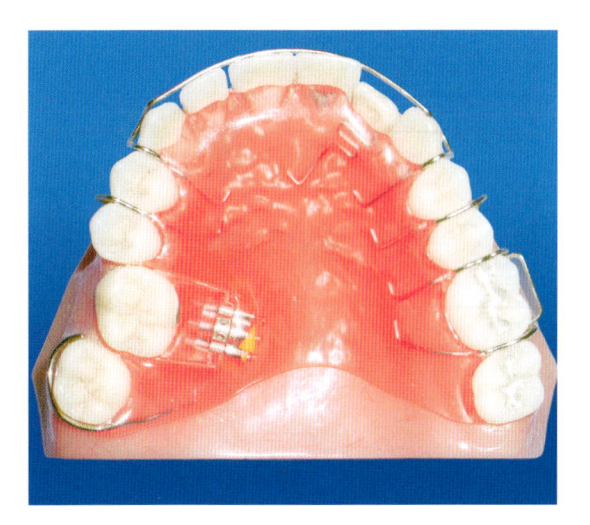

1334 Buccal Molar Uprighting L

It is not unusual to have one molar erupt in lingual version. This special expansion screw is designed to upright the lingually inclined molar. It affords a precisely controlled tipping of the crown without bodily movement. A key is provided with the appliance for the weekly adjustments.

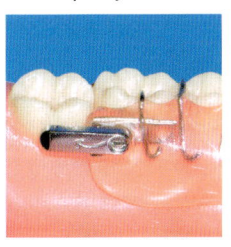

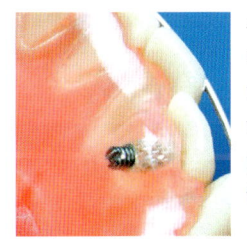

As is the case with all crossbites, it may be necessary to open the bite with an anterior or posterior bite plane to facilitate this movement.

Note - This appliance also shows a micro-screw. This screw is very effective in moving a single tooth labially.

CROSSBITES

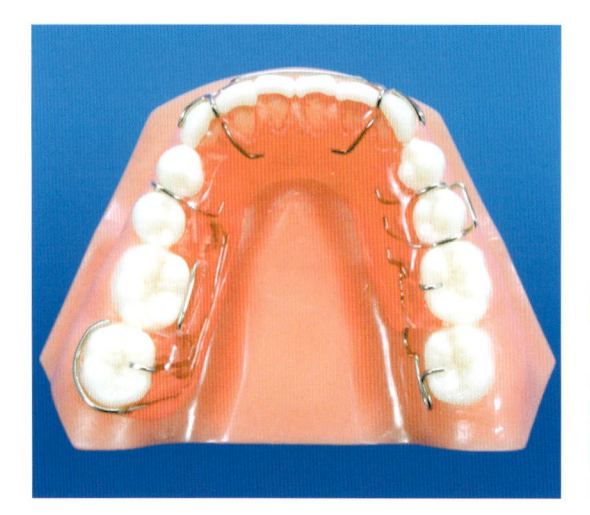

1076E Multi-Spring Molar Crossbite Correction   U/L

This appliance illustrates two very useful uprighting springs: the mushroom spring and the distal recurve. These springs are easy to adjust and can effectively upright tipped molars, usually with only two or three adjustments. The rest, placed on the molar with the distal recurved spring, aids in prohibiting super-eruption when an opposing tooth is missing.

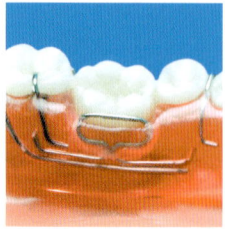

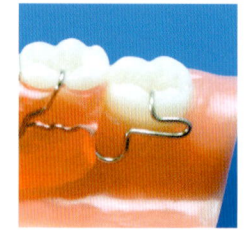

If a lingually positioned molar is locked in position due to occlusal interferences, remember to supply the lab with upper and lower models and a wax bite so occlusal coverage can be added to the appliance to open the bite.

Note - Again, when using "C" clasps, as on the left second molar, consider the use of a composite ledge for superior retention.

1082 Unilateral Posterior Crossbite   U

Most crossbites that seem to be unilateral are, in fact, bilateral. They appear to be unilateral because the mandible shifts to avoid an occlusal interference. So, before beginning to treat a unilateral posterior crossbite, it is essential to make sure that it is truly unilateral. This can be done by observing the relationship of the upper and lower teeth to each other, first out of and then in occlusion. If no shift is observed and there is not a change anywhere in the occlusal relationship, then a true unilateral crossbite exists.

The removable appliance shown here is particularly useful for moving an entire posterior segment that is in a unilateral crossbite. It is designed to utilize the entire part of the arch that is not in crossbite for anchorage, so that by turning the expansion screw, the segment that is in crossbite will move out buccally.

The bite is opened with a posterior bite plane to clear the occlusion. The stationary side of the bite plane is usually ground into occlusion for extra stability while the moving side is left smooth.

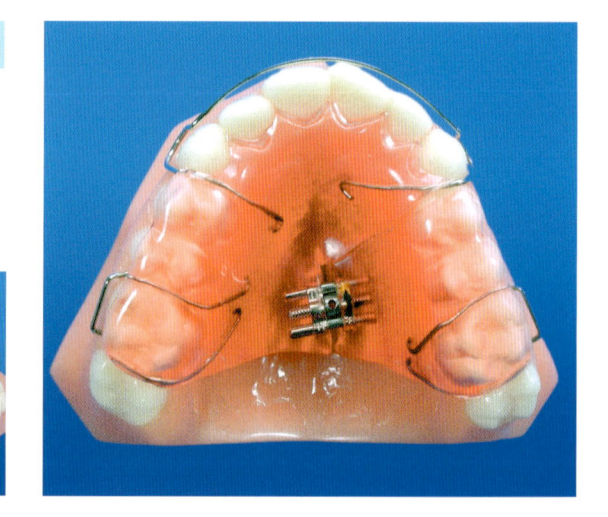

CROSSBITES

1082A Witzig Crossbite Appliance   U

Early loss of the primary molars in an upper quadrant can lead to the mesial eruption of the bicuspids and first molar. Because the anterior part of the arch is narrower, these teeth will often end up in crossbite.

The mesial migration of these teeth also creates enough loss in the arch length that the cuspid either remains impacted or is forced to erupt labially from its normal position. To correct the crossbite and make room for the cuspid, the posterior segment needs to be moved distally and buccally. This can be accomplished with the appliance shown here.

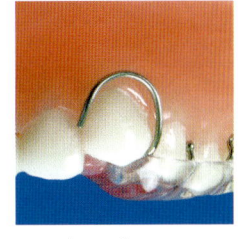

In this design, the expansion screws are angled to provide a disto-buccal movement. The use of two screws is recommended to provide enough force to expedite the crossbite correction. To clear the occlusion, the bite is opened with a posterior bite plane. The stationary side of the bite plane is usually ground into occlusion for extra stability while the moving side is left smooth. A cuspid retraction wire is often added to this appliance to begin guiding the cuspid back to its normal position.

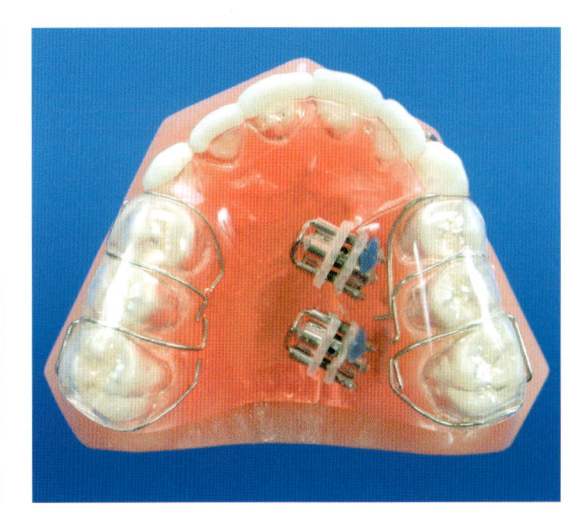

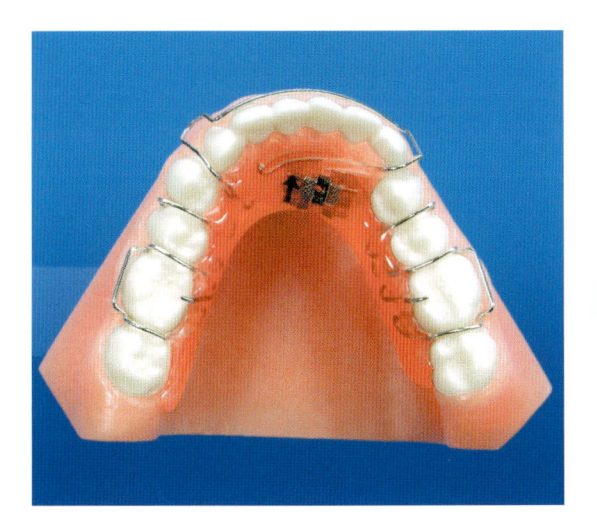

1083 Uprighting Lower Posteriors   L

On occasion, a single lower posterior segment will end up being lingually tipped. By placing the expansion device shown here, it is possible to upright this segment.

In this instance, the labial arch wire is incorporated into the non-moving section to create additional anchorage. The expansion screw is adjusted one-quarter turn once each week, providing 1mm of movement a month. This design is used to move one posterior quadrant buccally, from the bicuspids distally.

Note - If the tipped segment is in crossbite, it will be necessary to either design the appliance with an occlusal plane or make an opposing appliance with an anterior bite plane or occlusal coverage.

Design Notes:

_____
_____
_____
_____
_____

CROSSBITES

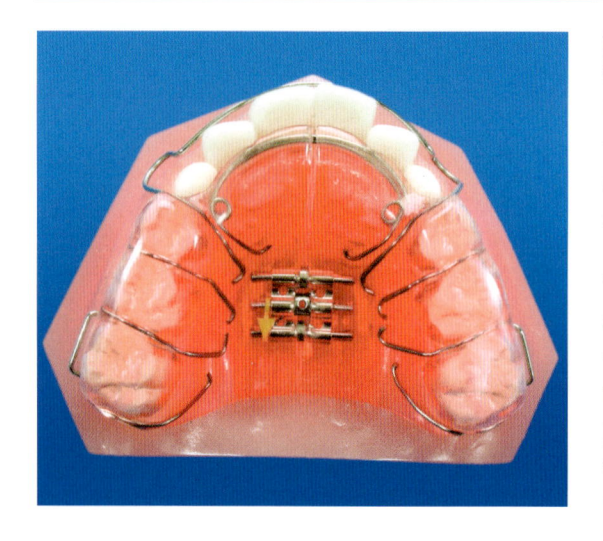

1095 Bilateral Crossbite   U

Bilateral posterior crossbites are usually the result of an underdeveloped maxilla. Some of the reasons that this occurs are an abnormal tongue posture, an irregular swallowing pattern, and an obstructed airway caused by allergies.

The appliance shown here is called a Standard Schwarz with Occlusal Coverage. It is designed with a smooth posterior bite plane to allow the posterior teeth to move free of any occlusal interferences. By turning the expansion screw one-quarter turn a week, a slow constant pressure is exerted on the teeth and bone. It is used to develop the arch and move both posterior segments buccally out of crossbite and, in the process, drop a high vaulted palate, opening the nasal airway. As the palate drops, it will be necessary to adjust the palatal acrylic throughout treatment.

Important - Recognition and treatment of a posterior crossbite early in a child's development is essential. When left untreated, it can lead to numerous serious medical complications. Some of them are a Class II skeletal deformity, TMJ dysfunction, and airway obstruction.

1073 Upper Anterior Crossbite   U

When an occlusal interference occurs in a child, they will often posture their mandible forward to avoid the interference. Although this allows them to maximize their ability to chew with their posterior teeth, it creates a pseudo Class III anterior crossbite or an end-to-end anterior bite.

Over time, this abnormal function will direct the mandible to grow forward, inhibit the growth of the pre-maxilla and create a skeletal Class III. Anterior crossbites of this nature need to be treated as early as possible. The simplest way to do so is to first eliminate the source of the interference and then move the inhibited pre-maxilla back to its normal position with an appliance like the one shown here.

In this appliance, the entire anterior segment is moved labially with an expansion screw placed in the sagittal position. The labial arch wire moves with the segment as a unit while the posterior teeth are used for anchorage. A posterior bite plane is necessary if the anterior teeth are already lingually locked behind the lower incisors.

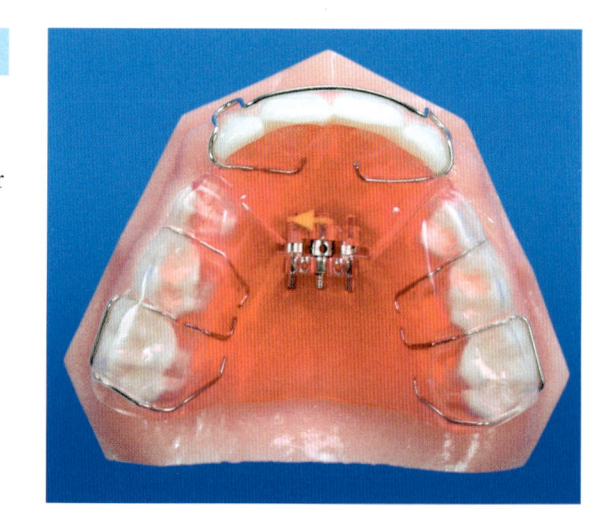

CROSSBITES

1074 Incline Plane   L

Constructed on the mandibular arch, this appliance utilizes an acrylic slide to guide the maxillary anteriors out of lingual version. Careful attention must be given during construction to the angle of the slide to keep the appliance as comfortable, and yet, as effective as possible. Clear acrylic may be used to make the appliance less conspicuous. No adjustment is usually necessary other than occasional spot grinding on the acrylic to facilitate movement.

This appliance requires a very cooperative patient as it is necessary to actively function against the incline in order to achieve results.

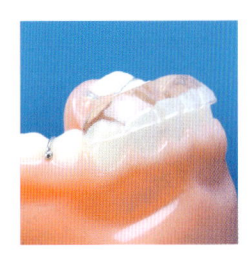

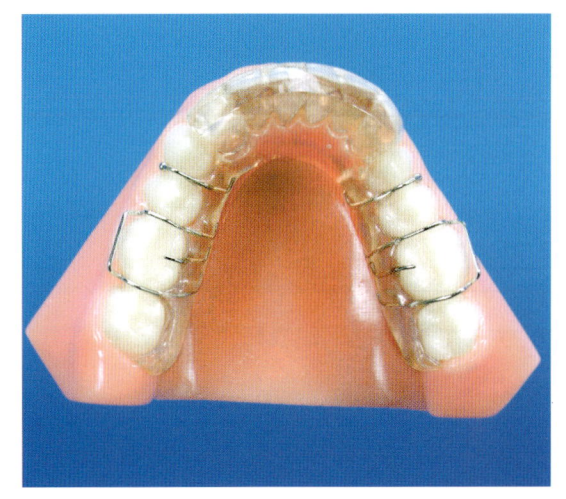

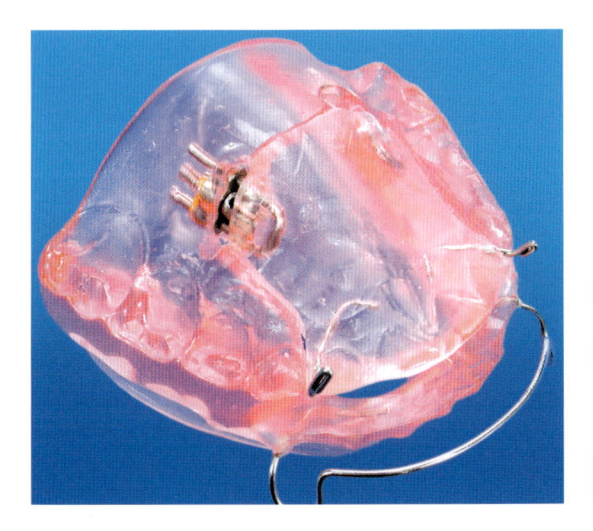

3504 Han Appliance

An anterior occlusal interference can lead to an underdeveloped pre-maxilla and retroclined maxillary anteriors that are locked lingually in crossbite to the lower anteriors. If left untreated over time, this pseudo Class III can become a permanent skeletal defect. The Han Appliance has been found to be an excellent tool for correcting this problem.

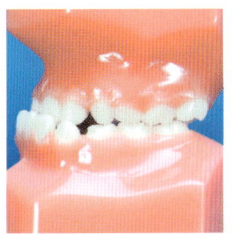

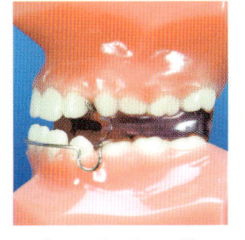

The Han appliance combines the stability and anchorage created by joining the posterior aspect of the maxilla and the entire mandibular arch with the effectiveness of an anterior-developing sagittal. By turning the screws, the pre-maxilla is developed and the anteriors are tipped labially.

Once the anterior segment is developed enough to create a positive overjet, the appliance can typically be replaced with a simple Hawley retainer.

7.7

CROSSBITES

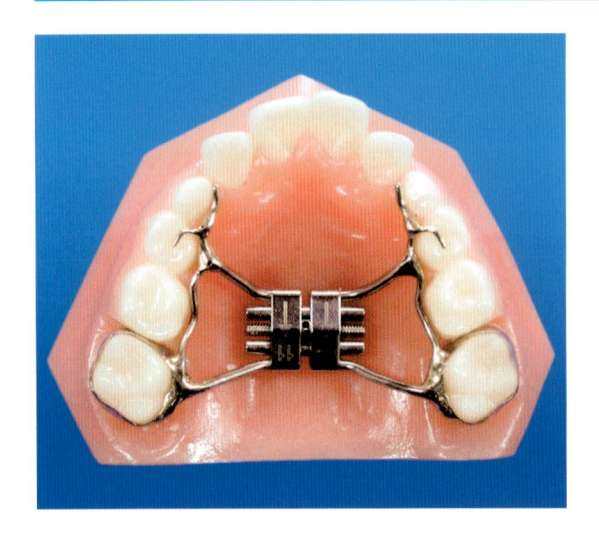

2155 High Palate R.P.E. U

Removable appliances, such as the Schwarz with occlusal coverage, correct crossbites by utilizing a slow constant pressure on the teeth and bone.

Another approach that has shown to be equally effective is the use of rapid expansion to open the mid-palatal suture. The rapid palate expansion hyrax design shown here can be used successfully in patients with mild to moderate transverse constriction when they are in the late mixed or early permanent dentition as the sutures are presumably still patent. This appliance works best when the crossbite is caused by a deficiency of the maxillary apical base. Rapid expansion is obtained with this design over a two to three week period by means of turning the expansion screw once a day. This creates enough pressure to separate the mid-palatal suture. The appliance is then worn for another three to five months to allow time for osseous healing.

This appliance uses an all-stainless metal framework. The expansion screw is positioned high in the palate for greater comfort. Bands are placed on the first molars and rests are bonded to the occlusal surface of the primary molars. This eliminates the path of insertion problem that occurs when four bands are used. Extra heavy support wires are also used to prevent the appliance from flexing as pressure is applied.

If you find that the posterior crossbite is locked due to a deep bite or tight intercuspation, it is recommend that a lower occlusal splint be placed temporarily to expedite treatment without affecting the mandibular dentition.

2343 Direct Bond Suture Expansion

This design uses direct bond occlusal pads for retention instead of banding 1st bicuspids and 6-year molars. This feature not only facilitates movement when a crossbite is present, but because it covers the buccal cusp tips, it prevents tipping from occurring. The design of this bonded bite plane, along with a rigid framework, creates a movement that is mainly orthopedic in nature.

This is an excellent design, especially for those patients who are still in mixed dentition. Besides correcting a crossbite, it has been shown that expansion of the maxilla during the early mixed dentition may lead to a spontaneous correction of other occlusal disharmonies. For example, expansion of the upper arch in a skeletal Class II can allow the mandible to come forward on its own.

Note - When delivering this appliance make sure to maintain a dry environment. Special instructions along with all the necessary supplies can be provided to you through Success Essentials.

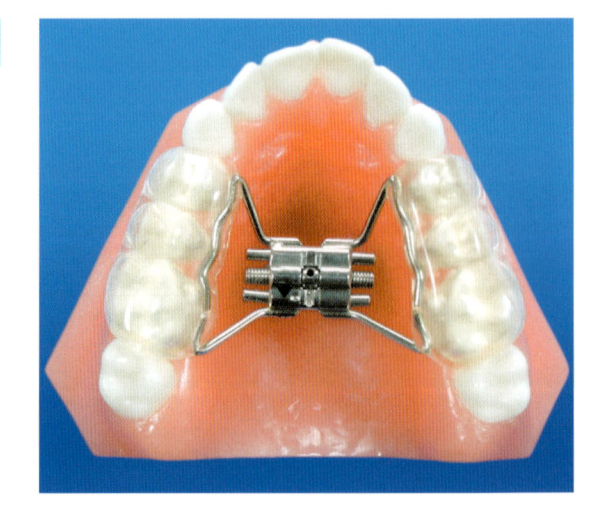

CROSSBITES

2154F Fan-Type R.P.E.

This appliance is used mainly in narrow, "V" shaped arches. It is possible to develop the upper arch laterally up to 9mm with the majority of the movement confined to the anterior region spanning from cuspid to cuspid. It is typically soldered to bands placed on the first permanent molars and the first bicuspids; however, it can be designed so that the anterior portion of the appliance is secured with bonding material over a wire.

If you find that the posterior crossbite is locked due to a deep bite or tight intercuspation, it is recommend that a lower occlusal splint be placed temporarily to expedite treatment without affecting the mandibular dentition.

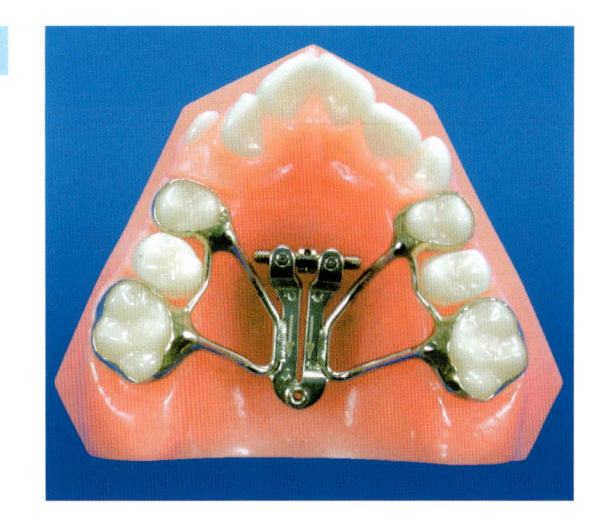

Design Notes:

Design Notes

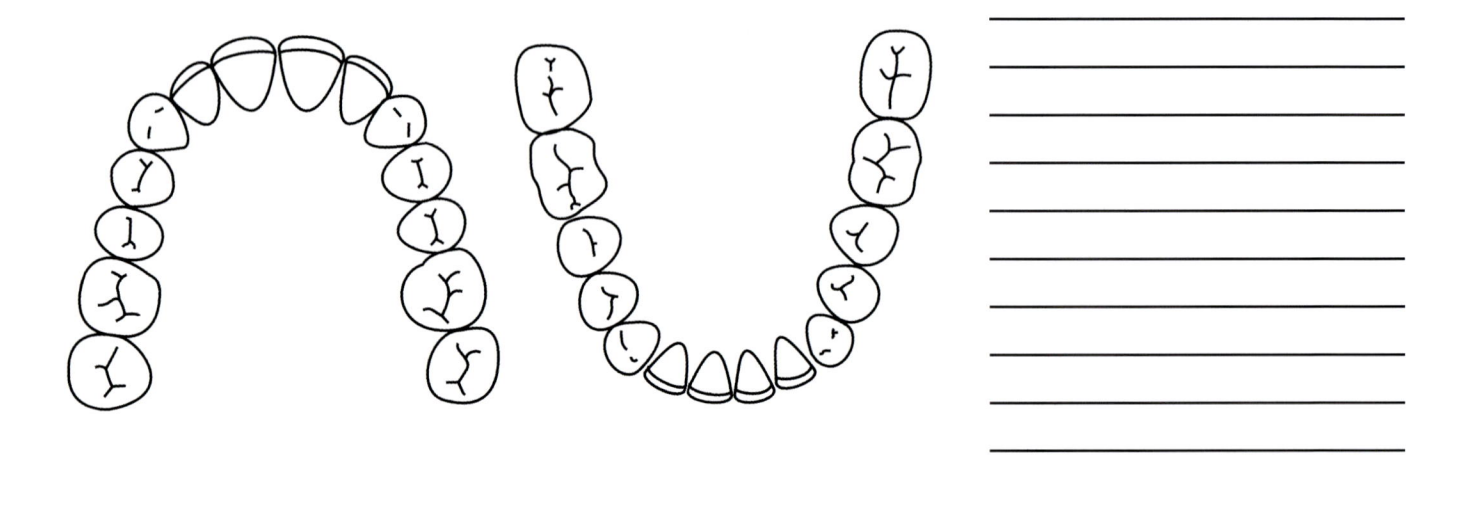

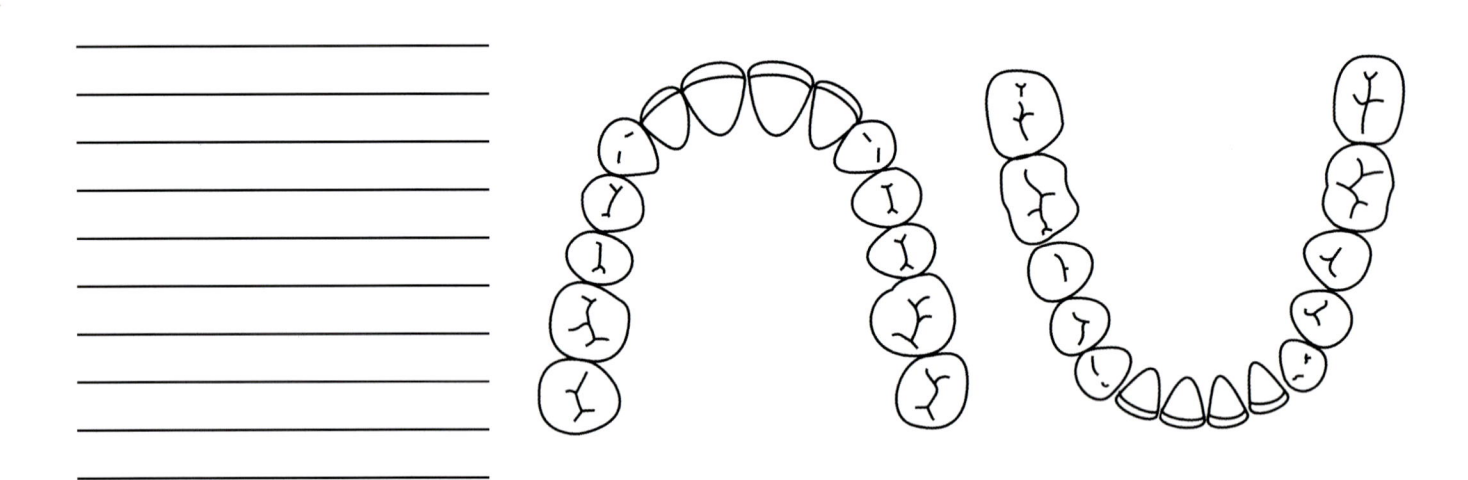

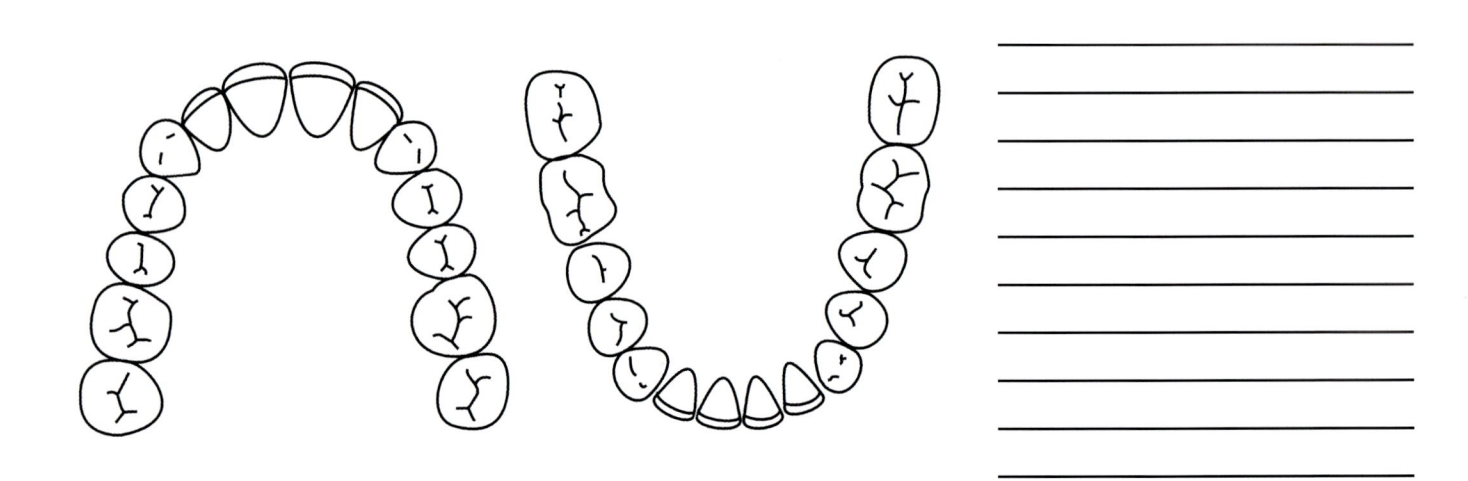

ARCH DEVELOPMENT

an overview: ARCH DEVELOPMENT

Chapter 8

Arch development is a collective term that describes a variety of appliances used to gain both arch width and arch length. These appliances range from the simple Schwarz appliance with lap springs to the high-speed, rapid palatal expanders. They may utilize orthodontic movement, orthopedic movement, or a combination of both and may be either fixed or removable.

With proper design, expansion appliances may be used to move teeth on either side of the arch unilaterally or bilaterally. They may be used to relieve crowding in the posterior segments, develop underdeveloped pre-maxillas, reposition retroclined anteriors, and relieve anterior crowding.

There are many indications for arch development. In children, the overwhelming majority of lateral expansion appliances are used to treat crossbites, crowded anteriors with an excessive overjet, or a combination of these conditions.

In adults, arch development appliances are mainly used to correct crowding in the anterior region, upright lingually tipped posterior segments back over the basal bone, distalize mesially inclined molars, correct retroclined anteriors, and, in conjunction with straight wire therapy, round out narrow arches and align the occlusal planes.

Arch development is also important for patients who need therapy to correct a skeletal problem. One of the main causative factors of a skeletal Class II relationship is an underdeveloped maxilla. In fact, it is rare to find a Class II case where the teeth are aligned and the arch is ideally shaped so that only a jaw-to-jaw alignment with a functional appliance is needed.

Even though the direction and the amount of the force applied are under complete control with these appliances, proper case selection is still essential. This is particularly true in a growing child. For example, in cases with a minimum overbite and a clockwise growth pattern, arch expansion can cause an increase in the vertical dimension and an open bite. These types of cases have to be monitored carefully. If the bite begins to open, treatment may have to be altered or abandoned. Whether you use a removable or fixed approach, a successful and stable result will depend on the patient's morphogenic pattern, muscular function, and simultaneous growth and development.

To help you choose the correct appliance, we have broken down the vast array of appliances into several distinct groups based upon their usage and type. The categories are:

- Lateral Development with Removable Appliances
- Lateral Development with Fixed Appliances
- Anterior/Posterior Development with Removable Appliances
- Anterior/Posterior Development with Fixed Appliances
- Combination Removable Appliances for AP/Lateral Development
- Combination Fixed Appliances for AP/Lateral Development
- Differential Development with Removable Appliances
- Differential Development with Fixed Appliances

ARCH DEVELOPMENT

Lateral Development With Removable Appliances

1093 Upper Schwarz Appliance   U

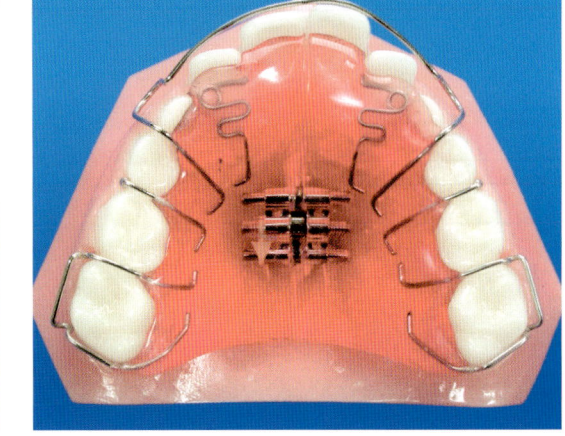

A narrow maxilla is one of the most common orthodontic problems seen in a developing child. Left untreated, it can lead to severe crowding and cause the occurrence of an anterior or posterior crossbite. It can also inhibit the normal development of the mandible, creating a skeletal Class II.

The Schwarz appliance is the most frequently used removable appliance to develop a narrow arch. This appliance works by turning the expansion screw in the center of the palate one-quarter turn once or twice a week. This slow expansion allows the acrylic to place pressure on both the palatal tissue and the teeth in a lateral direction. As the arch develops the palate will drop, so adjustment of the acrylic in the palatal region will be necessary throughout treatment.

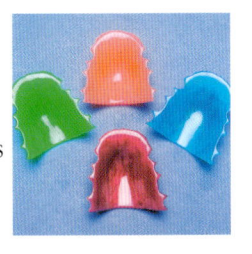

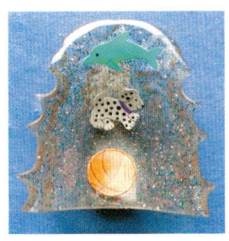

Although removable appliances tend to tip teeth as they are moved buccally, expansion is slow enough that normal occlusal function is usually sufficient to maintain their normal inclination. In this example, individual recurved springs are used to move #7 and #10 into position as space is created.

Note - These appliances can be made in different colors, designs and with decals. This is a great way to motivate your patients.

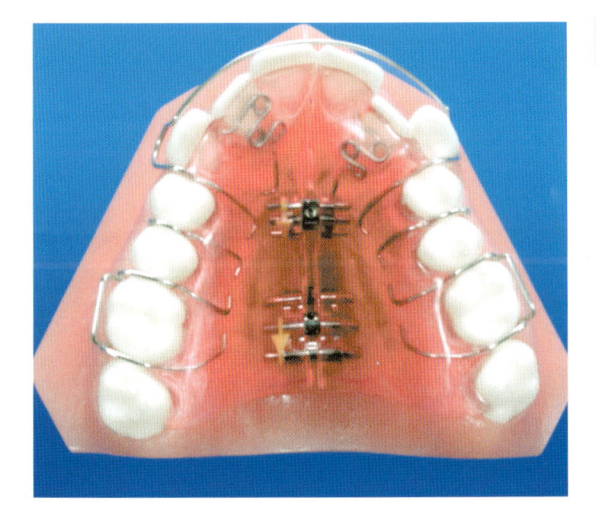

1097 Upper Adult Expansion   U

Although arch development is more commonly used when treating developing children, arch expansion appliances can be successfully used to treat adults. They are particularly effective when the posterior teeth are lingually tipped in conjunction with the arch being narrow. A typical scenario, consisting of lingually tipped posteriors and crowded anteriors, is shown here.

When using an appliance like this on an adult, lateral development can be greatly enhanced by the addition of a second expansion screw. This ensures uniform anterior-posterior pressure and affords more stability as the screws reach the limits of their threads.

Note - A small amount of differential expansion can be accomplished by adjusting these screws at a different rate. However, care must be taken when doing this to avoid cracking the appliance.

ARCH DEVELOPMENT

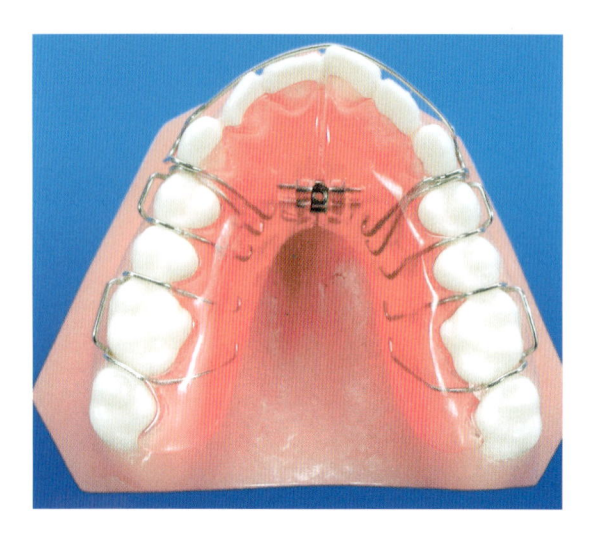

1231 Reduced Acrylic Schwarz   U

Some patients simply cannot tolerate the normal acrylic extensions found in the standard Schwarz. The design modification shown here is ideal for patients who have a severe gag reflex or a serious difficulty speaking while wearing a full coverage maxillary appliance. The horseshoe shape of the palatal acrylic allows more space for the tongue while still providing the necessary anchorage for lateral arch development.

1095 Schwarz with Posterior Bite Plane   U

Bilateral posterior crossbites are usually the result of an underdeveloped maxilla. Some of the reasons that this occurs are an abnormal tongue posture, an irregular swallowing pattern, and an obstructed airway caused by allergies.

When a patient presents a bilateral crossbite, a Schwarz appliance with posterior occlusal coverage can be used. The occlusal coverage opens the vertical and is typically finished flat to allow for the quick resolution of the crossbite without affecting the opposing dentition. By wrapping the occlusal acrylic over the buccal cusp tips, tipping of the dentition will be kept to a minimum.

Turning the expansion screw one-quarter turn a week will exert a slow constant pressure on the teeth and bone. This arch development will move the posterior segments buccally out of crossbite and, in the process, drop a high-vaulted palate opening the nasal airway. Once the crossbite is corrected, the occlusal coverage should be removed to allow the patient to function into a normal occlusion.

Note - As the high vault drops with expansion of the arch, adjustment of the acrylic on the palatal side of the appliance may be necessary to ensure proper seating of the appliance.

Important - Recognition and treatment of a posterior crossbite early in a child's development is essential. When left untreated, it can lead to numerous serious medical complications. Some of them are a Class II skeletal deformity, TMJ dysfunction, and airway obstruction.

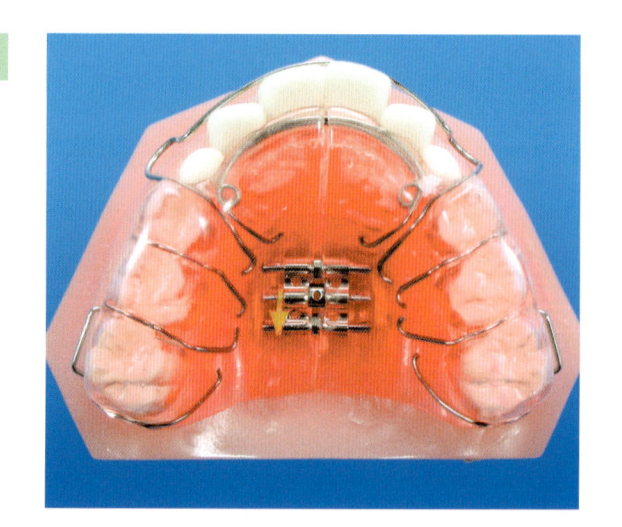

ARCH DEVELOPMENT

4183E Arch Expanding Temporary Partial   U/L

Patients of all ages who are undergoing orthodontic therapy may also be missing teeth. In this instance, a constricted maxillary arch with a lingually positioned left lateral incisor can be treated with a removable lateral expansion appliance while temporarily replacing two missing centrals.

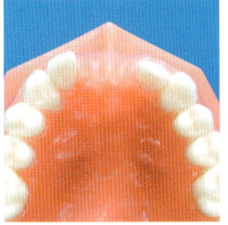

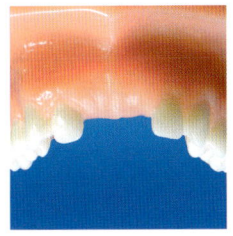

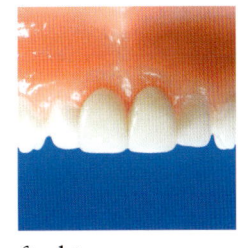

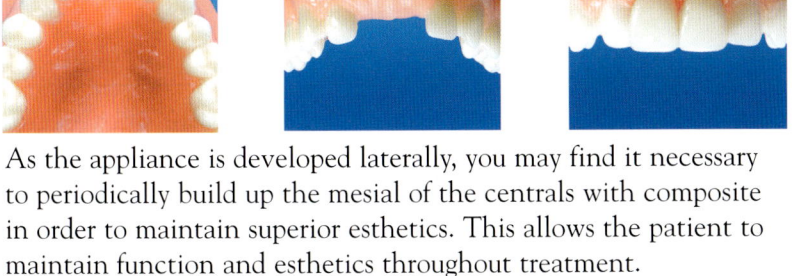

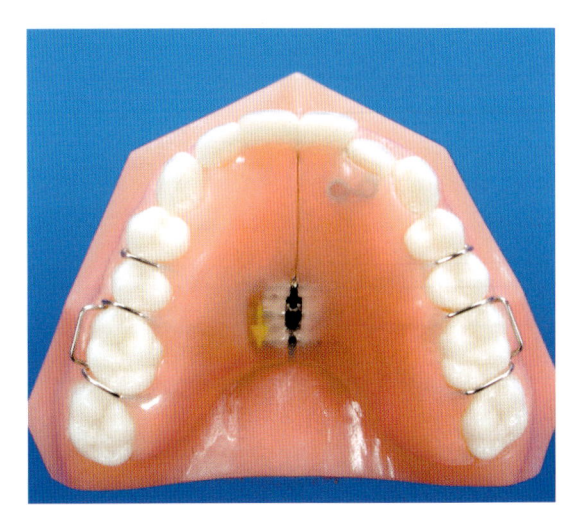

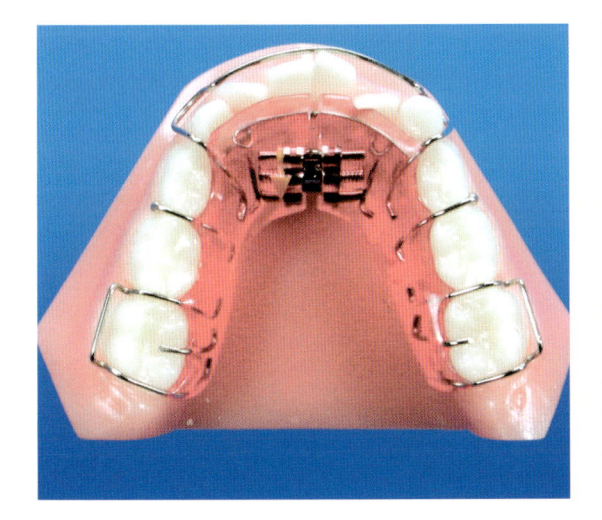

As the appliance is developed laterally, you may find it necessary to periodically build up the mesial of the centrals with composite in order to maintain superior esthetics. This allows the patient to maintain function and esthetics throughout treatment.

1094 Lower Schwarz Appliance - Mixed Dentition L

An underdeveloped maxilla is usually the causative factor leading to a crowded narrow mandible. When this occurs, arch expansion with a lower Schwarz appliance is the easiest way to correct the crowding and upright the lingually tipped posterior segments.

Taking the time to properly design the appliance to meet the patient's specific needs is critical to achieving a successful result. For example, the labial arch wire usually passes over the occlusion either distal to the cuspid or distal to the first bicuspid. Selecting the best position will depend upon the available occlusal clearance.

As the appliance is activated, the adjustment loops of the labial wire should be opened, permitting development in the anterior area. Once sufficient space is available, the lap springs can be activated to complete the alignment of the anteriors along the esthetically-formed labial arch. The labial loops can then be tightened to hold the aligned teeth in place.

Note - Maxillary and mandibular development are usually done at the same time. Care must be taken not to over expand the maxillary arch as it responds about twice as fast as the mandibular arch.

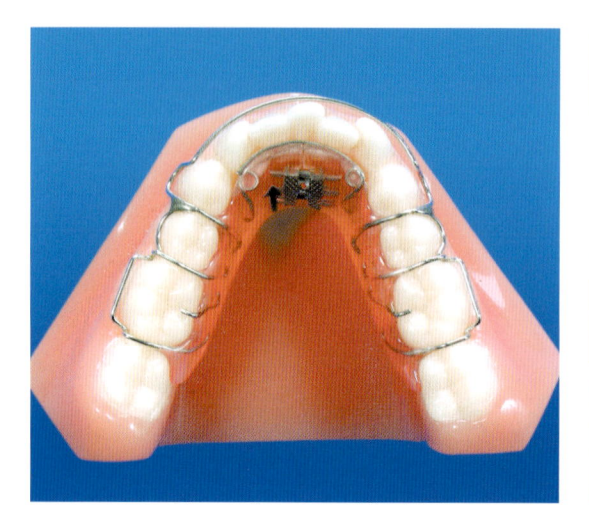

ARCH DEVELOPMENT

1094A Lower Schwarz Adult Dentition with "C" Clasps on the Bicuspids   L

When lower posterior segments (cuspids to molars) are tipped lingually, you will usually find that the anteriors are also significantly crowded. This can still be corrected in the adult dentition with a Schwarz appliance; however, to successfully accomplish this, some simple modifications to the basic appliance design must be done. For example, instead of leaving the labial bow distal to the cuspids where it can encroach upon the space needed for them to move, the bow can be carried back to the bicuspids. To get the adequate retention needed to activate the springs, a "C" clasp can be soldered to the labial bow and placed on the second bicuspids as illustrated. By placing composite ledges, you can even gain more retention.

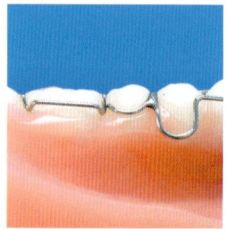

1094B Lower Schwarz with Alternate Methods of Retention   L

The lower Schwarz shown here illustrates two options for retention that are very helpful when the first permanent molars are not erupted sufficiently to use the standard Adams or Delta clasps.

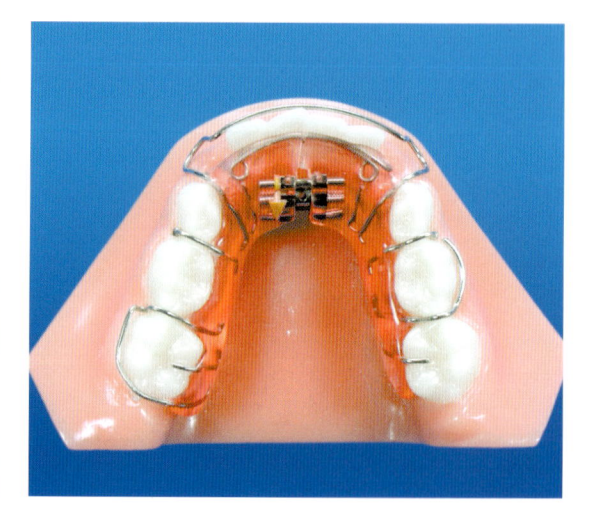

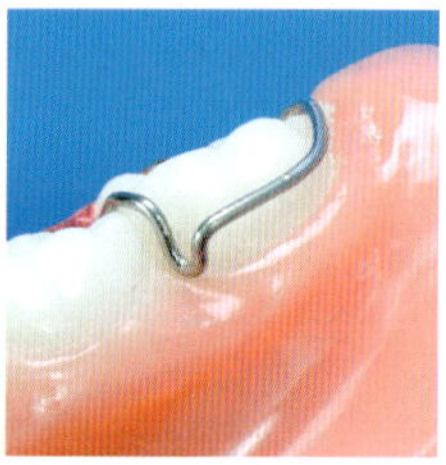

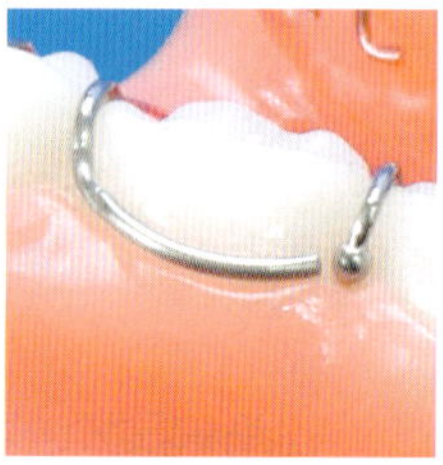

On the left first permanent molar, the use of a half Adams clasp is demonstrated. This is an excellent choice when the distal marginal ridge is still covered with tissue and no distal-buccal undercut exists. A retentive "arrowhead" is placed as usual on the mesial of the tooth, while the remainder of the clasp is contoured around the distal of the tooth as a circumferential clasp.

The next alternative clasp design is demonstrated on the right second primary molar. It is composed of a combination ball clasp and "C" clasp. The ball clasp can be used by engaging the interproximal undercut of either molar, while the "C" clasp is most effective when used in conjunction with a composite ledge placed just occlusal to the contact point of the clasp. Once the molar is lost, retention can still be maintained with the ball clasp.

ARCH DEVELOPMENT

1094C Lower Schwarz with Midline Correcting Spring   L

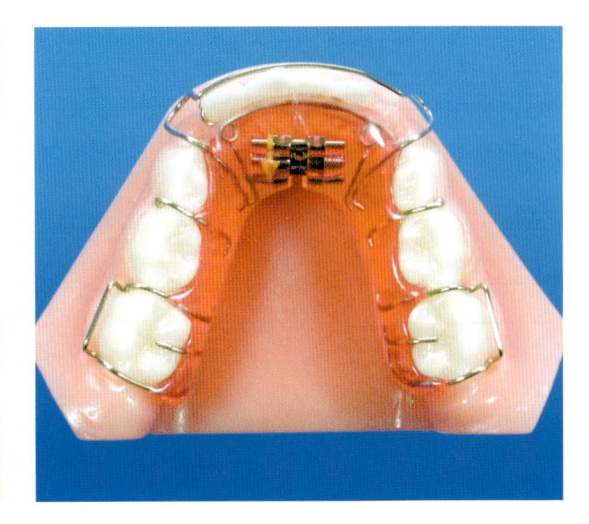

When a primary cuspid is lost prematurely during the mixed dentition stage, the anteriors can shift off of the midline. This will create a loss in arch length in that quadrant and block the eruption of the adult cuspid. It is not uncommon to see this type of arch length loss associated with a deficiency in arch width. When this occurs, it is possible to correct both of these problems with one appliance.

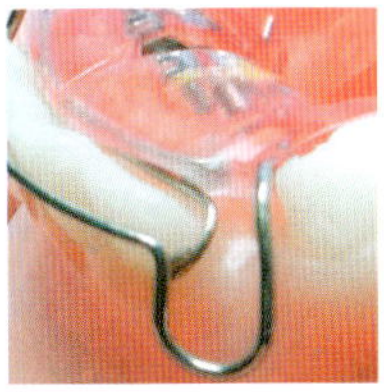

To correct a narrow arch and a midline shift with a removable appliance, simply add a midline correction spring to a standard Schwarz appliance.

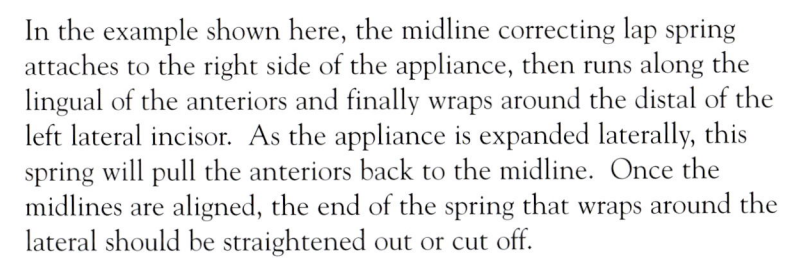

In the example shown here, the midline correcting lap spring attaches to the right side of the appliance, then runs along the lingual of the anteriors and finally wraps around the distal of the left lateral incisor. As the appliance is expanded laterally, this spring will pull the anteriors back to the midline. Once the midlines are aligned, the end of the spring that wraps around the lateral should be straightened out or cut off.

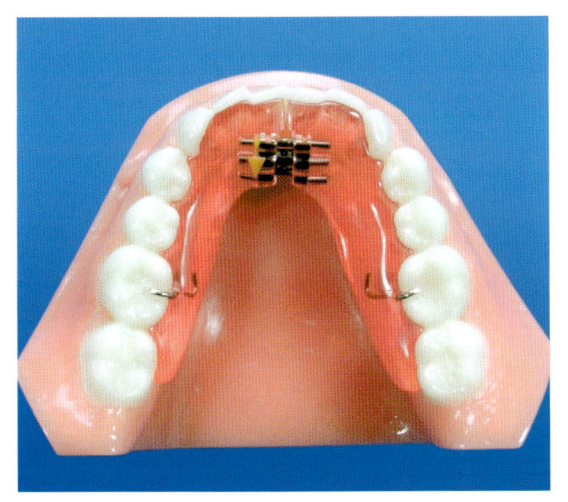

1162E Lower Bowbeer   L

The lower Bowbeer appliance is a popular modification of the Schwarz design. It is most commonly used when treating adults who have both a narrow arch and lingually tipped posteriors. Since it is designed without clasps, it is often used in conjunction with full arch bracketing in order to expedite treatment.

The design is extremely esthetic and its small size makes it less likely to affect the patient's speech. For all of these reasons this appliance is often preferred over other designs.

Design Notes:

ARCH DEVELOPMENT

Lateral Development With Fixed Appliances

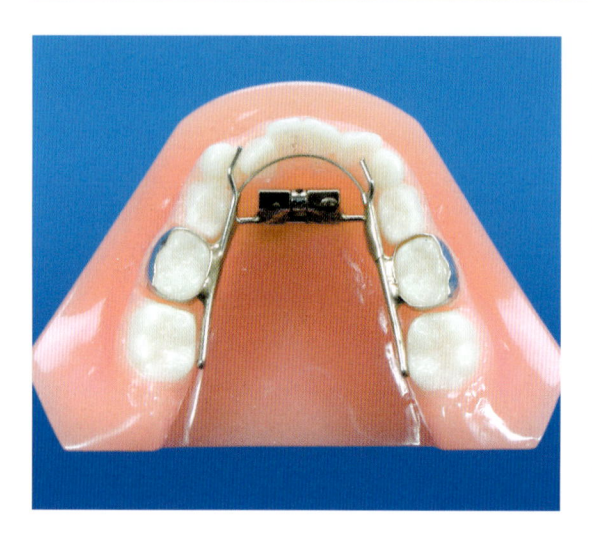

2156 Williams Expander   L

An underdeveloped maxilla, abnormal tongue posture and aberrant swallowing patterns are some of the causative factors leading to a crowded narrow mandible. In conjunction with maxillary appliance therapy that directly addresses these factors, appliances are available that will develop the constricted mandible and unravel the lower anterior crowding.

The Williams Expander is a fixed appliance that is used during the early mixed dentition stage. It is designed to develop the lower arch and create normal spacing for the alignment of the permanent lower incisors and cuspids.

The framework of the appliance consists of a specially designed midline expansion screw soldered to two long sections of hollow tubing that run along the lingual aspect of the posterior segments. This tubing accepts a preformed .016 or .018 NiTi arch wire that rests against the lingual of the incisors. As the expansion screw is activated and the appliance widens, the NiTi wire expresses itself labially and aids in un-crowding the incisors.

2155F Fixed Lingual Expansion Appliance (F.L.E.A.)   L

When lower posterior segments (cuspids to molars) are tipped lingually you will usually find that the anteriors are also significantly crowded. This can still be corrected in the adult dentition.

This transverse appliance is excellent for controlled lateral development in cases where poor retention is present or patient cooperation is of concern. Anterior lingual lap springs can be added as needed to aid in improving incisor rotations.

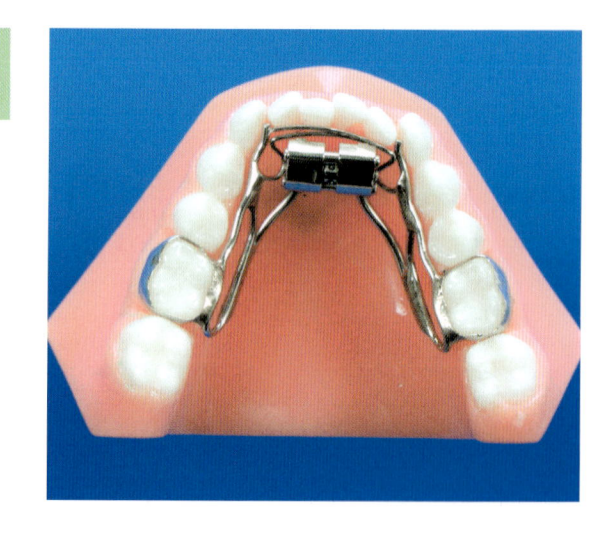

8-2.1

ARCH DEVELOPMENT

2092 Arnold Expander / E Arch   U/L

When patient compliance is an issue, a fixed appliance is always preferred. This fixed expansion appliance develops the arch using a spring-loaded split-lingual arch, housed in a tube. The tension on the spring coil is set before the appliance is initially placed and further adjustment is not usually necessary.

Once the desired space has been created, the appliance can be made passive by carefully pinching the tube tight against the wire with a pair of heavy wire cutters or a tube crimping plier. This appliance is often used in conjunction with a full arch, fixed technique. When this is the case make sure to ask the lab to fabricate the appliance with molar tubes soldered to the bands.

Hint - It is always difficult to cement a pre-activated spring loaded appliance. To make it easier, ask the lab to return the appliance to you on the model. This will allow you to tie the appliance together with floss and control the spring action prior to cementation.

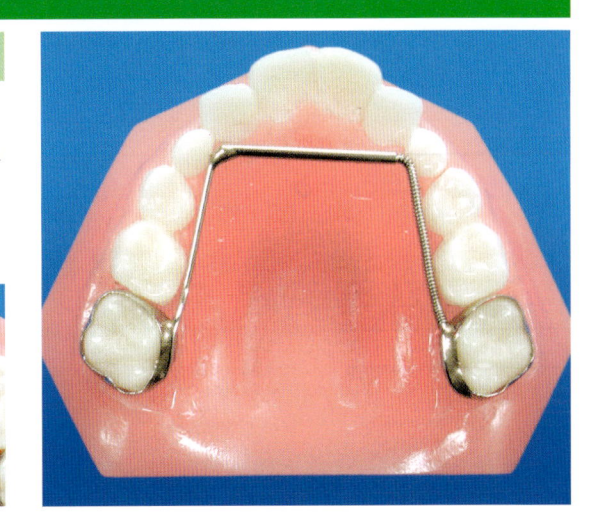

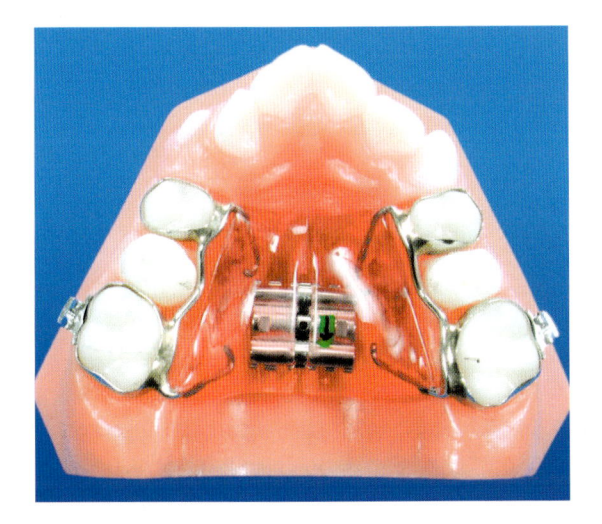

2153M The Haas "Memory" Transverse Expansion Appliance U

This appliance utilizes acrylic to support a spring-loaded expansion screw. By adjusting the spring-loaded expansion screw three 90-degree turns once every three days, it will supply a continuous positive biologic force of about 500g over a distance of 0.8 to 1mm. Many practitioners prefer this appliance over the coil-spring activated RPEs.

Because the appliance has acrylic closely contacting the palatal mucosa, more bodily movement and less tipping occurs as the forces generated by the appliance are applied to the teeth and the palatal tissues. One negative to this design is that the acrylic can cause a serious inflammation problem if hygiene is not carefully monitored.

Note - Bands may be custom fit, or pre-formed bands may be selected and sent with the prescription. Because this appliance uses four bands for retention, seating this appliance can have its challenges. To overcome these challenges, we recommend the following:

- Make sure to leave separators in place until the delivery appointment.
- When the path of insertion is a problem, gentle pressure will often allow it to seat over time.
- Cement the bands with a glass ionomer cement.

8-2.2

ARCH DEVELOPMENT

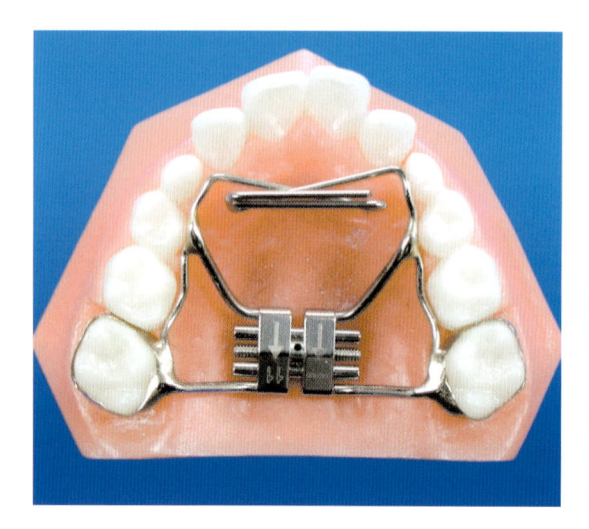

2150H Dillingham Habit-Expansion Appliance U

A tongue thrusting habit is often the cause of a narrow maxilla. When this is the case, simply correcting the narrow arch through lateral development is often not enough to assure a stable result. To maintain the correction, everything must be done to address the muscle imbalance that caused the problem in the first place. In other words, you cannot ignore the tongue habit.

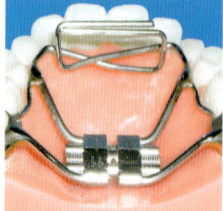

The Dillingham design not only functions as an expansion appliance, it also discourages tongue thrusting and/or thumb sucking with the use of adjustable habit loops.

When the appliance is delivered, these habit loops will prevent the tongue from thrusting forward against the anteriors. Instead, the tongue pressure is placed against the anterior loops. This has the effect of flexing the framework laterally and actually aids in developing the maxillary cuspid region. The expansion screw used in this appliance is the same type of screw used to expand the maxilla rapidly. In fact, this appliance can be used effectively in either a slow expansion or rapid expansion approach.

Note - Always send both upper and lower casts along with a construction bite to assure proper appliance fabrication.

Suture Expanding Appliances

When a crossbite is due to a deficiency of the maxillary apical base, the use of a rapid expansion appliance can be a very effective tool to correct the skeletal deformity. In fact, rapid palatal expansion is commonly used to correct a crossbite, increase arch perimeter, level the curve of Wilson, broaden the smile and increase airway patency.

Unlike slow expansion where the appliance is adjusted one turn every week, rapid expansion is obtained by means of turning the expansion screw one turn per day. This generates 3-10 pounds of force, which is enough pressure to separate the mid-palatal suture.

Indeed, the research shows that the whole circummaxillary sutural system is affected. The actual correction will generally occur within a two to three week period, but the appliance is worn at least for another three to five months to allow time for osseous healing.

The best time to use this technique to accomplish an orthopedic change is during the mixed dentition and early permanent dentition. After that time, fewer skeletal and more dentoalveolar adaptations will be observed.

Because this appliance is adjusted by the patient and cannot be removed to do so, a special expansion key has been designed to accomplish this movement. Please contact Success Essentials to order extra keys.

ARCH DEVELOPMENT

2153 Haas Suture Expanding Appliance   U

In patients with severe maxillary constriction in early permanent dentition or who have moderate maxillary constriction in late adolescence, the Haas appliance is the appliance of choice.

This suture-expanding appliance utilizes acrylic to support the screw and add extra stability to the appliance. The acrylic closely contacts the palatal mucosa because Haas believed that more bodily movement and less tipping occurred with the presence of the palatal coverage. This occurs as forces are generated not only against the teeth but also against the soft and hard palatal tissues.

One negative aspect of this design is that the acrylic can cause a serious inflammation problem if hygiene is not carefully monitored.

Note - Bands may be custom fit, or pre-formed bands may be selected and sent with the prescription. Because this appliance uses four bands for retention, seating this appliance can have its challenges. To overcome these challenges, we recommend the following:

- Make sure to leave separators in place until the delivery appointment.
- When the path of insertion is a problem, gentle pressure will often allow it to seat over time.
- Cement the bands with a glass ionomer cement.

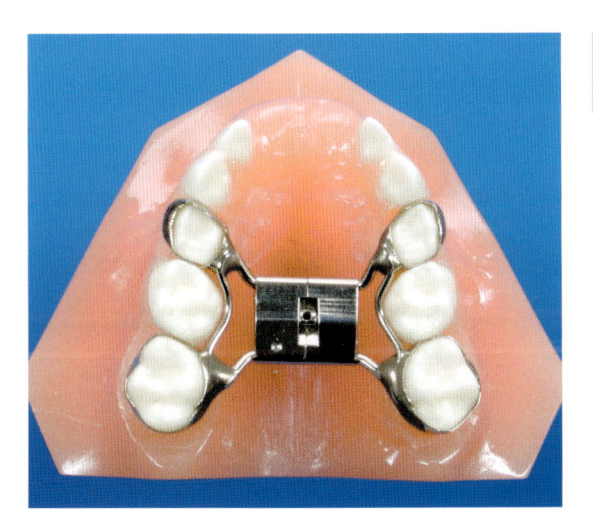

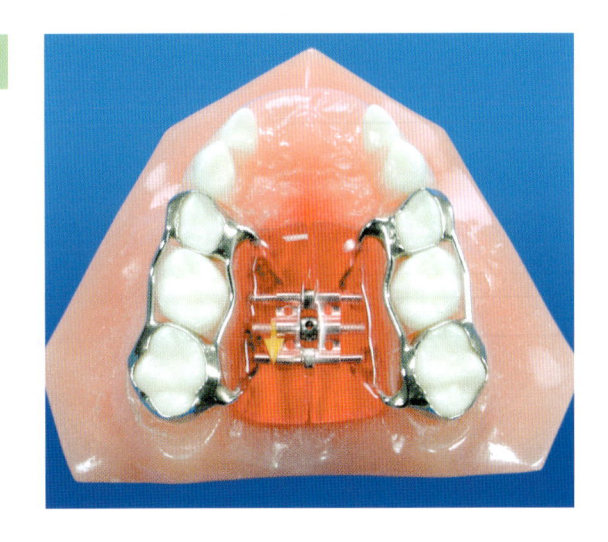

2154 Rapid Palate Expansion (R.P.E.) 4-Banded Hyrax   U

The rapid palate expansion hyrax design, shown here, can be used successfully in patients with mild to moderate transverse constriction when they are in the late mixed or early permanent dentition as the sutures are presumably still patent. This appliance eliminates the palatal acrylic and uses an all-stainless metal framework instead. Although this design makes it much easier for the patient to keep clean, there is a greater chance that fewer skeletal and more dentoalveolar adaptions will be observed.

Note - Bands may be custom fit, or pre-formed bands may be selected and sent with the prescription. Because this appliance uses four bands for retention, seating this appliance can have its challenges. To overcome these challenges, we recommend the following:

- Make sure to leave separators in place until the delivery appointment.
- When the path of insertion is a problem, gentle pressure will often allow it to seat over time.
- Cement the bands with a glass ionomer cement.

8-2.4

ARCH DEVELOPMENT

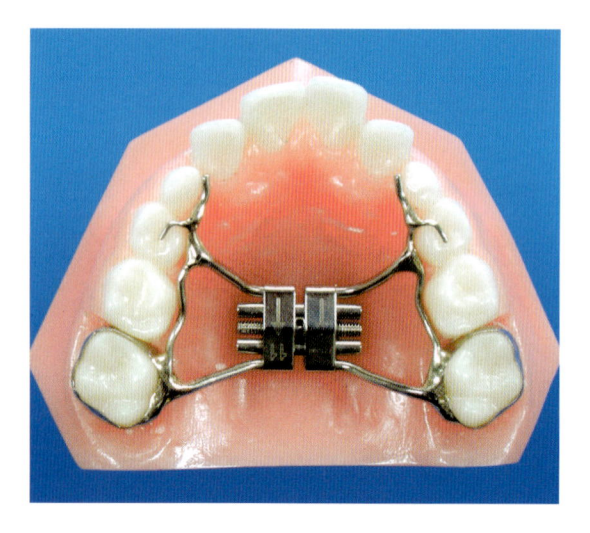

2155R High Palate (R.P.E.) Hyrax Type   U

In this particular design, the expansion screw is positioned high in the palate for greater comfort. Bands are placed on the first molars and rests are bonded to the occlusal surface of the primary molars. This eliminates the path of insertion problem that occurs when four bands are used. Extra heavy support wires are also used to prevent the appliance from flexing as pressure is applied.

If you find that a posterior crossbite is locked due to a deep bite or tight intercuspation, it is recommended that a lower occlusal splint be placed temporarily to expedite treatment without affecting the mandibular dentition.

2154S R.P.E. Super Screw   U

When a significant amount of lateral development is needed, the expansion provided by a Standard R.P.E. screw is often not enough. When this is the case, a second appliance frequently needs to be placed. To avoid having to place a second appliance, we recommend the use of a "Super Screw" R.P.E.

Although the dimension across the arch of a small Super Screw is the same as a standard R.P.E., it expands significantly wider. In fact, it can be opened a full 12mm, compared to 7-8mm for the standard screw. Some of the other benefits of using this screw are:

- It is easy to adjust from the front of the mouth with a small hex wrench.
- It has a clearly visible graduated scale milled into the body of the screw making it very easy to monitor the amount of lateral development achieved.
- It is quite comfortable due to its smooth rounded shape.

Note - The Super Screw comes in a larger size as well. The 16mm screw will give you up to 18mm of expansion.

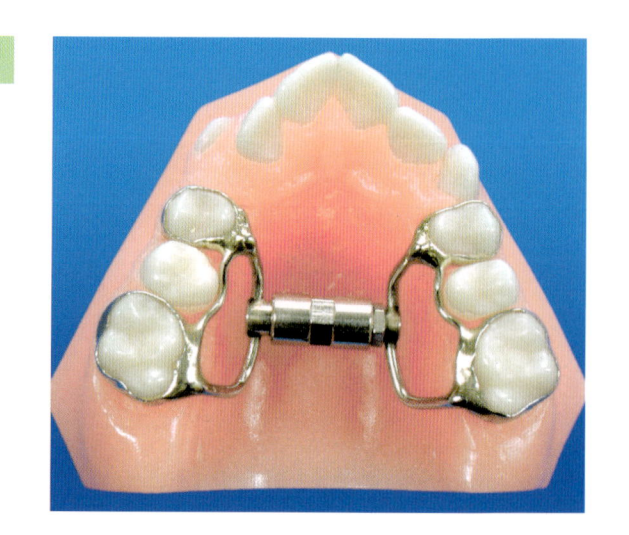

ARCH DEVELOPMENT

1343 Direct Bond Suture Expansion   U

This design uses direct bond occlusal pads for retention instead of banding 1st bicuspids and 6-year molars. This feature not only facilitates movement when a crossbite is present, but because it covers the buccal cusp tips, it prevents tipping from occurring. This, along with a rigid framework creates a movement that is mainly orthopedic in nature.

This is an excellent design, especially for those patients who are in the early mixed dentition stage or in the early adult dentition stage as seen here. It is not recommended for patients who are in the late stage of mixed dentition as loose or exfoliating teeth will greatly compromise the anchorage of the appliance.

Note - When delivering this appliance make sure to maintain a dry environment. Special instructions along with all the necessary supplies can be provided to you through Success Essentials.

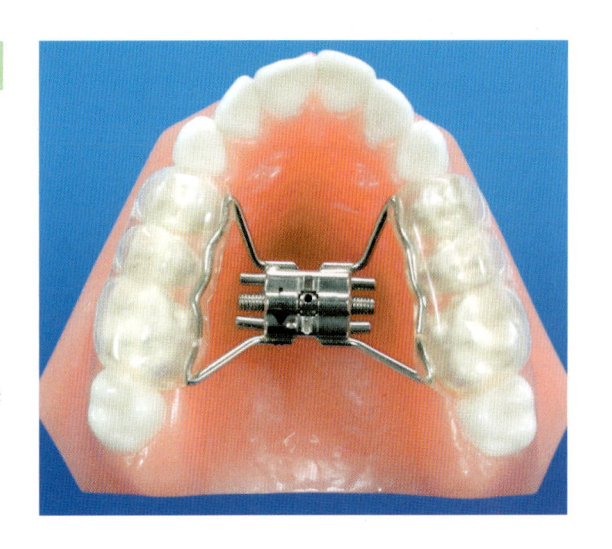

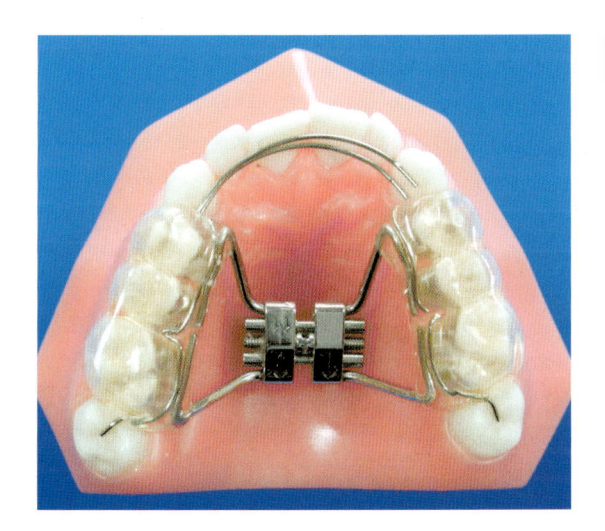

1343SR Bonded R.P.E. w/Lap Spring and Rests   U

During the early stage of the adult dentition, second molars are often still erupting. When placing a Bonded R.P.E. during this time, you will typically want to leave the partially erupted second molars free from the occlusal acrylic. To control their vertical development, simply prescribe occlusal rests as illustrated here. These rests can be adjusted or removed at any time.

By adding anterior lap springs, anterior crowding can be resolved. This is especially important when the anteriors are in an end-to-end or mild crossbite. These springs can be adjusted intraorally with the use of a three-prong plier.

Hint - Only apply bonding agent to the buccal and lingual surfaces. Do not apply the bonding agent to the occlusal surface as it makes the appliance difficult to remove.

ARCH DEVELOPMENT

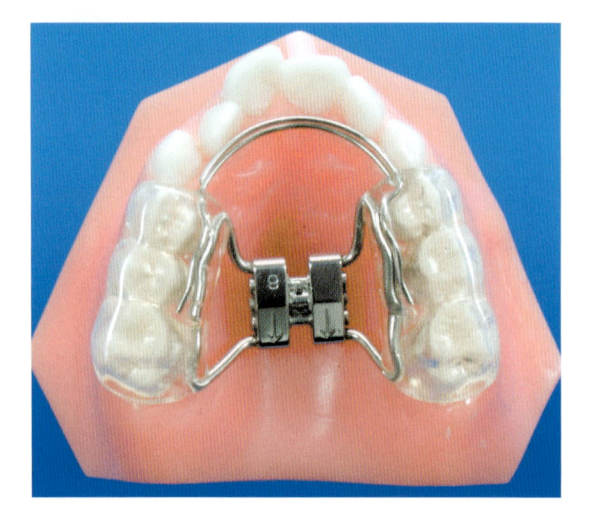

1343LS Bonded R.P.E. w/Lap Springs   U

This example illustrates the placement of a Bonded R.P.E. with Lap Springs in a mixed dentition patient. This is the best time to use a Bonded R.P.E. Besides correcting a crossbite, it has been shown that expansion of the maxilla during the early mixed dentition stage may lead to a spontaneous correction of other occlusal dis-harmonies. For example, expansion of the upper arch in a skeletal Class II can allow the mandible to come forward on its own.

By adding anterior lap springs, anterior crowding can be resolved. This is especially important when the anteriors are in an end-to-end or mild crossbite. These springs can be adjusted intraorally with the use of a three-prong plier.

A Bonded R.P.E. is not recommended for patients who are in the late stage of mixed dentition as loose or exfoliating teeth will greatly compromise the anchorage of the appliance.

Design Notes:

ARCH DEVELOPMENT

Anterior/Posterior Development With Removable Appliances

1105   Class II Division 2 Sagittal Appliance   U

Patients with a Class II Division 2 skeletal relationship usually have a combination of a retroclined premaxilla, lingually tipped centrals with overlapping labially placed laterals and a posteriorly placed mandible that is locked into this position by a deep bite. The first step in correcting this problem is to treat the maxilla by developing the arch in an anterior-posterior direction.

The primary objective of the Sagittal appliance shown here is to develop the premaxilla. This is accomplished by the activation of the expansion screws and by utilizing extra anchorage created by intercuspating the opposing arch with the posterior bite plane. Once this is accomplished the laterals can be guided lingually into place with T-springs.

Note - A combination of anterior and posterior occlusal bite planes are commonly used in Sagittal appliances. A wax bite allowing about 1 to 1-1/2 mm of vertical opening, measured between the most posterior teeth in the arch, is needed to properly fabricate the appliance. This bite should be taken in the patient's natural centric position.

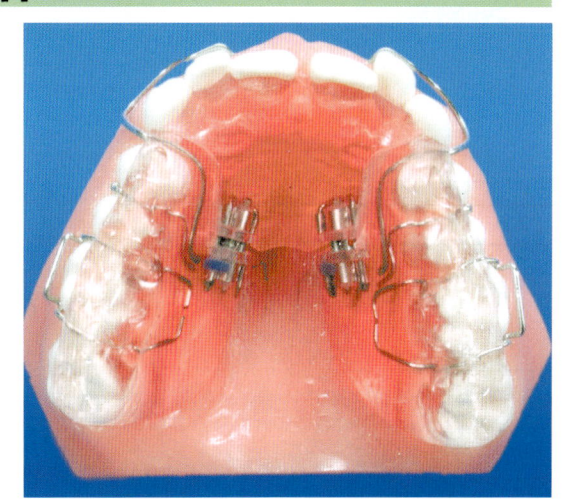

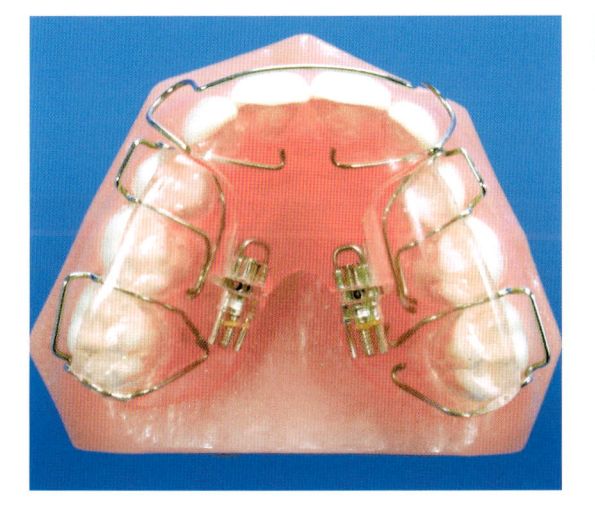

1261   Pre-Maxillary Development Sagittal   U

This Sagittal appliance is designed to move the pre-maxillary segment labially to regain lost cuspid space and correct an anterior crossbite. Success is dependent upon excellent retention and setting up the proper anchorage. Multiple posterior clasps usually provide enough retention, but a labial arch wire can be added if more retention is needed.

Occlusal coverage aids in appliance retention and can also be indexed heavily to take advantage of inter-arch anchorage. Opening the vertical dimension with occlusal coverage is essential when treating anterior crossbite cases.

8-3.1

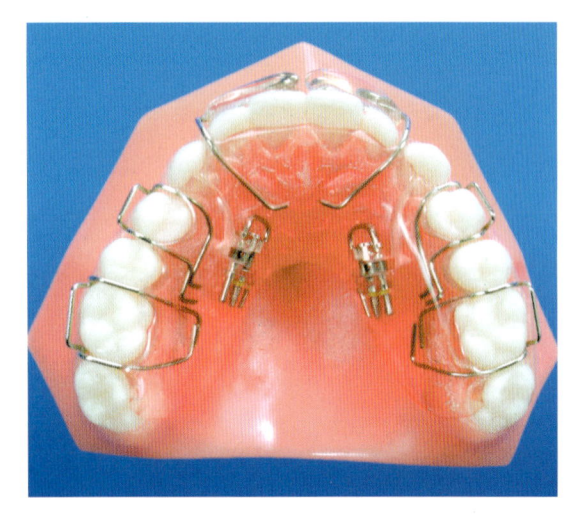

ARCH DEVELOPMENT

1263 Pre-Maxillary Development Sagittal with Frankel Pads U

This Sagittal appliance is designed to move the pre-maxillary segment labially to regain lost cuspid space. Frankel pads have been added to eliminate lip pressure on the anteriors and facilitate alveolar development of the maxilla. Holding the upper lip forward creates the tension needed to stimulate the periosteum over the maxillary labial plate.

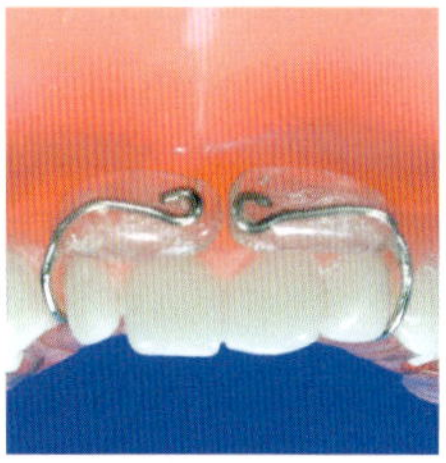

Note - Many clinicians like to add occlusal coverage to these appliances as it aids in the retention of the appliance. The occlusal coverage can also be indexed heavily to take advantage of inter-arch anchorage.

1265 Sagittal with Recurved Springs   U

Pre-maxillary development alone is not always sufficient to correct a Division 2 malocclusion. Sometimes the anteriors need to be tipped labially to gain additional arch length. Recurved springs lingual to the centrals provide a controlled labial force, tipping the centrals and increasing arch length. Placing small composite buttons or ledges on the lingual aspect of these teeth is often helpful in maximizing spring effectiveness.

Note - Many clinicians like to add occlusal coverage to these appliances as it aids in the retention of the appliance. The occlusal coverage can also be indexed heavily to take advantage of inter-arch anchorage.

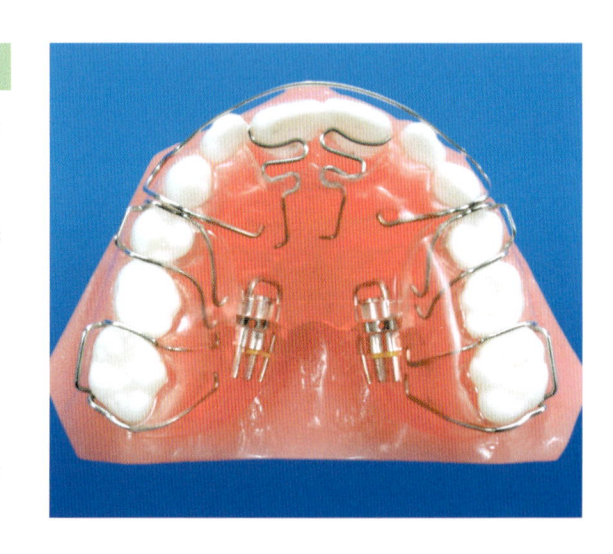

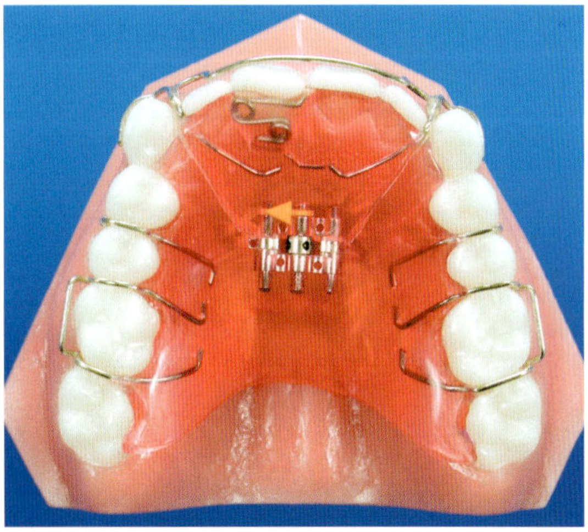

1073B Upper Anterior Developer   U

When upper anteriors are lingually positioned, the upper cuspids are often blocked out of the arch form. To gain room for the cuspids, the anteriors must first be moved back into their normal position. This design employs the use of a single expansion screw to uniformly torque the four incisors labially. A labial bow is placed from lateral to lateral to aid in appliance retention and to provide an attachment point for the T-springs that will be used to move the cuspids back into the arch form. As with all appliances, sequencing the movements is important. The incisors must be moved to gain space prior to activating the T-springs.

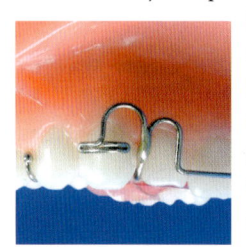

Note - The labial bow is carefully bent so that the distal crossover point will not interfere with your ability to reposition the cuspid.

8-3.2

ARCH DEVELOPMENT

1251 Upper Sagittal to Distalize Molars — U

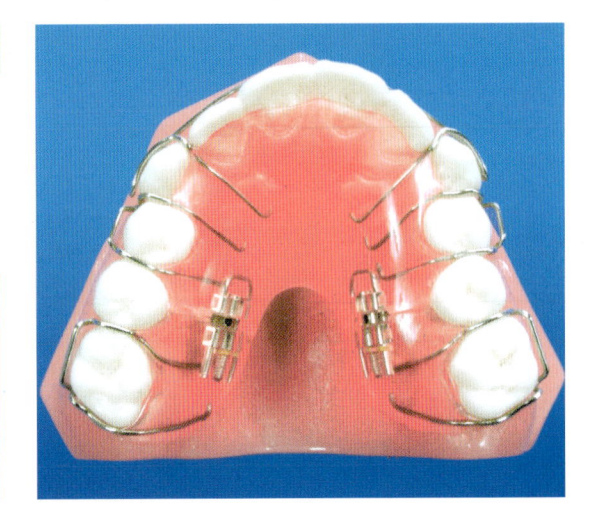

Sagittals employed to distalize upper first molars are primarily used to treat Skeletal Class I dental Class 2 cases and and Skeletal Class II dental Class 2 cases. Adequate anchorage is the key to successfully moving molars. The anterior teeth, along with the palatal acrylic, labial bow and Adams clasps, make up this anchorage unit. When it is possible, the anchorage unit should even include the bicuspids. Doing so will make it unnecessary to cover the occlusal surfaces with acrylic.

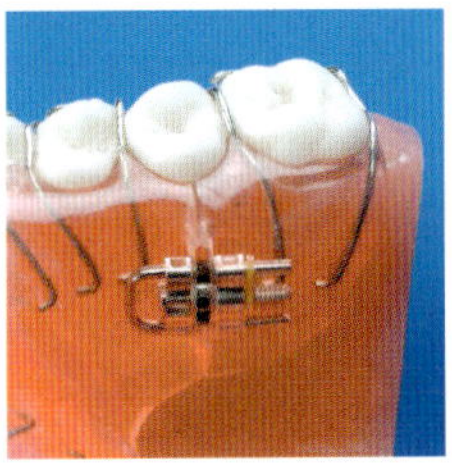

Warning - Distalizing molars can cause the patient's bite to open. This is great for skeletal deep bite cases but often very difficult to manage in open bite scenarios.

Note - Distal movement of the molars is much easier when the second molars have been removed or when they have not yet erupted. When second molars are not yet erupted, it is important to check their position to be certain that first molar distalization will not create an impaction. This can easily be accomplished by taking an x-ray of the second molars. In some cases, removal of the second molars may be indicated.

Design Notes:

_____

_____

_____

1252 Lower Molar Distalizing Sagittal — L

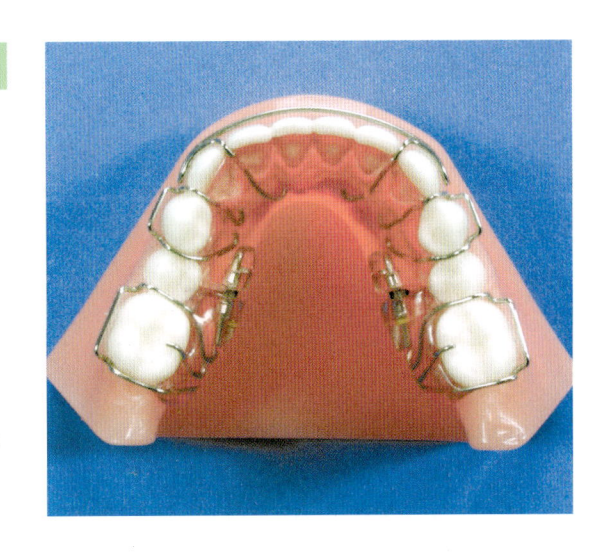

Early loss of primary teeth can allow first molars to drift mesially and block the eruption of the bicuspids. This removable sagittal uses two expansion screws with the acrylic cuts placed just mesial to the molars. By adjusting the expansion screws 1/4 turn once each week, the part of the appliance mesial to the screws acts as an anchor while the molars are moved distally.

When second molars are not yet erupted, it is important to check their position to be certain that first molar distalization will not create an impaction. This can easily be accomplished by taking an x-ray of the second molars. In some cases, removal of the second molars may be indicated.

8-3.3

ARCH DEVELOPMENT

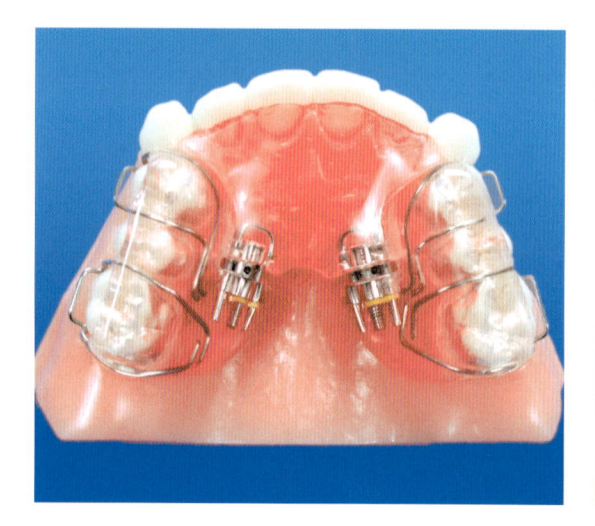

1105D Upper Sagittal to Distalize Posterior Segments   U

When primary molars are lost prematurely, bicuspids will often erupt mesially eliminating the space in the arch needed for the cuspids. When this occurs, the bicuspids and the first molars need to be moved distally to regain the cuspid space. This can be accomplished using the sagittal appliance design shown here.

This appliance uses two sagittal screws with the cut in the acrylic just mesial to the first bicuspids. By the nature of the design, some reciprocal movement of the anteriors will occur. To assure that the majority of the movement is in the distal direction, it is imperative that the second molars are removed and smooth occlusal bite planes be placed over the posteriors to eliminate any occlusal forces that might interfere with the distal movement.

Appliance anchorage is of primary concern and is achieved by using multiple clasping, as illustrated by the use of four Adams clasps. This appliance is best used when the molars and bicuspids are fairly well aligned along the posterior arch.

Note - Many practitioners like to add cuspid retraction hooks to this appliance. This allows them to retract the cuspids at the same time that the space for them is created.

1105L Lower Sagittal to Distalize Posterior Segments   L

When there is not a sufficient amount of space for all the teeth to erupt into their ideal position, it is important to determine the cause for the deficiency. In this example, arch length is less than ideal because the patient lost his primary molars and cuspids early, and the first molars and bicuspids erupted mesially. To regain the room for the cuspids, the posterior segments need to be moved back to their normal position. This can be accomplished using the appliance design shown here. This sagittal design uses two screws with the cut in the acrylic just mesial to the first bicuspids to regain the lost space. Then, as the space is regained, cuspid retraction springs are used to guide the cuspids into position.

It should be noted that second molars are not present. Once second molars have erupted, distalization of the posterior segments becomes very difficult with this design. Therefore, when your evaluation indicates that the arch length needs to be gained in a distal direction, second molar removal should be part of your treatment plan. However, by the nature of the appliance design, some reciprocal movement of the anteriors will always still occur.

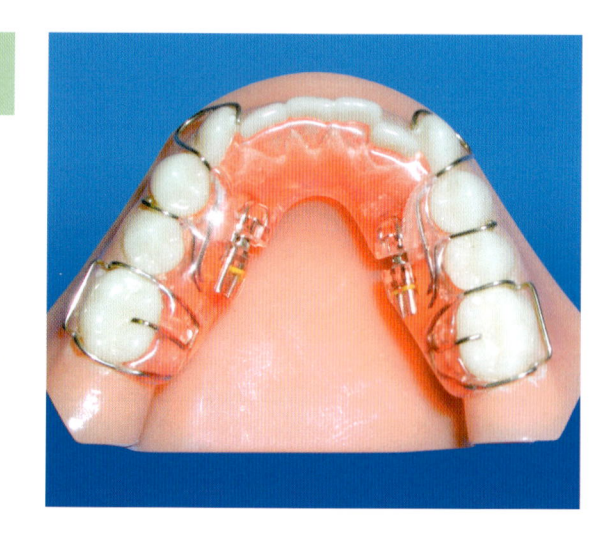

ARCH DEVELOPMENT

Anterior/Posterior Development With Fixed Appliances

2158 A/P Fixed Sagittal   U

A Fixed Sagittal can be used when arch length increase is required in a non-compliant patient, or a patient that may have speech difficulties when wearing an acrylic removable Sagittal. With the second molars removed, as illustrated in this photo, the arch length gain will be achieved predominantly by distalization of the posterior segments. With the second molars in place, movement of both the anteriors and posteriors will occur. If movement of the anteriors alone is desired, the cuspids will need to be combined with the bicuspids and molars to create a posterior anchorage unit.

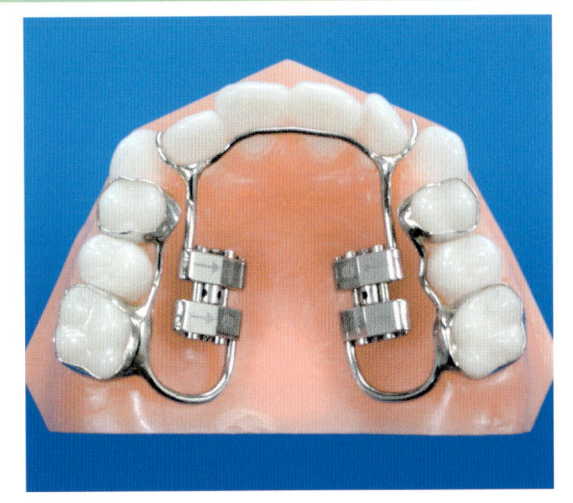

Design Notes:

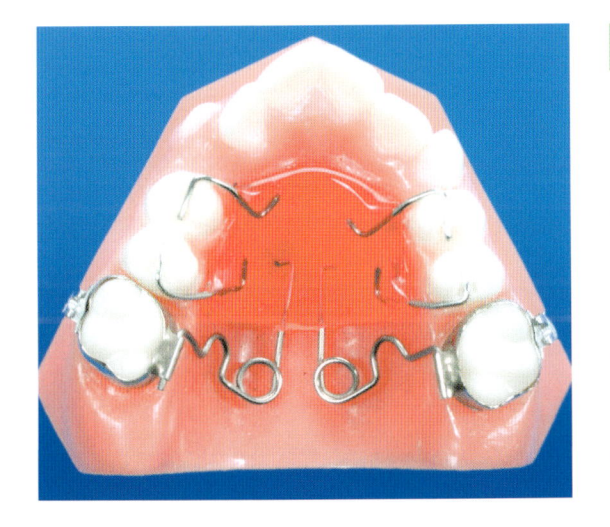

_____
_____
_____
_____
_____

2085M The M Pendulum   U

This appliance produces AP changes by distalization and rotation of the maxillary first molars. To accomplish this, .032 TMA springs are engaged into .036 lingual tubes that are soldered to the molar bands. This delivers a light continuous force to the molars.

The anterior anchorage needed to accomplish this movement is gained through the use of occlusal bonded rests on the pre-molars. Bands can be used on the bicuspids in place of these rests if added retention is desired.

It should be noted that this appliance incorporates the innovative M-Pendulum spring design. This spring utilizes an inverted horizontal loop placed half way between the spring helix and the .036 molar tubes. This unique design overcomes the standard Pendulum spring's tendency to cause crossbites and leave the molar roots mesially inclined. By simply opening the horizontal loop, a buccal and/or distal uprighting force is created producing a bodily movement of the molars.

8-4.1

ARCH DEVELOPMENT

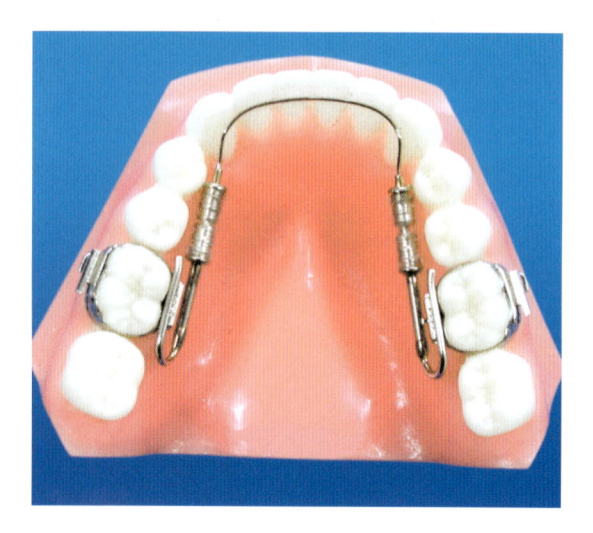

2511 Lower Trombone   L

The principal goal of this appliance is to manage a loss in arch length by using a pre-activated system. The original design of this appliance used coil springs to provide the necessary force, and chain elastic attached to mesial and distal hooks to control the force.

In the new design shown here, the AP force is provided through a unique Compression Tube Activator that is comprised of fine bore silicone tubing. Replacing the springs and hooks with this new material has greatly improved the stability and safety of the appliance.

The advantages of this appliance are that it is removable from the bands, giving the doctor complete control. It is virtually invisible and it can be used in conjunction with any conventional fixed appliance technique.

2154D Fixed Unilateral Distalizer

This appliance utilizes a unique expansion screw and fixed anchorage system to allow you to move a single molar distally on only one side of the arch. So, when space has been lost unilaterally, you can easily distalize the offending molar up to 8mm. This appliance is easy to keep clean and is also ideal for the non-compliant patient.

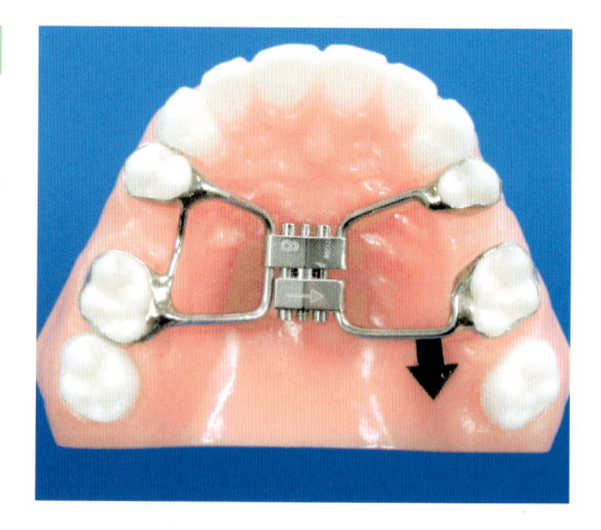

Design Notes:

ARCH DEVELOPMENT

2045 CD Distalizer U/L

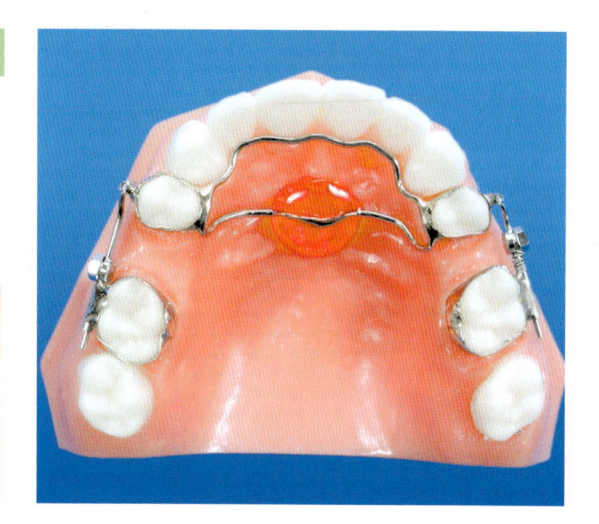

This photo illustrates the original design of this popular molar distalizing appliance. It, of course, can be used on either arch and can be used in a unilateral or bilateral configuration. It can also be used to move banded second molars by carrying the distalizing mechanism back to them. The anterior portion typically attaches to the first bicuspid bands with a Nance button and often an additional lingual wire to act as anchorage. Vertical tubes on the buccal aspect of these bicuspid bands accept the .032 guide wires that run back through the horizontal tubes on the molar bands. Gurin locks and open coil spring are placed as illustrated to provide the necessary distalizing force to the molars. Adjustments are made approximately every three to four weeks.

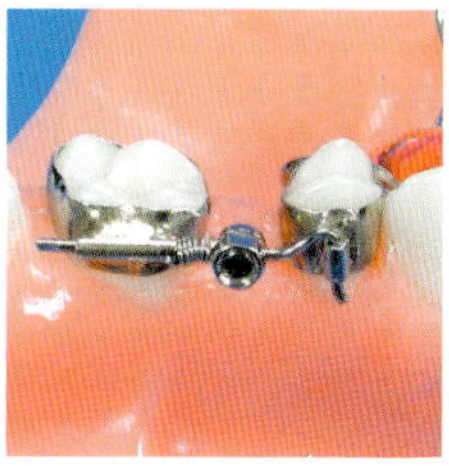

The vertical tubes on this appliance allow it to be placed segmentally, by first cementing the anterior segment, and then by placing the molar bands with the .032 guide wires inserted in the tubes as individual units. The appliance shown here illustrates the force module necessary to distalize #14 and the use of the Gurin lock to maintain the already distalized #3.

Note - When selecting this appliance please provide the lab with detailed instructions.

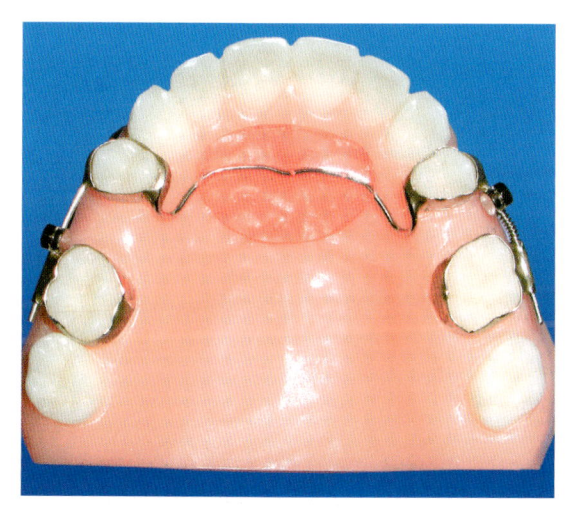

2045M Modified CD Distalizer

This appliance works the same way as the CD Distalizer (appliance #2045). However, the design has been modified so that the guide wires are soldered to the first bicuspids rather than using the vertical tube assembly to attach them to the bicuspids. The advantages to this design are superior strength as well as added comfort to the patient as the attachments to the bicuspids are smooth and reduced in overall bulk. Although this design requires all four bands to be seated at once, this is typically not a problem.

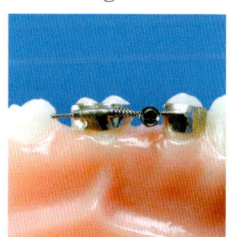

8-4.3

ARCH DEVELOPMENT

Combination Removable Appliances For AP/Lateral Development

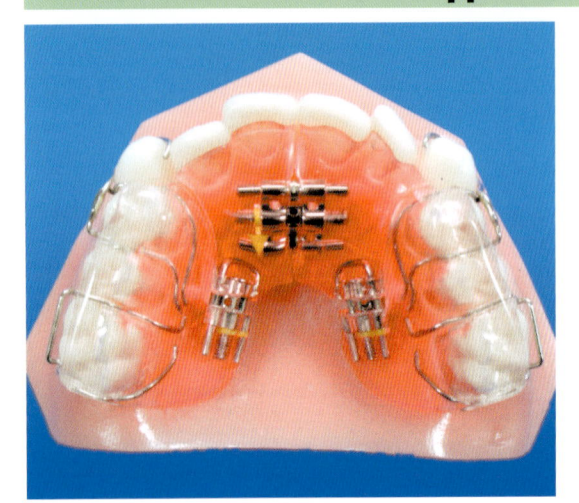

1106 Three Screw Sagittal

It is not unusual to see cuspids blocked out of the arch form. To properly select an appliance to treat this problem, it is imperative to understand the underlying cause of a malocclusion. In this example, arch length is deficient because the patient lost her primary molars early and the first molars and bicuspids erupted mesially. The arch is also slightly underdeveloped laterally because of a finger habit. To make room for the cuspids, both arch length and width need to be regained. Specifically, arch length needs to be gained by distalizing the posterior segments. This can be accomplished using the appliance design shown here.

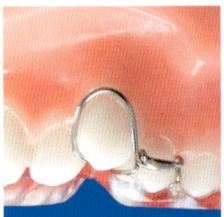

This three screw Sagittal uses a third (midline) expansion screw. As a general rule, the midline screw is activated first. Engaging this screw will give the additional arch width desired and create enough lateral force to set up the anchorage needed to move the posterior segments distally. It should be noted that second molars are not present. Once second molars have erupted, distalization of the posterior segments becomes very difficult with this design.

Note - Many practitioners like to add cuspid retraction springs to this design so they can guide the cuspids into position as the space for them is made available.

1102 3-Way Expander

This unique device features three independently expanding sections in one housing for transverse as well as sagittal anterior development. Each section can be independently activated. When an equal amount of lateral development is desired, turn the two lateral sections at the same time. If a differential amount of lateral development is needed, by turning one of the lateral sections the rest of the appliance will act as an anchorage unit allowing you to get unilateral movement. This is an excellent appliance when the size of the palate is large enough to handle the dimension of the screw. Due to its considerable bulk, it is not suited for narrow palates or younger patients.

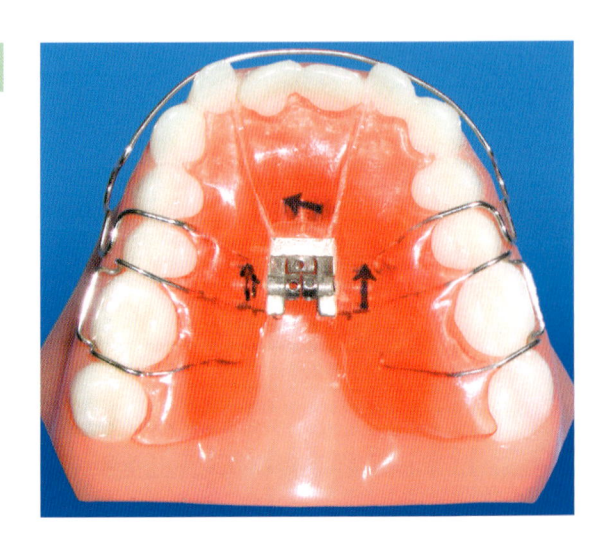

ARCH DEVELOPMENT

Combination Fixed Appliances For A/P Lateral Development

2046A Magill Sagittal to Advance

When both anterior and lateral development are needed, but patient compliance is a problem, the fixed Magill Sagittal to Advance is an excellent solution. In this example, second molars are present and an anchorage unit is created by joining the bicuspids and molars together with metal tubing on the lingual aspect. This tubing accepts a sliding wire that allows the anteriors to move forward when the appliance is activated. Activation is accomplished by engaging the unique buccal drive tubes with an Allen wrench. Lateral development can be achieved by turning the central screw one turn a week.

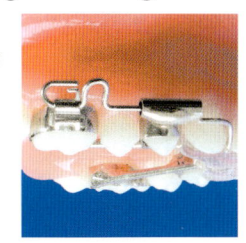

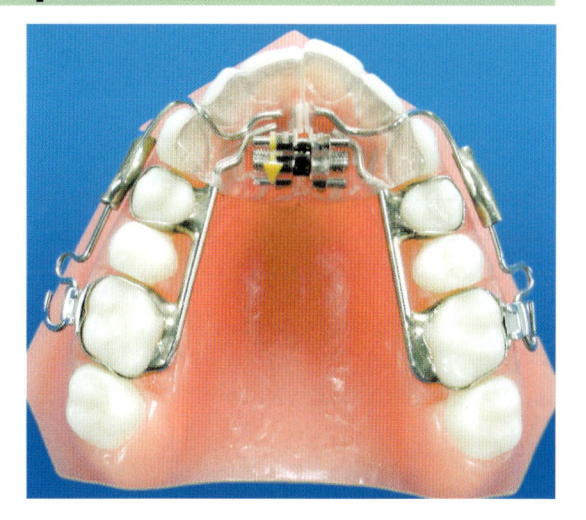

Design Notes:

_____
_____
_____
_____

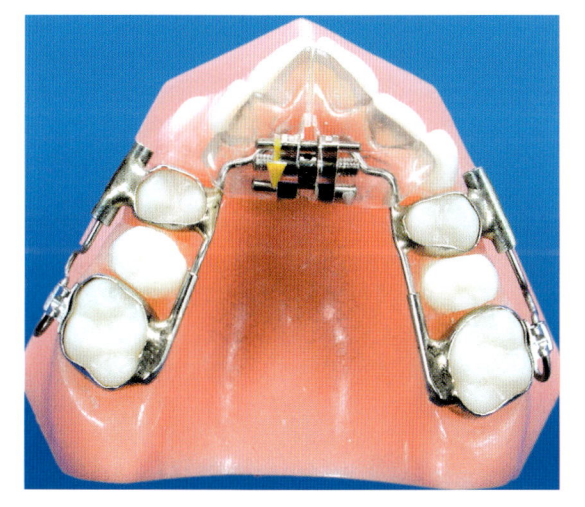

2046B Magill Sagittal to Distalize

When posterior and lateral development are needed, but patient compliance is a problem, the fixed Magill Sagittal to Distalize is an excellent solution. This design is essentially the reverse of the sagittal to advance that is illustrated in the preceding example. Here, the drive tubes are anchored to the bicuspids instead of the anterior lingual acrylic. This set-up change allows the anteriors to be used for anchorage by first activating the central screw and expanding the acrylic segment laterally. When this is done, activation of the buccal drive tubes will distalize the posterior segments. Notice that in this example the second molars have been extracted. As with all Distalizing Sagittals, always evaluate the vertical dimension and consider second molar removal to expedite treatment.

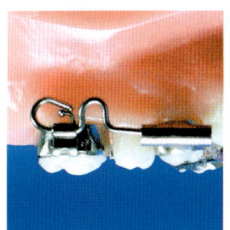

8-6.1

ARCH DEVELOPMENT

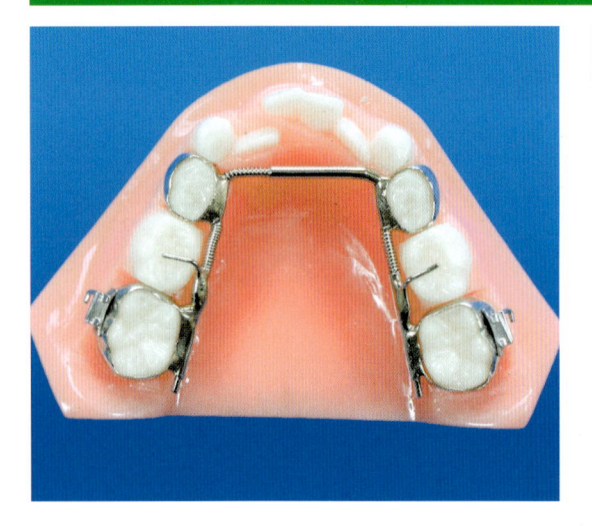

2092D Modified Lateral & AP Arnold Appliance U/L

The Modified "Arnold" expansion appliance has been a standard in the industry for many years. The use of compressed "open-coil" spring as part of a fixed appliance has allowed arch development to be accomplished in those patients who simply will not wear a removable appliance. As can be clearly seen in this photo, the Modified Arnold can produce both lateral and AP development. The introduction of NiTi coil spring added a new dimension to this design by providing a lighter, yet more continuous force over a greater range of motion. Because of the continuous force provided by the coil, the patient needs to be monitored carefully to prevent over-development in both planes.

Hint - It is always difficult to cement a pre-activated, spring-loaded appliance. To make it easier, ask the lab to return the appliance to you on the model. This will allow you to tie the appliance together with floss and control the spring action prior to cementation.

2085E Pendex/Hilgers Pendulum   U

The original pendulum appliance was designed to both distalize and rotate the maxillary molars. Once both of these movements were accomplished and the molars were in their ideal position, straight wire mechanics would be used to guide the bicuspids into their proper position in the arch. Hilgers took this concept and modified the appliance by adding an expansion screw in the palatal acrylic. With this simple change in design, lateral arch development could also be accomplished.

In this example, the distalizing springs are fashioned to fit into horizontal sheaths rather than round tubing. This is done because the horizontal sheaths add a degree of control that limits any buccal or lingual tipping.

To place this appliance, first pre-activate the springs by bending them to a 90° angle, then cement the appliance in two separate units. The anterior portion of this appliance, which uses bands on the bicuspids for retention, is cemented first, followed by the cementation of the molars. Once the cement has set, the activated springs are pulled forward and inserted into the lingual sheaths. These TMA springs can produce about 5mm of distal movement in three to four months without the need for interim re-activation.

Note - When an increase in arch length and width are both needed, many practitioners prefer to idealize the position of the molars at the same time that they expand the arch. Others prefer to initiate molar distalization several weeks (2 to 4) after transverse changes begin. Either way, once these movements are accomplished, the bicuspids and cuspids will have to be brought back in the arch form one at a time using fixed mechanics.

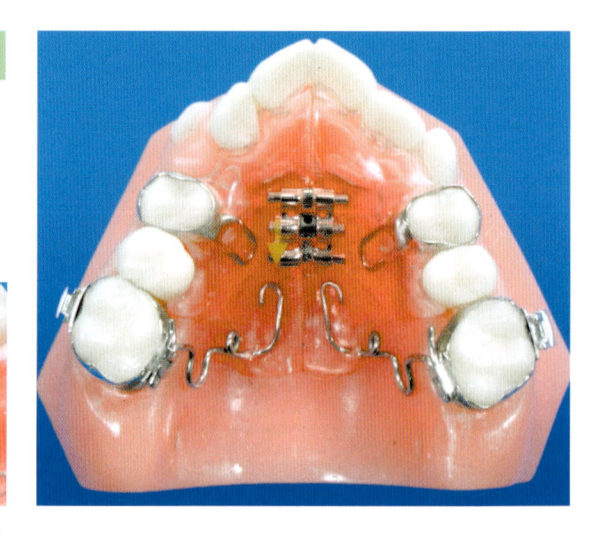

ARCH DEVELOPMENT

2085MX The "M" Pendex   U

This fixed appliance is used to increase arch width and length. The anterior anchorage needed to accomplish this movement is gained through the use of occlusal bonded rests on the pre-molars just like the Hilgers/Pendex design. However the addition of the "M Pendulum Spring" makes this design unique.

This innovative spring utilizes an inverted horizontal loop placed in the spring half way between the helix and the .036 lingual sheath on the molar band. This inverted loop overcomes the standard Pendulum spring's tendency to cause crossbites and leave the molar roots mesially inclined after distalization.

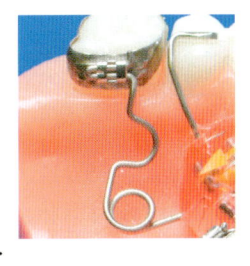

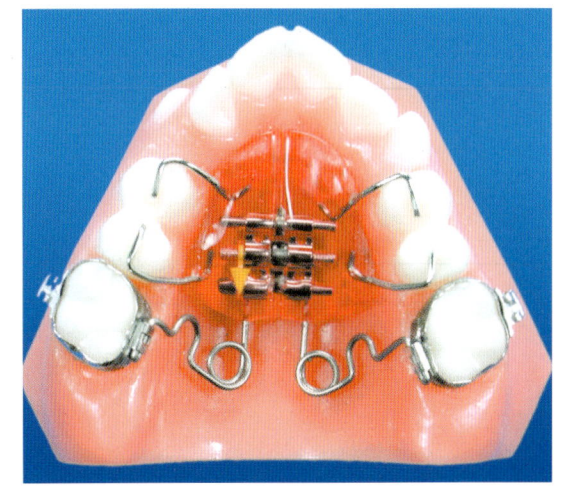

By simply opening the loop, a buccal and/or distal uprighting force is placed on the molar roots. The result is true bodily movement of the molars. The midline screw can be activated as needed to develop the lateral arch width and/or aid in correcting posterior crossbites.

Note - When an increase in arch length and width are both needed, many practitioners prefer to idealize the position of the molars at the same time that they expand the arch. Others prefer to initiate molar distalization several weeks (2-4) after transverse changes begin. Either way, once these movements are accomplished, the bicuspids and cuspid will have to be brought back in the arch form one at a time using fixed mechanics.

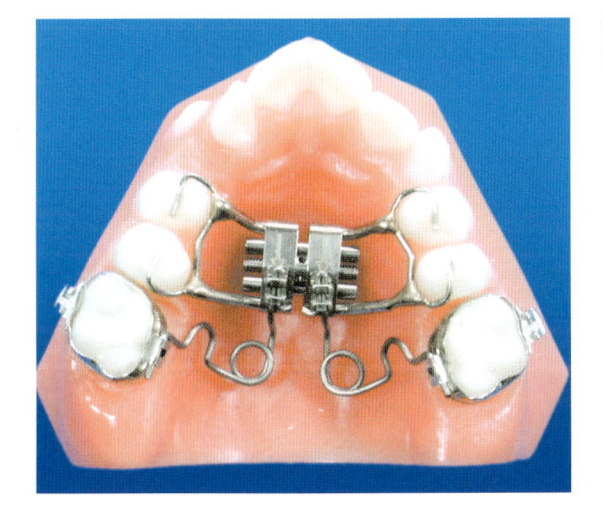

2085F Grumrax   U

The Grumrax Appliance can develop an arch laterally while being able to distalize and rotate the molars at the same time. This makes it similar to the Hilgers/Pendex appliance in both its use and design. However, there are a few design modifications that make this appliance quite unique. The first change is the use of an R.P.E. screw and the obvious absence of any palatal acrylic. The second modification is the attachment of the distalizing springs to the body of the R.P.E. screw via horizontal sheaths. These springs are fully removable making them easier to initially activate and reshape throughout treatment. They can also be unilaterally activated. This design is also more hygienic making it an excellent choice for patients exhibiting compromised dental hygiene. For the other advantages provided by the M Pendulum spring, see the M Pendex appliance.

Note - When an increase in arch length and width are both needed, many practitioners prefer to idealize the position of the molars at the same time that they expand the arch. Others prefer to initiate molar distalization several weeks (2 to 4) after transverse changes begin. Either way, once these movements are accomplished, the bicuspids and cuspid will have to be brought back in the arch form one at a time using fixed mechanics.

8-6.3

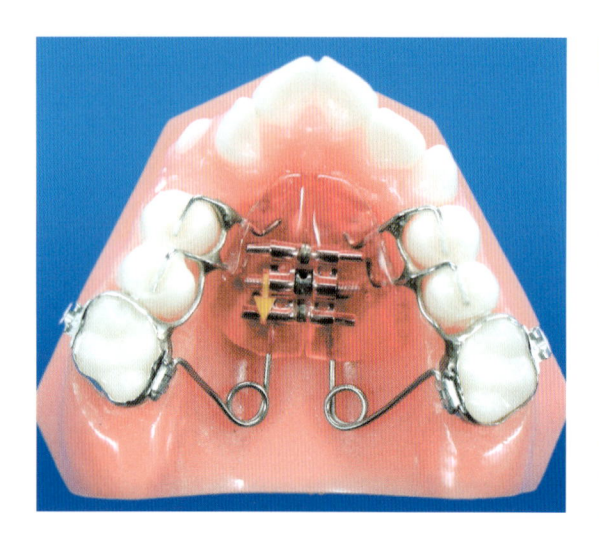

ARCH DEVELOPMENT

2085G Snodgrass

The Snodgrass appliance incorporates a Rapid Palatal Expansion feature into the Hilgers Pendulum design. It is used in the mixed and permanent dentition as an adjunct to treat Class II malocclusions that require expansion, molar rotation, and molar distalization. As can be seen in the photo, heavy wires from the anterior portion of the appliance are soldered to the molar bands. This makes the entire appliance rigid for rapid palatal expansion.

The initial adjustments involve twice daily activation of the midline screw until the desired lateral expansion is achieved. This usually takes about two weeks. The appliance should then be left in place for at least one month after expansion before activating the pendulum springs.

Activating the pendulum springs requires intraoral cutting of both solder joints mesial to the six-year molars using a 557 bur. These springs can be pre-activated by the lab, while additional activation is possible using a Weingart plier. This is usually done once a month. The illustrated appliance here shows the standard Pendulum spring design. The addition of the "M Pendulum" spring is often preferred to aid in more bodily molar distalization.

Note - Once molar position is established, the bicuspids and cuspids will have to be brought back in the arch form one at a time using fixed mechanics.

2154CD Multi-Action Hyrax

Another method to accomplish distal bodily movement of the first molars while expanding the arch laterally is seen here. The CD Multi-Action Hyrax incorporates the use of NiTi coil spring compacted onto buccal and lingual bars that run from the bicuspids to the molars. These bars are soldered to the bicuspid bands and run through tubes that are soldered to the molar bands. As the coil expresses itself, the molars will slide distally along the bars in a bodily fashion.

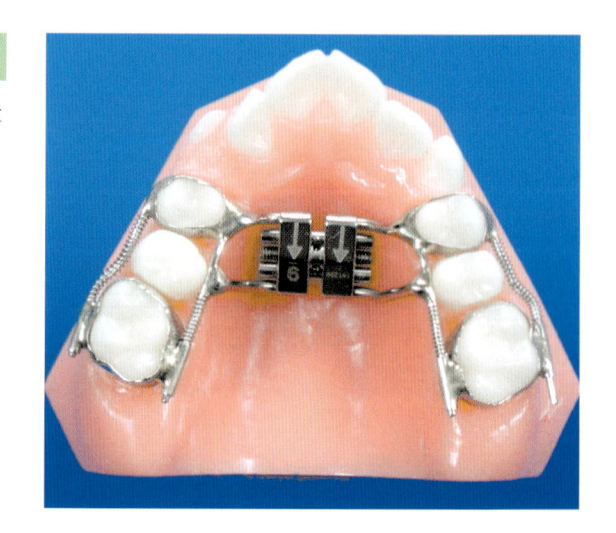

Note - Once molar position is established, and the arch is expanded, a holding arch is usually placed and the bicuspids and cuspids will be brought back in the arch form one at a time using fixed mechanics.

ARCH DEVELOPMENT

2153LD Modified Haas Expander

The Haas suture-expanding appliance utilizes acrylic to support the screw and add extra stability to the appliance. The acrylic closely contacts the palatal mucosa because Haas believed that more bodily movement and less tipping occurred with the presence of the palatal coverage. This occurs as forces are generated not only against the teeth but also against the soft and hard palatal tissues.

In this design, the Haas Expansion appliance is modified by adding a component of force to distal drive the molars. This is accomplished by using sliding lingual bars that are attached to the molars via horizontal sheaths and compressed nickel titanium coil spring packed along the bar.

Note - Bands may be custom fit, or pre-formed bands may be selected and sent with the prescription. Because this appliance uses four bands for retention, seating this appliance can have its challenges. To overcome these challenges, we recommend the following:

- Make sure to leave separators in place until the delivery appointment.
- When the path of insertion is a problem, gentle pressure will often allow it to seat over time.
- Cement the bands with a glass ionomer cement.

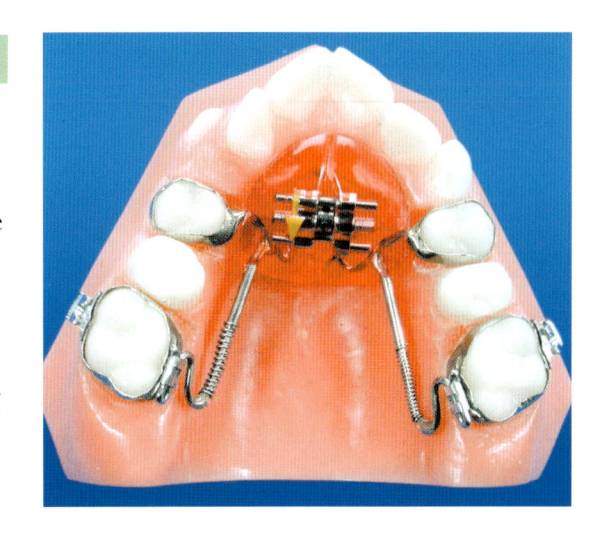

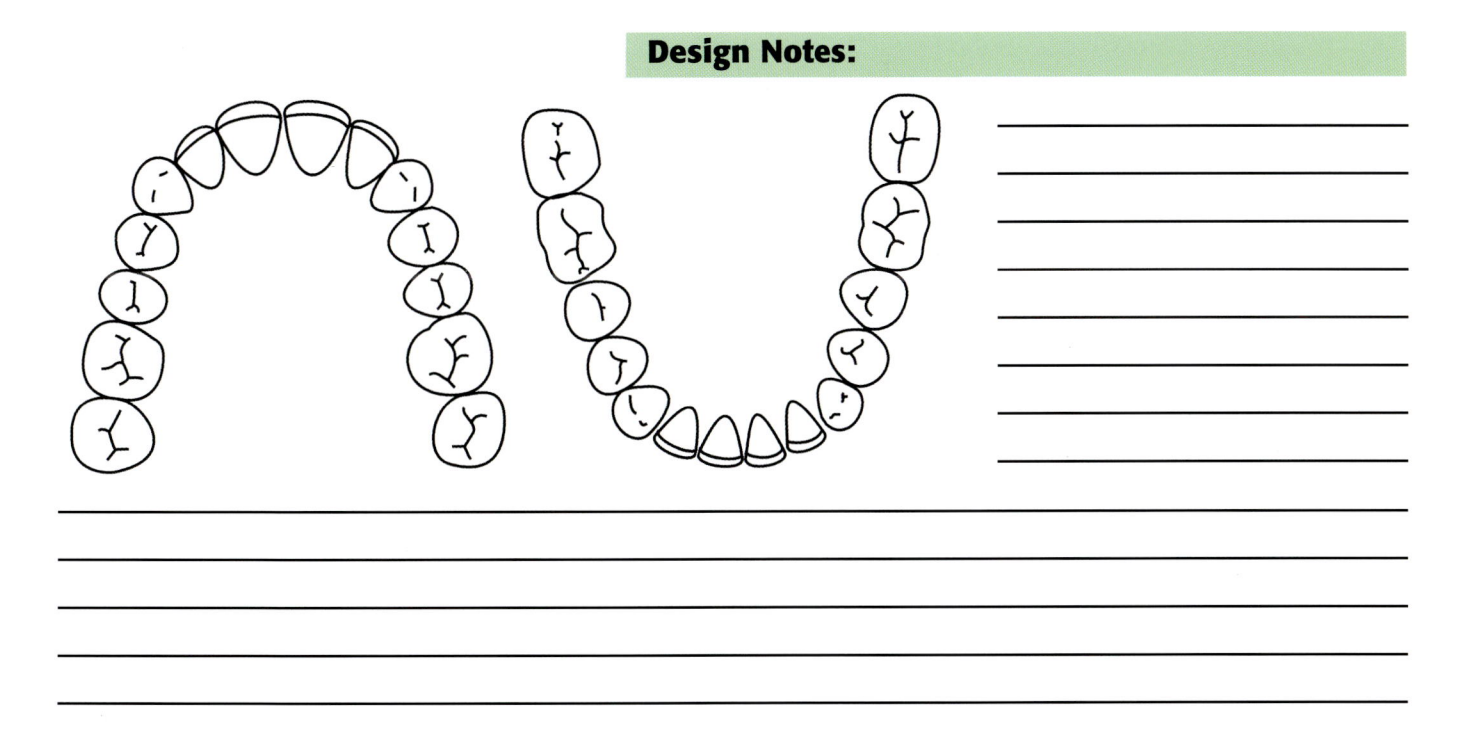

Design Notes:

ARCH DEVELOPMENT

Differential Development With Removable Appliances

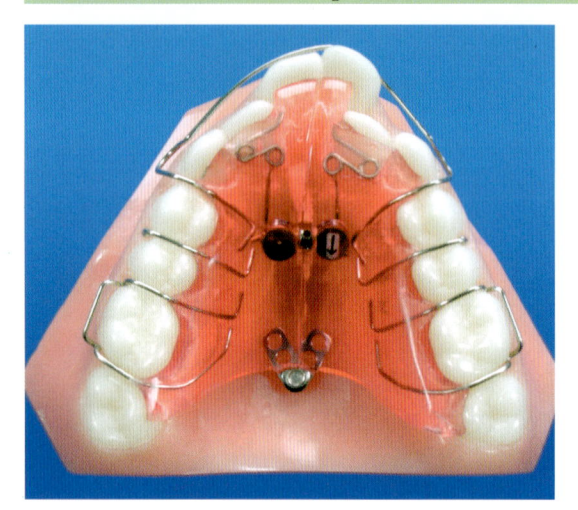

1103 Swing Lock Expander

Many patients exhibit a V-shaped or Gothic arch form as a result of an abnormal habit or an airway problem during development. When this occurs, the arch may only be narrow in the anterior region. Therefore, use of an expansion appliance that expands equally in the posterior and anterior region would be contraindicated. To overcome this problem, an appliance that uses an expansion screw in conjunction with a posterior hinge has been designed. It gains anterior space without disturbing the posterior bite relationship. Since the expansion screw and the hinge are separate pieces, it is possible to keep the palatal acrylic thickness at a minimum for patient comfort.

This design is only effective for a limited amount of expansion (up to 4mm). If additional expansion is required, either plan for making a second appliance or utilize an appliance with a larger fan screw such as the one seen in appliance #1104.

Note - As in all removable expansion appliances, activation of any of the springs should take place after space has been created through the expansion process.

1104 Wipla Swivel Plate

When the maxilla is significantly more narrow in the anterior region than in the molar region and crowding is severe, the use of a "Wipla" screw can make it possible to expand the arch and correct the crowding without disturbing the posterior bite relationship. The expansion screw is hinged in the posterior segment, confining the expansion to the anterior region. The anterior portion of the screw pivots, allowing up to 8mm of expansion.

Note - Since this screw is available in only one size, it may not fit all cases needing this type of development. Appliance #1103 would be a viable alternative when this is the case.

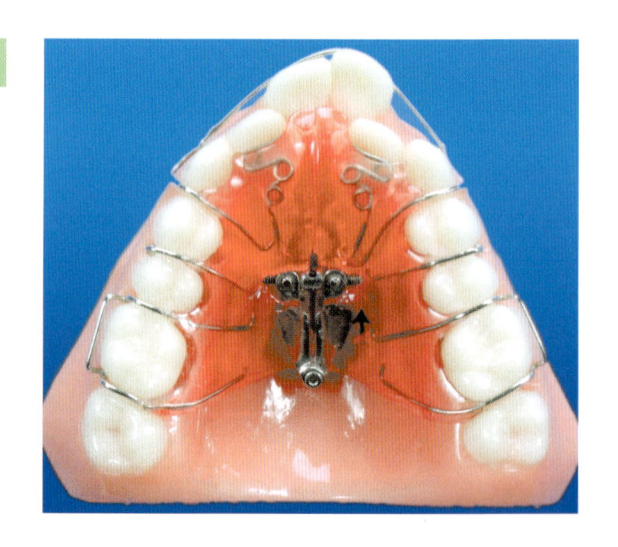

Design Notes:

_____
_____
_____
_____
_____

ARCH DEVELOPMENT

1096 Upper Jackson

The upper Jackson appliance was one of the original removable expansion appliances. Because it requires careful adjustment of the body wire, it has not been popular for this purpose since the development of the simple-to-adjust expansion screw.

Regardless, it is still an excellent appliance when a differential amount of development is needed throughout the arch. This appliance can be adjusted at the body wire with a 139 bird beak plier or a three prong plier and at the acrylic extensions. The lap springs can control the anteriors while the open palate promotes proper tongue position helping to maintain any lateral development.

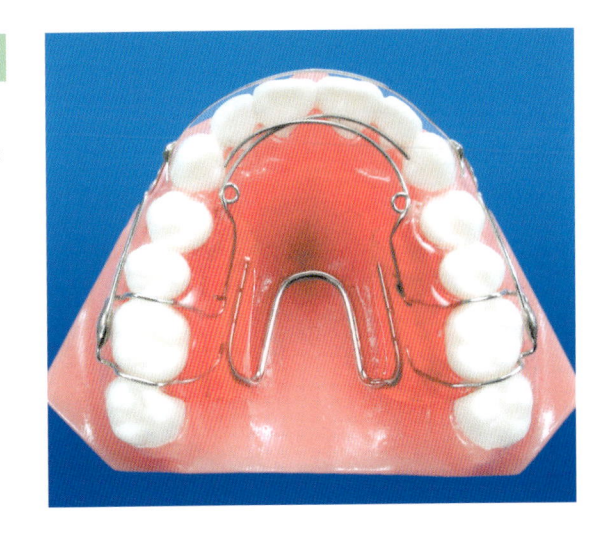

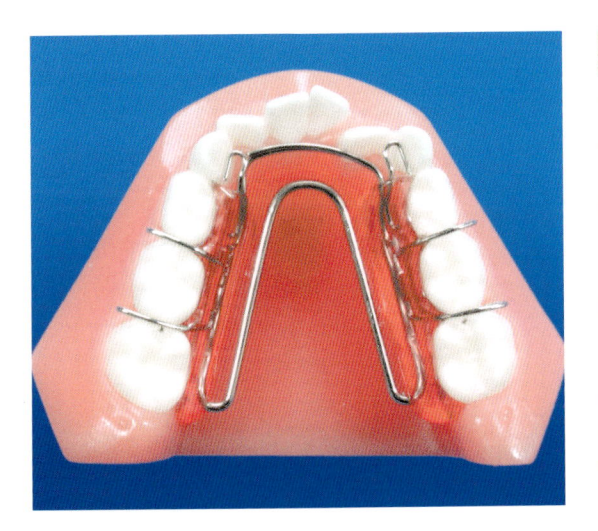

1098 Lower Jackson

This active expansion appliance is well suited for the mixed dentition stage of growth where lateral development of the lower arch is indicated. The "pumping" action of this appliance makes it particularly effective and produces rapid results. Since the upper arch develops faster than the lower, it is not uncommon for a doctor to prescribe an upper Schwarz and a lower Jackson to keep pace with the upper.

The typical activation of this appliance is to add a uniform 3mm to 4mm lateral adjustment to the body wire. However, the unique design of this appliance gives you the ability to differentially expand the arch in the anterior and posterior regions.

Note - Some patients find this appliance uncomfortable if care is not given to relieve the acrylic from the lingual-inferior undercut.

1342 Lower Posterior Expansion

The tongue plays an important role in the normal development of the upper and lower arch. When a tongue thrust exists and/or an abnormal swallowing pattern is exhibited, the posterior segments of the arches can collapse lingually.

Uprighting the posteriors in the mandible can be accomplished with this unique appliance. Its screw mechanism is designed to initiate expansion in the lower molar region without corresponding expansion in the anteriors. Since it operates on a fan principal, with the distal lingual flanges opening toward the buccal, activation will cause more expansion to occur in the molar region than in the premolar area.

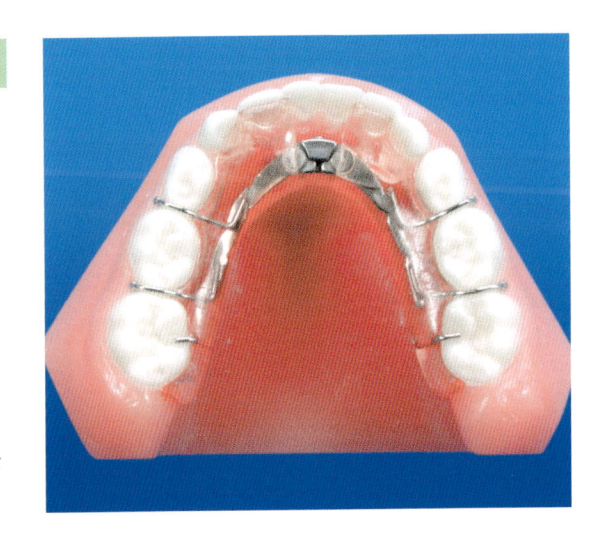

ARCH DEVELOPMENT

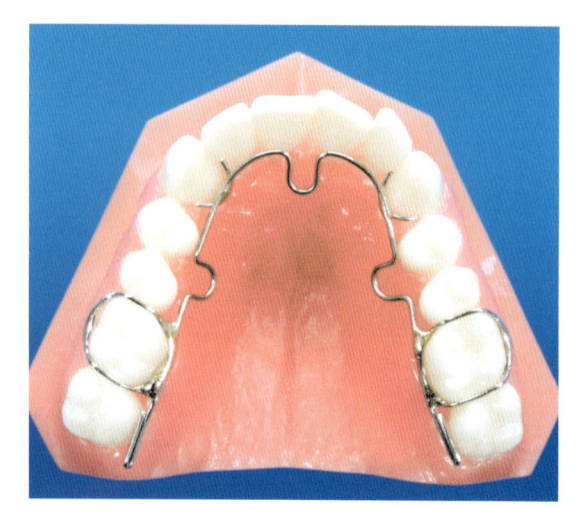

3106 ALF (Alternative Lightwire Functional)

The ALF is a light wire (.025 being used for the body wire itself) removable appliance that is capable of delivering a differential amount of development in both arches. It works by providing a physiologic force that is consistent with the Arndt-Schulz Law: "Weak stimuli will increase physiologic activity while very strong stimuli will inhibit or abolish physiologic activity." This appliance is incorporated in the treatment of a variety of malocclusions, however "ALF trained" practitioners often use it to treat chronic pain and TMD patients because of its ability to align the maxilla (cranial base) and correct cranial and upper cervical structural distortions.

Developed by Dr. Darick Nordstrom, this appliance provides excellent development of both the inter-cuspid area and the posterior segments. It is easy to adjust, does not hamper speech, and can be worn comfortably while eating.

The Crozat Technique

The Crozat technique offers a number of advantages to those who are familiar with the appliance's applications and adjustments. The Crozat has proven to be an excellent method of treating a wide variety of malocclusions.

This technique, when applied carefully, can accomplish the following objectives: treat cases on a non-extraction basis; develop arches laterally; stimulate alveolar bone growth; correct crossbites; control vertical development; direct and control skeletal growth changes; establish a proper plane of occlusion; maintain a balanced relationship between the joint, teeth, and muscles; and finally, position individual teeth for good esthetics and function.

From the patients' point of view, there are several advantages to the Crozat approach. Esthetically, the appliance is very inconspicuous and therefore is widely accepted by both children and adults. Being acrylic free and easy to take in and out, patients find it easier to maintain their oral hygiene. There also seems to be less interference with normal speech.

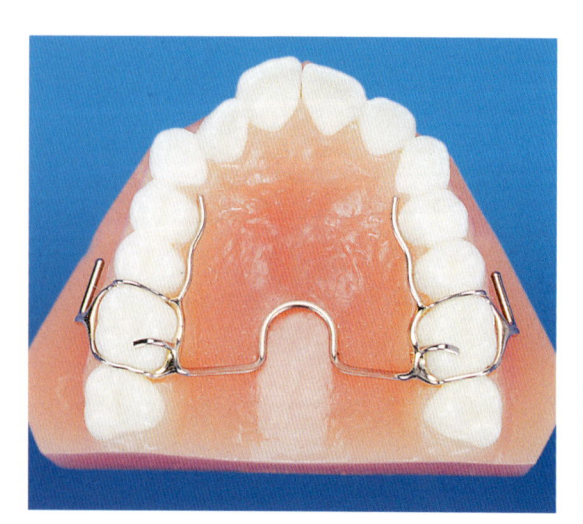

3101 Basic Maxillary Crozat

The Basic Maxillary Crozat typically clasps the first permanent molars and is used primarily for lateral development. Once this is accomplished auxiliary attachments, i.e. lap springs, labial bows, pins, putters, and appropriate inter-maxillary elastic hooks, can be added to the basic appliance to continue treatment as required.

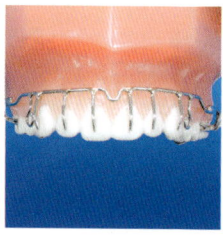

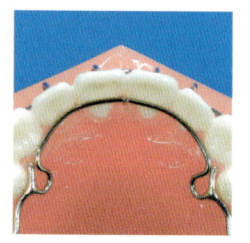

Note - The key to success with the Crozat technique is careful and accurate appliance adjustment.

ARCH DEVELOPMENT

3102 Basic Mandibular Crozat w/Lingual Springs

This appliance is used simultaneously with the maxillary Crozat for lateral arch development. As with the maxillary appliance, auxiliaries can be attached to the basic appliance as required. The appliance illustrated here has the added lingual lap springs to align the incisors and the distal extensions to help develop the second molars.

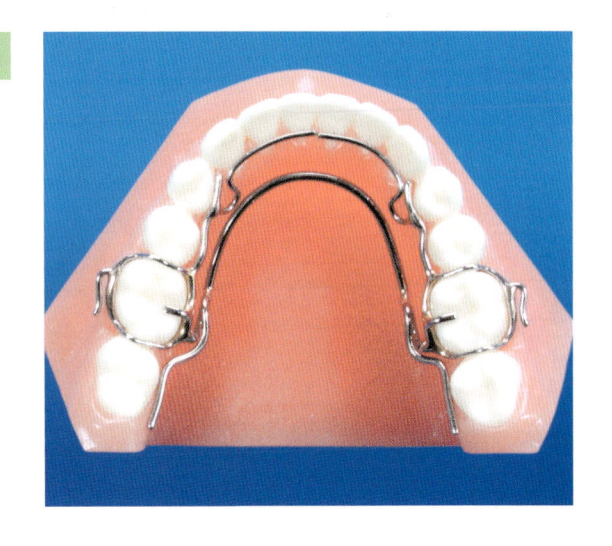

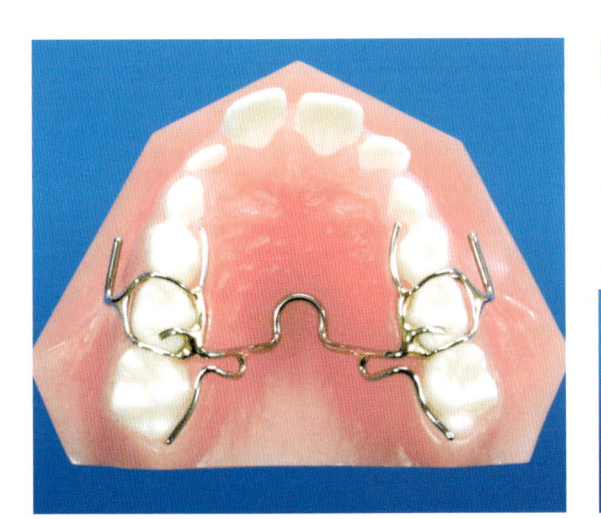

3103/3104 Interceptive Crozats   U/L

Crozats can be used for treating the young patient in mixed dentition. Here Crozat clasps are attached to the primary second molars, with extensions to the erupting six-year molars. It is the extensions that are used to develop the arches by moving the permanent molars buccally. To effectively use these appliances, it is essential that the primary second molars have substantial root structure still present.

3105/3106 Phase I Crozats   U/L

These Crozats are used primarily for the arch development phase of a comprehensive treatment plan that will include Straight Wire fixed appliances for the final alignment of the individual teeth. In these illustrations, the upper appliance has Class II hooks added while the auxiliary springs on the lower appliance are soldered to the body wire rather than the mesial extension. Some prefer this for ease of adjustment. Note that the lower lap springs only effect the incisors while individual push springs are placed on the cuspids. This provides more individual tooth movement.

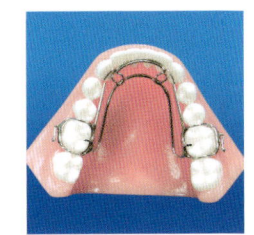

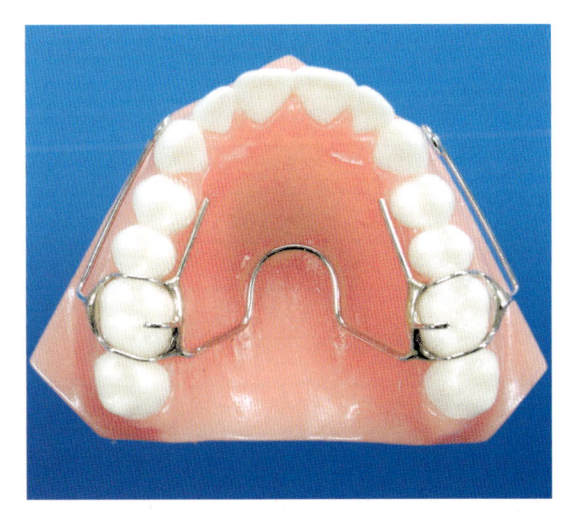

8-7.4

ARCH DEVELOPMENT

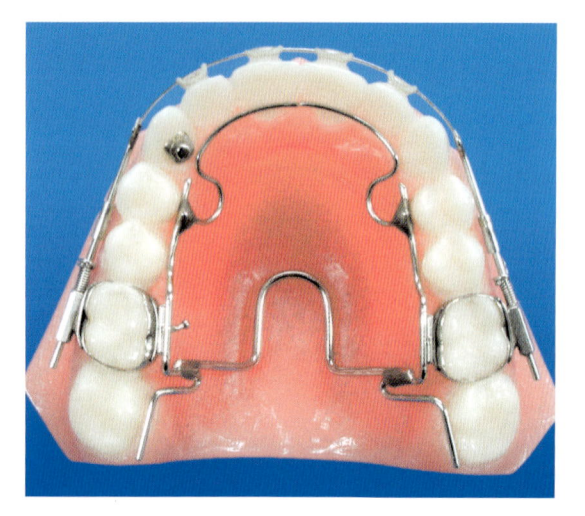

3810/3820 The FR (Fixed/Removable) Crozats U/L

The FR Crozat appliance eliminates some of the compliance problems from uncooperative or careless patients. This appliance utilizes the Wilson 3D® modular system* to attach the Crozat to bands cemented on the molars. All the regular Crozat additions

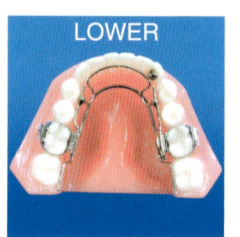

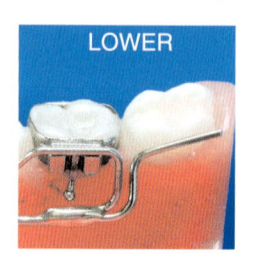

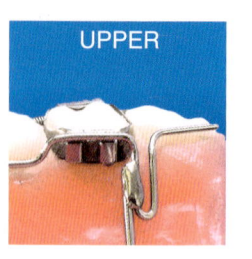

LOWER LOWER UPPER

and auxiliaries as well as other 3D® components can be integrated into this appliance. It can even be used in conjunction with the Straight wire technique.

The #3810 is an upper and #3820 is the lower.

*3D® is a trademark of Rocky Mountain Orthodontics.

Design Notes:

8-7.5

ARCH DEVELOPMENT

Differential Development With Fixed Appliances

2101 Porter Appliance   U

The fixed Porter appliance is designed to allow for a differential amount of expansion in the molar and cuspid/bicuspid region of a constricted maxillary arch. Lateral pressure is placed on the banded molars by adjusting the loop with the flat side of a #139 plier. The primary molars, bicuspids and cuspids can be adjusted independently by adjusting the lingual arms. Since it is usually easier to adjust an appliance out of the mouth, sliding vertical or horizontal brackets (as shown) can be fitted on the lingual aspect of the molar bands. This facilitates the removal of the wire without disturbing the banded teeth.

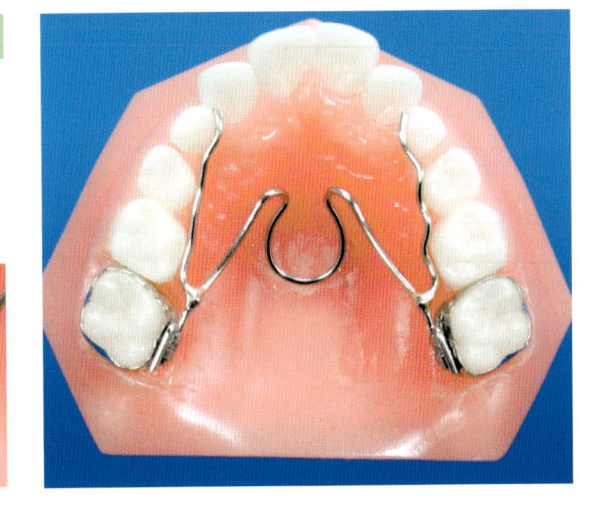

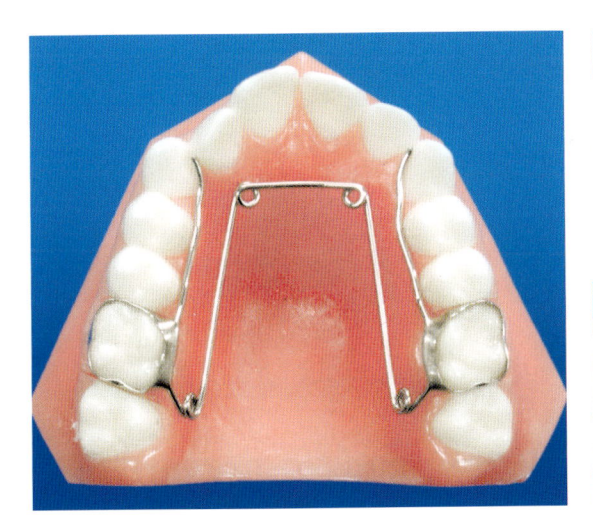

2084 Quad Helix   U

This appliance provides continuous controlled force for a variety of applications. It may be used for rotation or stabilization of molars, expansion or contraction of the arch, and even to assist in thumb, finger or tongue habit control. However it is mainly used because it allows for a differential amount of expansion in the anterior and posterior region of the arch.

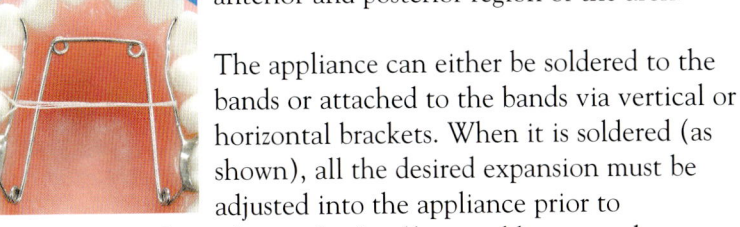

The appliance can either be soldered to the bands or attached to the bands via vertical or horizontal brackets. When it is soldered (as shown), all the desired expansion must be adjusted into the appliance prior to cementation. If you choose the fixed/removable approach, adjustments can be made throughout treatment.

Hint - If you choose to use the soldered design, always request that the working model be returned with the appliance. The appliance can then be activated out of the mouth, seated back on the model, and tied with dental floss across the arch from lingual arm to lingual arm into a passive position. Once the appliance is fully seated and the cement has set, the dental floss can be cut and removed.

ARCH DEVELOPMENT

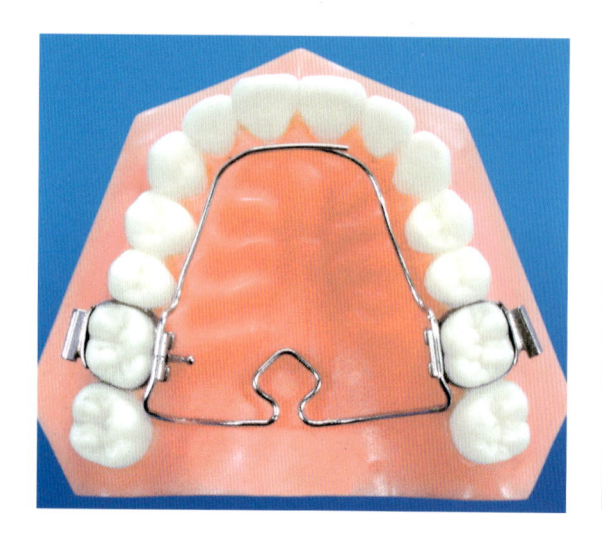

2505 Wilson 3D® Multi-Action Palatal Appliance U

The 3D® Multi-Action Palatal Appliance offers an alternative to using the Quad-Helix appliance. It, too, offers a simple, inexpensive alternative to numerous sagittal and transverse removable appliances. Often used in conjunction with the Quad-Action Mandibular appliance, this appliance produces rapid arch expansion or contraction, unilaterally or bilaterally; expansion or contraction of the bicuspids; advancement or retraction of the incisors; and tip, torque, and rotation of the molars.

Buttons placed on the cuspids are used to keep the lingual wires (termed "extenders" in the 3D® system) functioning in a horizontal plane and not riding up the lingual incline when activated.

2503 Wilson 3D® Quad-Helix U

The 3D® Quad-Helix Appliance is a multi-purpose maxillary arch development appliance. The appliance plugs into the 3D® Lingual Tube and the twin posts produce a tight friction-lock, with no free play. The .036" Tru-Chrome™ (RMO) stainless steel construction assures both stability and flexibility. In addition to being used for the traditional lateral arch development, this appliance can be used for unilateral expansion, molar rotation, molar buccal or lingual tip, molar buccal or lingual torquing, as well as anterior advancement.

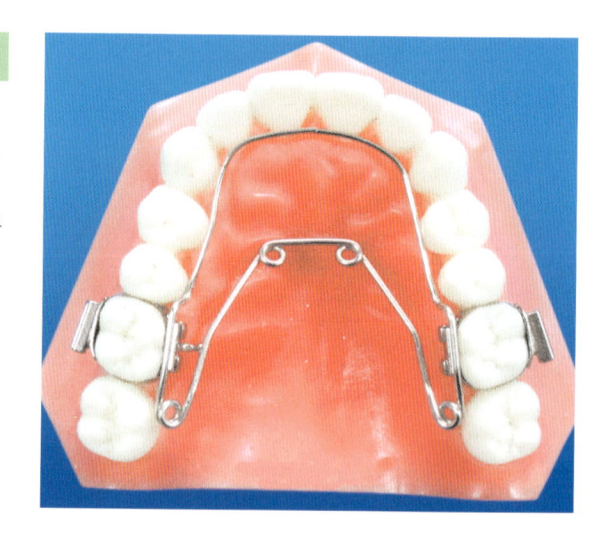

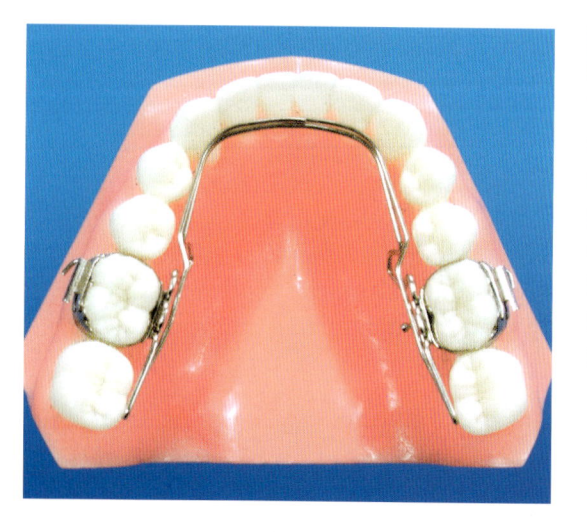

2504 3D® Quad-Action Mandibular Appliance L

The 3D® Quad-Action Mandibular Appliance offers simple, inexpensive alternatives to more than 20 different sagittal and transverse removable appliances. This versatile appliance can produce unilateral or bilateral rapid arch expansion or contraction; can expand or contract bicuspid position; can advance or retract incisors; and can rotate, tip, or torque the molars. The adjustments necessary to accomplish these movements are easily made since the arch wire is simple to remove from the molar bands.

ARCH DEVELOPMENT

2157 Nitanium Palatal Expander[2]   U

The Nitanium Palatal Expander[2] (NPE[2]) is a fixed/removable nickel titanium appliance, attached to molar bands via horizontal lingual sheaths. The main body wire of this appliance is fabricated from heat activated, nickel titanium wire with shape memory. It is formed to a set shape that it maintains when heated above its thermal transition temperature of 94° F. The appliance comes prefabricated in several sizes. The appropriate size for the patient is determined by comparing measurement of the patient's existing arch width to the ideal arch width chosen as your treatment goal.

Clinically, before appliance delivery, the NPE[2] is chilled and becomes extremely flexible and easy to insert. As the mouth begins to warm the appliance, the body wire becomes stiffer as the shape memory is restored. This exerts a continuous low force on the teeth and mid-palatal suture to produce expansion.

Appliance adjustment of the body wire is not necessary but the extension arms can be adjusted to provide a differential amount of expansion in the bicuspid region if it is needed.

Note - Initially, the patient may experience slight pressure that can be relieved by sipping a cold fluid or sucking on an ice cube. This feature makes the appliance very "patient friendly" because they can mitigate the pressure response.

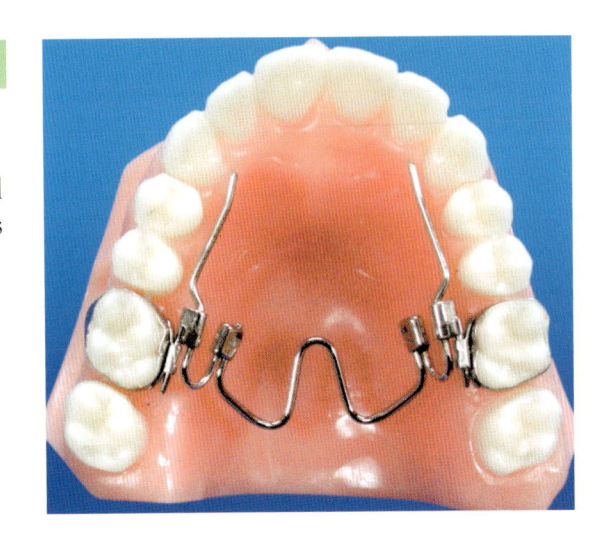

2154F Fixed "Fan-Screw" R.P.E.   U

Many patients exhibit a V-shaped or Gothic arch form as a result of an abnormal habit or an airway problem during development. When this occurs, the arch may only be narrow in the anterior region. Therefore, use of an expansion appliance that expands equally in the posterior and anterior region would be contra-indicated.

The Fixed Fan Screw appliance can produce up to 9mm of lateral arch development, confining the majority of movement to the anterior/cuspid region. It is typically soldered to bands placed on the first permanent molars and the first bicuspids.

Some practitioners prefer to band just the molars. When this is done, it is recommended that the anterior portion of the appliance be secured by placing bonding material over a wire rest.

ARCH DEVELOPMENT

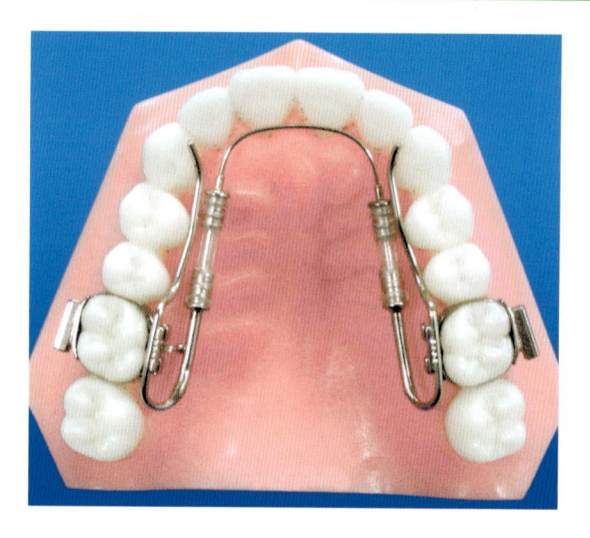

2521 Clark Trombone & Lingual Arch Developer (LAD)

The principal goal of this appliance is to manage a loss in arch length by using a pre-activated system. The original design of this appliance used coil springs to provide the necessary force, and chain elastic attached to mesial and distal hooks to control the force. In the new design shown here, the AP force is provided through a unique Compression Tube Activator that is comprised of fine bore silicone tubing. Replacing the springs and hooks with this new material has greatly improved the stability and safety of the appliance.

By simply adding extensions to this design, lateral arch development can also be accomplished. With proper adjustment, both molars and bicuspids can be moved buccally. For example, bayonet bends can be placed mesial to the molar tubes to expand the arch transversely in the bicuspid region when extra pressure needs to be applied to align a palatally displaced bicuspid.

Design Notes:

FUNCTIONAL ORTHOPEDICS

an overview: FUNCTIONAL ORTHOPEDICS

Chapter 9

The three major components of the stomatognathic system are the teeth, the bone, and the musculature. A balanced stomatognathic system exists when there is normal expression of a person's hereditary pattern, without the influence of unfavorable internal or external forces.

Abnormal forces cause malocclusion. Most patients' malocclusions entail more than just the malposition of teeth alone. Often there are orthopedic discrepancies and muscular dysfunctions as well. In treating these patients, equal importance must be placed to correcting both the dental and skeletal abnormalities.

Functional appliances are used to control and direct orthopedic and muscular forces in an effort to prevent or correct a malocclusion. They are designed to influence the growth and development of the facial skeleton in a vertical plane, a horizontal plane or both.

Functional appliances are designed to work hand-in-hand with nature. The uniqueness of functional appliances is their mode of force application. They do not act on teeth like conventional appliances, using springs and elastics, but rather transmit, eliminate or guide forces. Some of the natural forces that can be controlled by functional appliances are: muscle activity from the tongue, lips, and cheek; tooth eruption; and growth direction of the maxilla and mandible.

Although functional appliances also exert an orthodontic effect on the dentoalveolar structures, improperly shaped, shortened, narrowed or crowded arches should first be prepared by one of the arch preparing appliances described in the arch development chapter of this book.

Functional therapy is usually used, when treating children, to give the patient's normal hereditary pattern a chance to express itself. Therapy must start early so it will have the greatest opportunity to use growth in its favor. For example, the best time to accomplish Class II corrections is between 9 and 11. At this age, the patient is usually mature enough to follow your instructions while there is still plenty of time left for growth. Also at this age, with the use of an appropriate cephalometric analysis, you should have a more accurate picture of the patient's growth pattern.

Diagnosis is the key to successful Functional Orthopedic care, as an abnormal jaw-to-jaw relationship can be due to multiple factors. For example, a Skeletal Class II relationship can occur because the maxilla is too protrusive, the mandible is too retrusive or both may be contributing in varying degrees simultaneously. What is needed from a cephalometric analysis is, not only whether or not the case is in fact a Class II, but also which member of the jaw-to-jaw complex is errant and to what extent. This knowledge is the key to choosing an appliance and technique to correct the problem.

Functional therapy may also be used when treating adult patients. Although the sequence of treatment and the types of appliances used may be different when treating an adult, the basic concepts remain the same:

- Always respect the health of the Temporomandibular Joint. This can best be accomplished by creating a harmonious balance between the muscles, bones, and teeth.
- Treatment direction will totally depend upon the diagnosis of the patient's existing skeletal, dental and muscular relationship. All three components must be addressed to achieve a stable result.

FUNCTIONAL ORTHOPEDICS

The Bionator

The Bionator is an arch positioning appliance that moves the mandible as a unit. Its main use is to produce a full functional occlusion by correcting a Skeletal Class II with a retruded mandible to a Skeletal Class I relationship. However, this myofunctional appliance can be used to treat a variety of conditions. It can increase vertical dimension and eliminate deep overbites, treat TMJ dysfunction by taking the condyle out of the a superior posterior retruded position, widen moderately narrow maxillary and mandibular arches, correct excessive overjet, correct improper upper and lower lip relationships, and eliminate tongue thrusting and sucking habits.

Bionators are intended for the treatment of reasonably uncrowded dental arches that are misaligned either horizontally or vertically. Although the appliance can accommodate arches that have some minor crowding, the more irregularities that are taken care of prior to using the Bionator, the easier the treatment.

Although the Twin Block has replaced the Bionator as the mainstay appliance for Class II corrections, it still has advantages over the Twin Block that make it a very valuable appliance. The first advantage is that it can be used throughout the mixed dentition stage of development, as it does not depend upon these teeth for retention. This is important because skeletal corrections are always easier when the patient still has the potential to grow. Having to wait for teeth to erupt so they can be used for anchorage can often cause you to miss the patient's greatest growth period.

Another reason Bionators have stayed popular is that in adult therapy it is a great appliance to wear as a night time retainer. Whether the patient has been treated for TMJ or orthopedically corrected surgically or non-surgically, the Bionator will hold the mandible forward throughout sleep and prevent a patient from clenching.

> Important - As with all functional appliances, the proper construction bite must be provided for laboratory construction of the Bionator.
> For a Class I closed-bite or a Class II malocclusion, the mandible must be brought forward until the lower anteriors are labial to the upper anteriors by 1-2 mm.
> Overbite cases require 4-6 mm of bite opening in the molar area.
> Open vertical patients need only 2-3 mm of opening in the molar area.
> In deep bite patients, the anterior teeth should also have a bite opening of 2 to 3 mm.

3021 Balters Bionator to Open

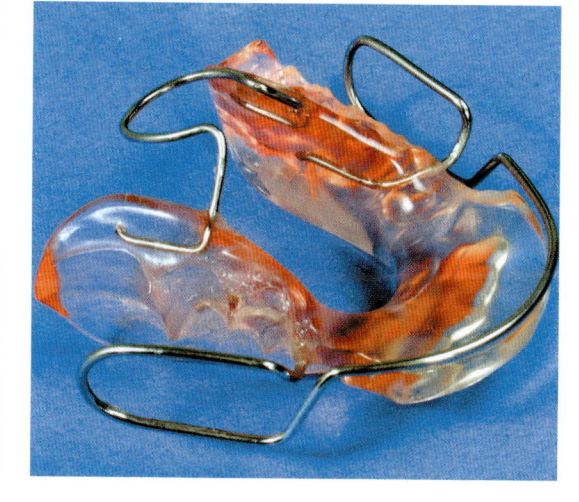

The Balters Bionators are the original Bionator designs. Their base of operation is the acrylic that is lingual to the dentition. This particular appliance is designed to open a closed bite in Class I and Class II malocclusions, and to correct Class II skeletal relationships.

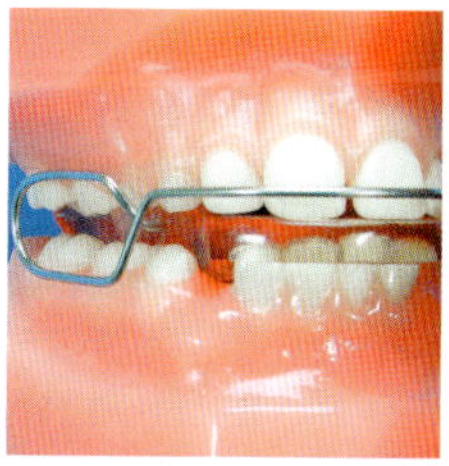

To accomplish this, the lower anterior teeth are covered with acrylic to act as a bite plane, hold the bite open, and to prevent anterior super-eruption. An extended labial bow acts as a buccal shield to keep the buccal musculature away from the posterior teeth. Controlling these muscles encourages eruption. The lingual acrylic prevents the tongue from interposing in the inter-occlusal space.

Upon delivery of the appliance, the posterior acrylic is carefully ground-in to permit controlled eruption of the molars and bicuspids until the closed bite is corrected.

9.1

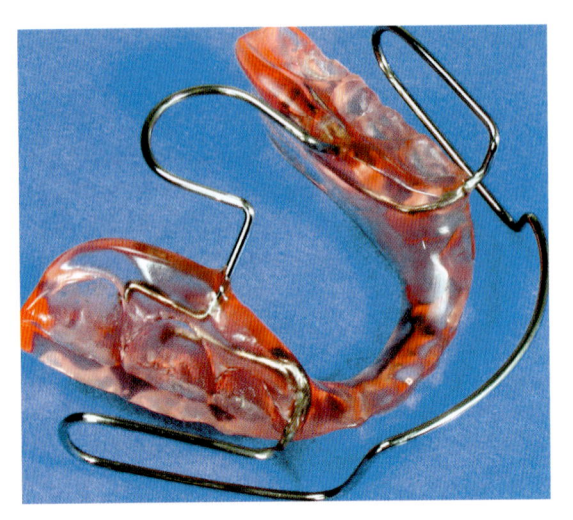

FUNCTIONAL ORTHOPEDICS

3022 Balters Bionator to Close

This Bionator is designed to correct skeletal and dental anterior open bites in Class I and Class II malocclusions. The posterior teeth are covered with acrylic to prevent their eruption while the acrylic is kept away from the incisors to permit closure of the open bite. Note that like the Balters Bionator to open, the appliance has an extended labial bow and no midline expansion screw. The enlarged coffin spring illustrated here is available on all designs.

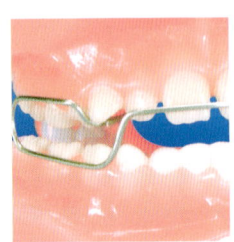

3023 Neutral Balters Bionator

This appliance is essentially a combination of the Balters Bionator to open and close. Its primary function is to correct skeletal Class II malocclusions without changing the vertical dimension. Acrylic covers both the anterior and posterior occlusal surfaces so that the vertical dimension will remain unchanged as you correct the skeletal problem.

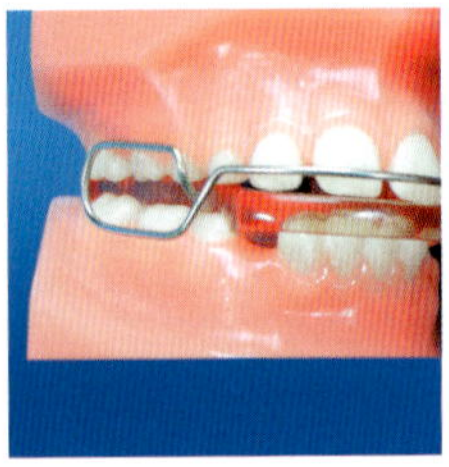

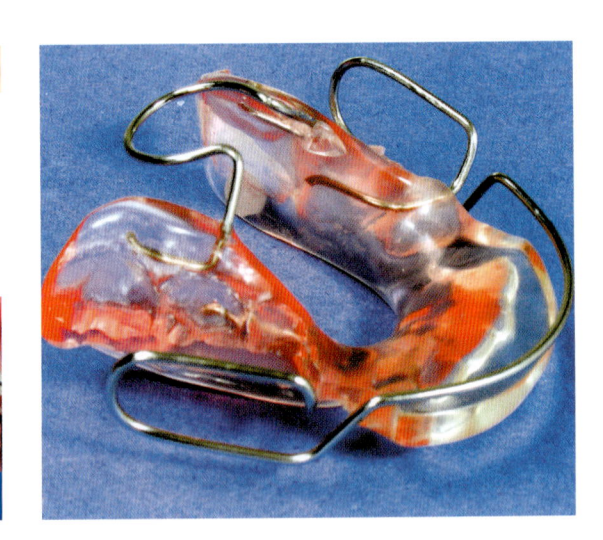

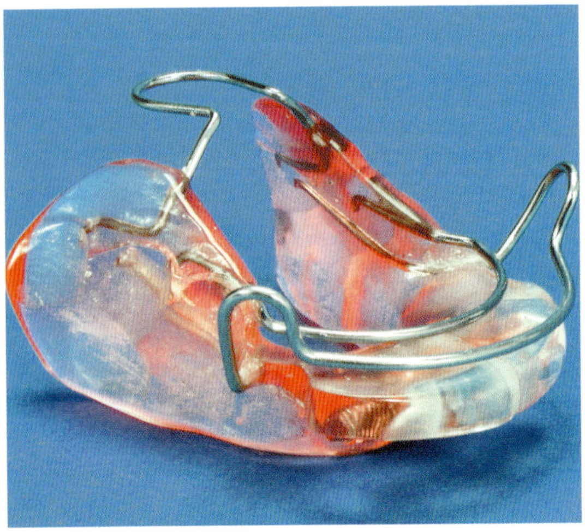

3011 Bionator to Open

This appliance, commonly referred to as the Bionator I, is designed to open a closed bite in Class I and Class II malocclusions and to correct Class II skeletal relationships. The lower anterior teeth are covered with acrylic to act as a bite plane, hold the bite open, and to prevent anterior super-eruption. The posterior acrylic is carefully ground-in to permit controlled eruption of the molars and bicuspids until the closed bite is corrected. Opening the midline expansion screw aids in posterior eruption by relieving tight interproximal contacts. It also allows for a limited amount of arch development when it is necessary.

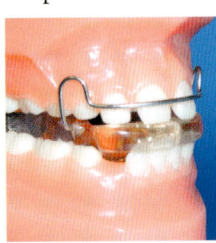

FUNCTIONAL ORTHOPEDICS

3012 Bionator to Close

This Bionator, commonly referred to as the Bionator II, is designed to correct anterior open bites in Class I and Class II malocclusions.

The posterior teeth are covered with acrylic to prevent their eruption while the acrylic is kept away from the incisors to permit closure of the open bite. The midline expansion screw can be used for arch development when it is indicated. Adding a "Balters Type" labial wire will also enhance lateral arch width development.

Note - If desired, the lower incisors can be capped with acrylic if you wish to prevent their eruption. If so, please be sure to include this on your lab prescription.

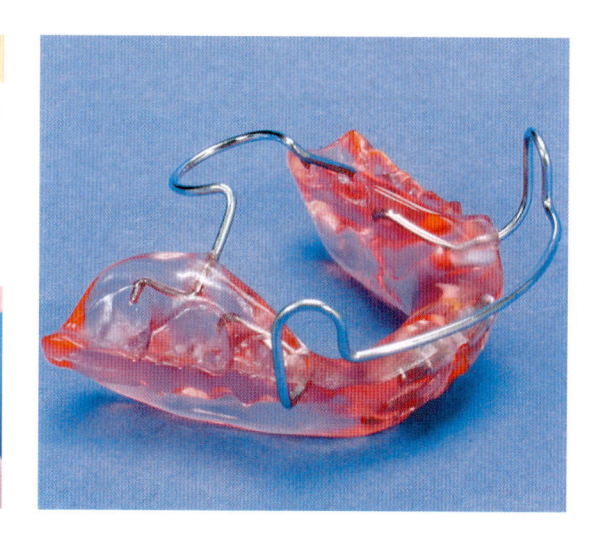

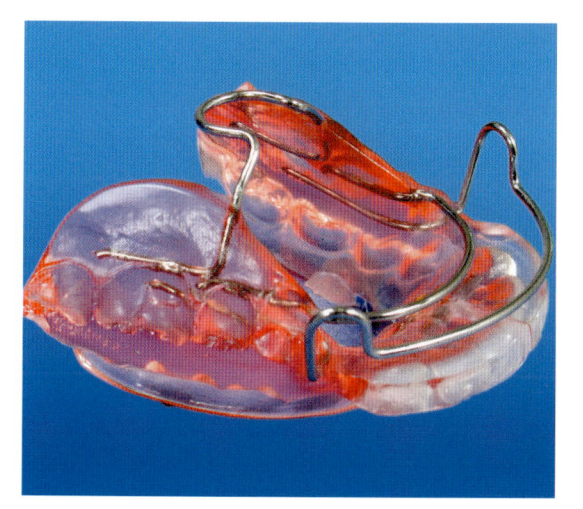

3013 Neutral Bionator

The Neutral Bionator has posterior occlusal coverage as well as acrylic coverage over the lower anteriors. Its primary function is to correct Class II malocclusions without changing the vertical dimension.

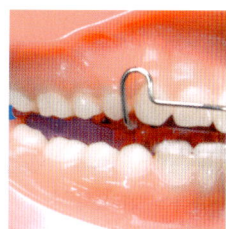

Note - The "Balters Type" labial wire can be used on any Bionator design and can act to enhance lateral arch width development when a midline expansion screw is included in the design.

Design Notes:

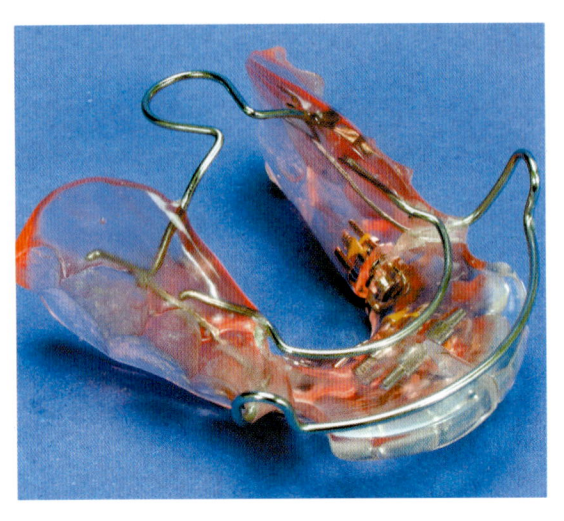

FUNCTIONAL ORTHOPEDICS

3026 Orthopedic Corrector

The Orthopedic Corrector is similar to a Bionator with the exception that there are two additional expansion screws added to the appliance. The addition of these screws prevents the need for the construction of a second appliance in severely retruded skeletal Class II or TMJ involved cases. After the third or fourth month of wear, when the patient's muscles have readjusted to their new position, the screws can be activated. Turning them in unison moves the anterior cap forward. This allows the mandible to be advanced even further as treatment progresses.

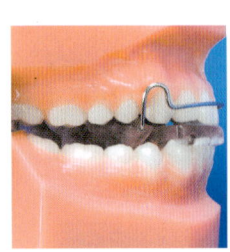

The Orthopedic Corrector I is used to increase the vertical in deep overbite cases, while the Orthopedic Corrector II is used to close open bites.

Note - Wax bite requirements for this appliance remain the same as for the regular Bionator.

Design Notes:

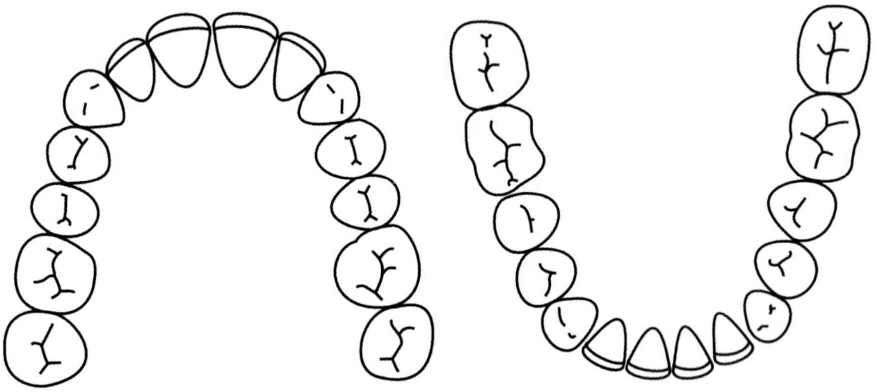

FUNCTIONAL ORTHOPEDICS

3032 Bio-Finisher

Functional treatment can be slow because the natural forces are not always enough to stimulate a rapid onset of measurable changes. This causes patients to experience "burnout" due to long treatment times. Dr. Lynn developed the Bio-Finishing appliances to help overcome this problem.

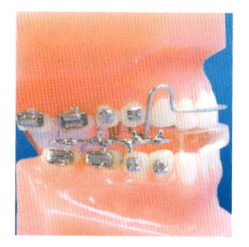

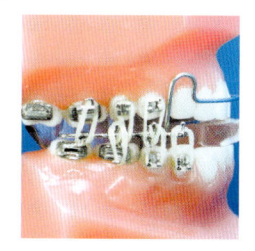

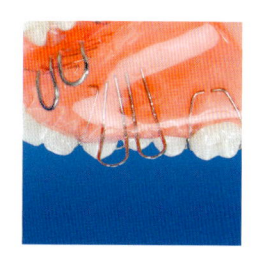

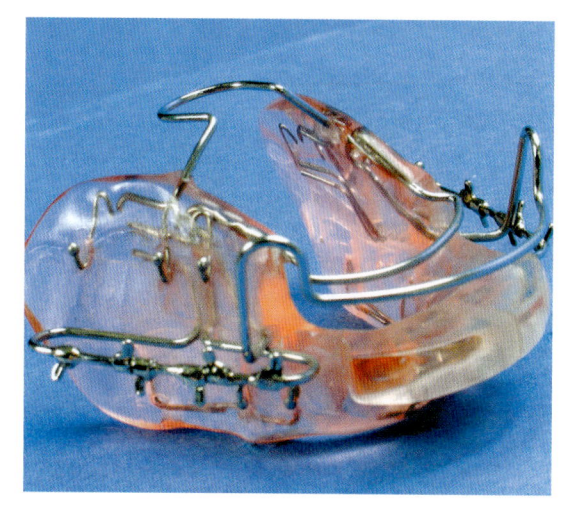

These very active appliances allow the doctor to control the time of treatment with much more accuracy and confidence than with many of the other functional appliances.

The Bio-Finisher is basically a Bionator with the addition of two buccal rakes placed into the body of the appliance at the plane of ideal occlusion. Small hooks are placed on the rake in line with the vertical axis of each of the opposing posterior teeth. Elastics (1/8") are then placed from each hook to the opposing bracketed tooth in order to extrude the teeth at a faster rate than is possible with the standard Bionator. This appliance offers excellent control of the direction and amount of posterior eruption. It is designed to be worn only at night.

A daytime appliance is to be used in conjunction with the Bio-Finisher and is to be worn all day, even while eating. The normal design of this appliance includes lingual ball clasps for retention and an anterior bite plane to encourage posterior vertical eruption. Because the bite is being held open, bilateral tongue cribs are used to prevent both a lateral tongue thrust and to stop the tongue from resting between the posterior teeth.

Design Notes:

9.5

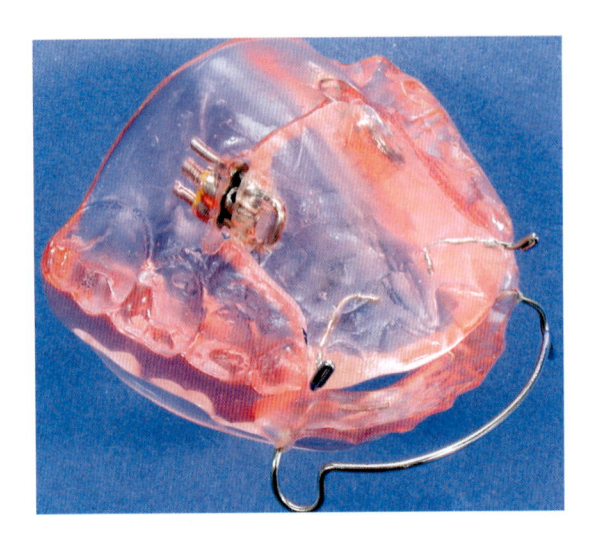

FUNCTIONAL ORTHOPEDICS

3504 The Han Appliance

An anterior occlusal interference can lead to an underdeveloped premaxilla and retroclined maxillary anteriors that are locked lingually in crossbite to the lower anteriors. If left untreated, over time this pseudo Class III can become a permanent skeletal defect. The Han Appliance has been found to be an excellent tool for correcting this problem.

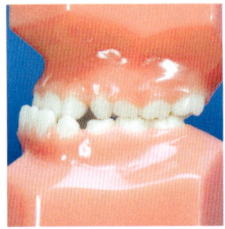

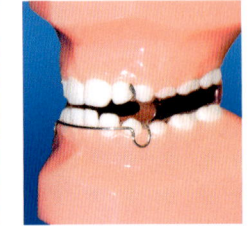

The Han Appliance ties the posterior aspect of the maxilla and the entire mandibular arch together to create enough anchorage to effectively use sagittally placed expansion screws to develop that premaxillary segment labially.

By turning the screws, the premaxilla is developed and the anteriors are tipped labially. Once the anterior segment is developed sufficiently to create a positive overjet, the appliance can typically be replaced with a simple Hawley retainer.

A carefully taken construction bite is essential for the proper fit and function of this appliance. The construction bite must be taken in the most retruded arc of mandibular closure that is possible making sure that the patient does not posture forward. This is important because these patients will want to posture their lower jaw forward to avoid the incisal interference that is created in an end-to-end bite.

Design Notes:

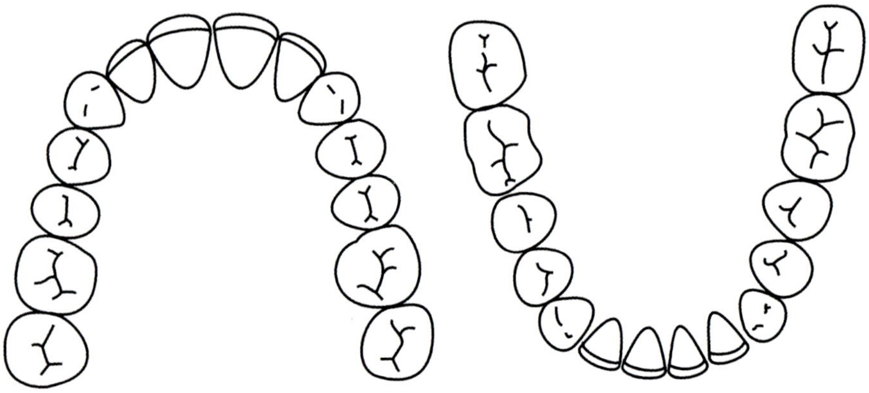

FUNCTIONAL ORTHOPEDICS

The Twin Block Appliance

It has been estimated that approximately 70% of all malocclusions are Skeletal Class II relationships. The majority of these have a constricted maxilla that is in a normal position relative to the cranial base, a retrognathic mandible, a normal or short lower face height, a large overjet and a deep overbite.

Although a wide variety of appliances have been successfully used to correct this type of problem and achieve a proper functional occlusion, most of them share one major disadvantage. The upper and lower components are joined together making it difficult for the patient to speak and function normally. The end result is poor patient compliance. The Twin Block is the one appliance designed to overcome these objections.

The Twin Block appliance has been described as "the most comfortable and the most esthetic of all the functional appliances." Unlike the other bulky, one-piece functional appliances, the Twin Block has separate unattached, upper and lower components. While this design can still hold the mandible forward like the other functional appliances, the mandible is free to move normally in both anterior and lateral excursions. It can be worn 24 hours a day, even while eating. This allows you to take advantage of all the functional forces applied to the dentition during mastication, which leads to faster results and shorter treatment plans.

Although its main use is to correct Class II Division 1 and Class II Division 2 cases, the appliance is versatile enough to also treat: Class I open bites, Class I closed bites, Class III lateral arch constrictions, and anterior/posterior arch length discrepancies. The Twin Block can also be used effectively in TMJ therapy.

Design Notes:

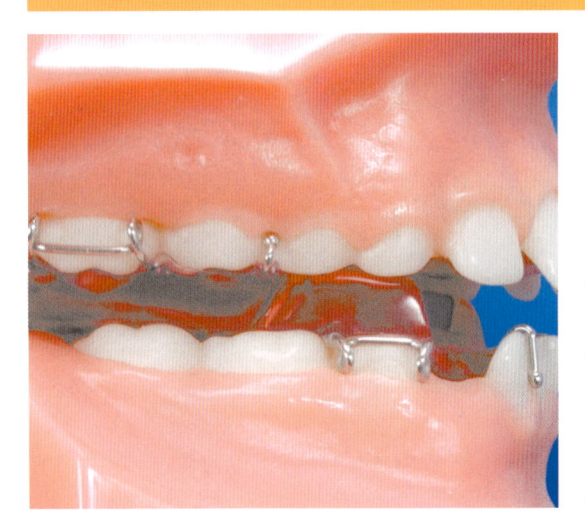

FUNCTIONAL ORTHOPEDICS

3610 Standard Twin Block to Open Bite Class II Division 1

The Twin Block is a removable functional appliance consisting of two bite blocks (twin blocks), upper and lower, that are designed to interlock at 70 degrees in such a manner that the mandible is held in a more protrusive position. Over time, the repositioning of the mandible forward eliminates the overjet and, when acrylic is removed from the upper block, eruption of the lower first molars occurs eliminating the overbite. When treatment with the Twin Block is complete, the first molars will be in contact and the maxillary and mandibular incisors will be nicely coupled. In the mixed dentition sample shown here, the lower molars will usually erupt passively. But in the permanent dentition, the lower molars often need to be actively erupted using vertical elastics.

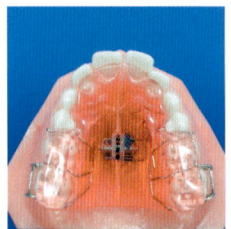

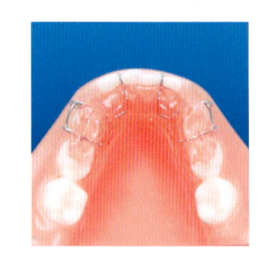

To ensure that the patient does not end up with a dual bite, the appliance must be worn a minimum of 7 to 9 months. When the patient's bite is stable, he should not be able to retrude the mandible without experiencing discomfort. Once the first phase of treatment is completed, i.e. the case is at the desired vertical and AP position, it will be necessary to place a Phase 2 or "Support Appliance". Detailed information on this appliance can be found in this chapter on page 9.18.

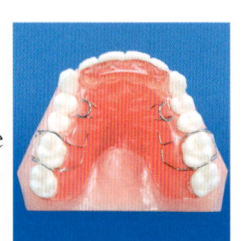

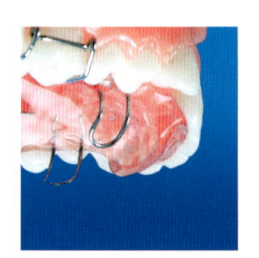

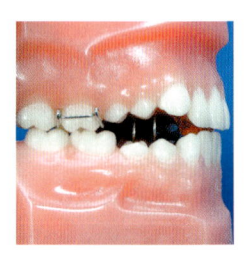

The Standard Twin Block seen here has an upper block that covers the second primary molar or bicuspid, first molar and second molar. The lower block covers the first primary molar and two thirds of second primary molar. It is vital to the success of the Twin Block treatment that the lower block is held ahead of the upper block at all times. To accomplish this, the blocks must be at least 5 to 6 mm thick. If they are not, adjusting them to allow for the eruption of the lower first molars will destroy the interlocking effect of the two blocks. Appliance retention is also critical to the success of this appliance. If you do not have first primary molars that are going to be present for 7 to 9 months or first bicuspids that are sufficiently erupted, it would be better to choose another appliance or delay the treatment until the first bicuspids have erupted and adequate retention is available.

Note - The expansion screw added to this design can be used at the same time to initiate lateral arch development.

Design Notes:

_____
_____
_____
_____
_____

FUNCTIONAL ORTHOPEDICS

3615 Twin Block to Close an Anterior Open Bite with spinner & tongue loops

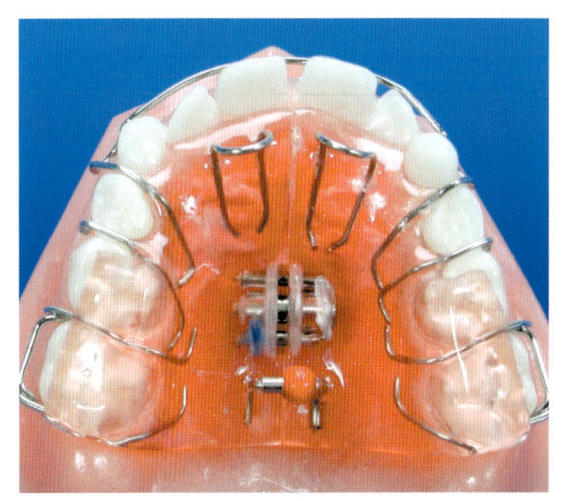

The Twin Block can also be used to close an anterior open bite. Here the design utilizes the standard 70° occlusal bite blocks to initiate a functional correction of a skeletal Class II while the anterior teeth are left slightly out of contact with the appliance to encourage reduction of the open bite.

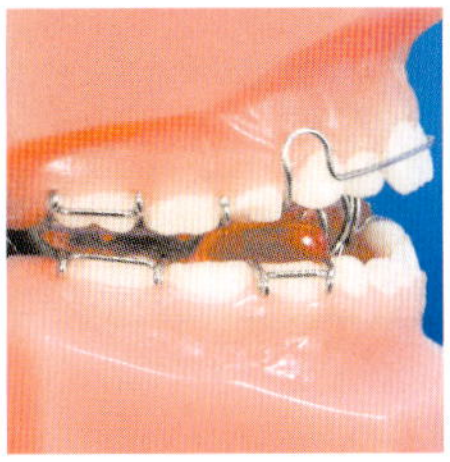

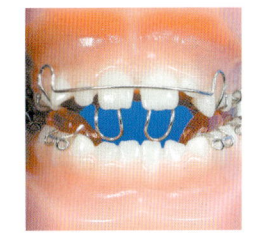

By leaving all the posterior teeth in contact with the blocks, their eruption will be prevented, and every time the patient swallows, lip action will work to close the open bite. The labial bow can also be adjusted to actively move the anteriors lingually.

In this example, the upper appliance has tongue loops positioned lingual to the upper anterior teeth to inhibit the effects of an anterior tongue thrust. In addition, a transpalatal wire with a spinner is added to help re-train tongue position and control the tongue thrust.

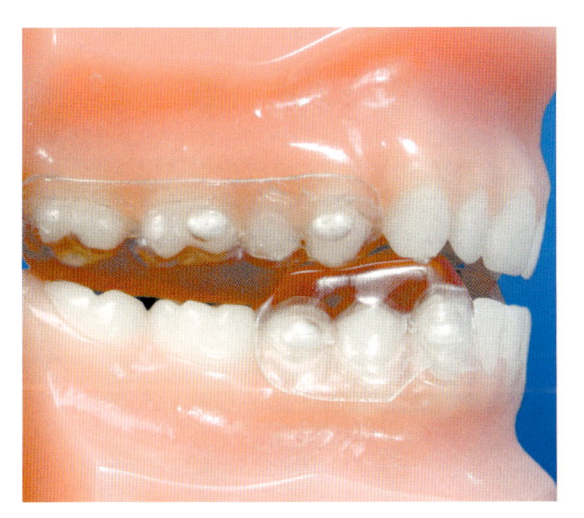

3804 Truax Twin Block

The Truax Twin Block is a claspless appliance that uses bonded "crown contours" to create uniform buccal undercuts for retention. The crown contours are carefully placed on the buccal/labial aspect of the retention teeth. Then, an impression is taken in the normal manner.

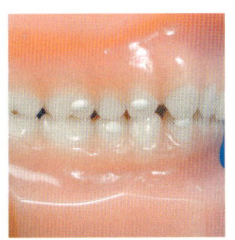

At the lab, a sheet of clear acrylic material is formed over the teeth, including the crown contours, and the remainder of the appliance is fabricated with traditional acrylics. The result is an appliance that "snaps" into place over the teeth thereby giving optimum retention without the use of wire clasping. This claspless technique is quite versatile and can be applied to a variety of appliances.

Note - It is essential that the crown contours are clearly represented on the working model, i.e. no bubbles or "drag" can be seen in the impression.

9.9

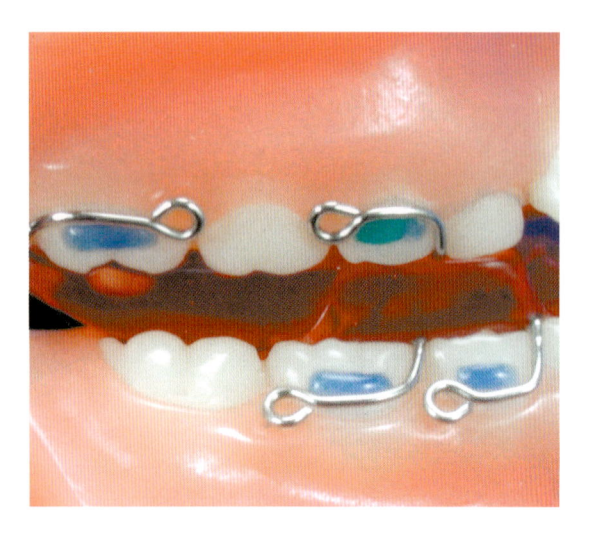

FUNCTIONAL ORTHOPEDICS

3907 Bonded Button Twin Block

This appliance uses the standard Twin Block approach for treatment mechanics, however the clasping is quite unique. Composite ledges, illustrated by the blue acrylic, create undercuts that provide superior retention for circumferential clasps. This technique is particularly useful when the teeth being used for retention have short clinical crowns. The free end of the circumferential clasps can be finished in a loop, if desired, to make it easy for the patient to remove the appliances for cleaning.

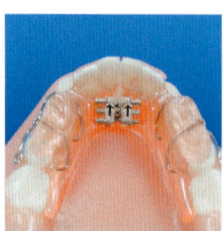

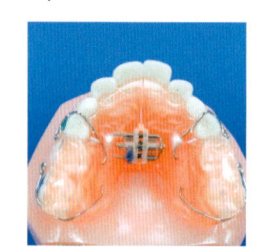

3610BC Evans Twin Block

This design is usually used in the adult dentition when the choice has been made to accomplish the majority of the orthodontic corrections needed prior to using the twin block to correct the patient's orthopedic problems. In the adult dentition, vertical changes are often easier when the majority of orthodontic corrections are done first. Because multiple ball clasps are used for retention, this appliance can be used while the patient is still in full brackets. The placement and number of ball clasps used on a given case is dependent upon the type of orthodontic corrections needed to finalize treatment. Of course, if needed, midline expansion screws can be added to the appliances.

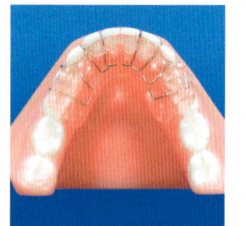

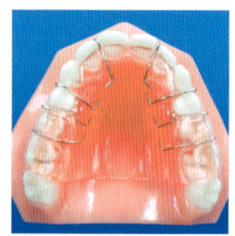

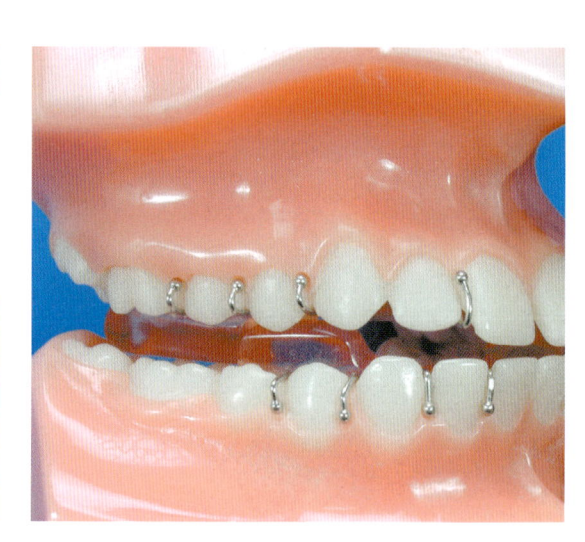

Design Notes:

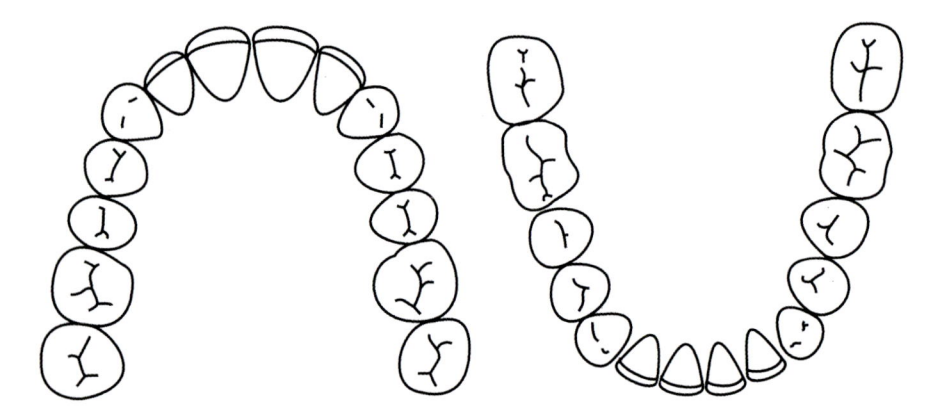

FUNCTIONAL ORTHOPEDICS

3616 Mahony Twin Block

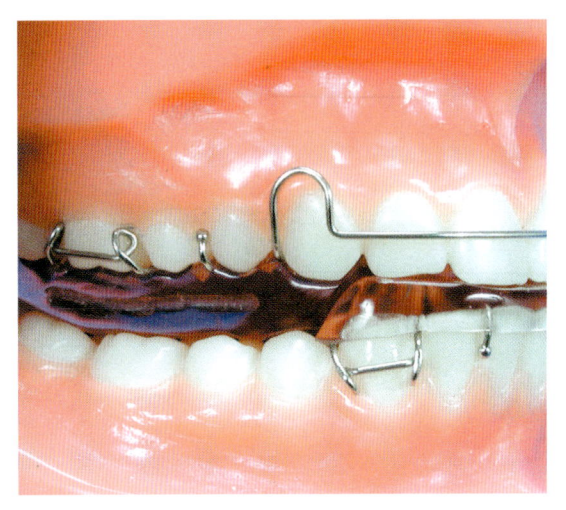

The Mahony Twin Block has several innovative features that are believed to enhance the skeletal corrections when compared to the standard Clark Twin Block. First, the lower 70° incline block is moved forward, just distal of the cuspids rather than distal to the second premolars. This results in less need for a support phase appliance because the premolars are allowed to erupt during the initial phase of treatment. To help the patient masticate, the lower incisors are covered with clear acrylic. Capping the incisors in this manner prevents lower incisor flaring and aids in overbite reduction by providing intrusion forces to the upper and lower incisors. Anchorage and stability of the lower block have also been improved by extending the lingual flanges distal of the terminal molar. Often, "C" clasps are placed around the distal of the terminal molar to further enhance retention. The anchorage unit of the upper block has also been improved by adding a labial bow. This results in adding the incisors and cuspids into the anchor system. Dr. Mahony also prefers using Delta clasps–it is felt that they are less prone to failure.

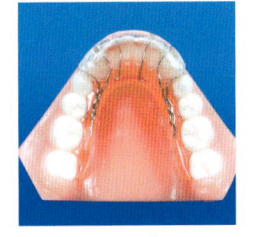

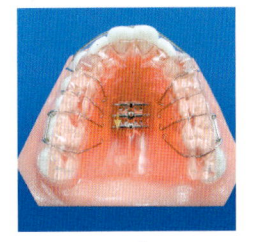

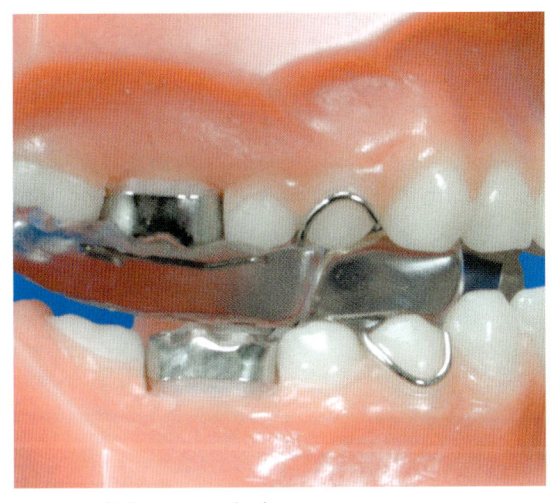

2640 The Fixed Twin Block

When patient compliance is a concern, the Twin Block can be delivered as a fixed appliance. The simplest design involves merely bonding the Twin Block Incline components directly to the posterior dentition. The teeth to be bonded must be secure. If the blocks are placed on primary molars, it is important that they are expected to be stable for at least 9 months. This technique is mainly used when only mandibular advancement is needed, as it is difficult to adjust the blocks intraorally to accomplish vertical changes.

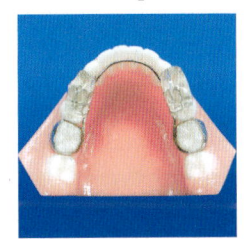

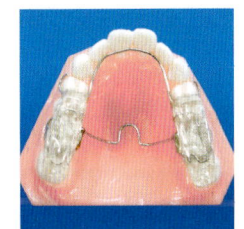

The more versatile design of the Fixed Twin Block is illustrated here. In this appliance, the molars are banded and "C" clasps are placed on the first bicuspids. This makes the appliance easy to seat (i.e. by eliminating any path of insertion problems) while adding the option of increasing retention by bonding the "C" clasps to the bicuspids. Since the Twin Block portions are not bonded to the occlusal surfaces, appliance removal after treatment is easy. Again, this fixed design is best used to accomplish mandibular advancement when the patient has adequate vertical dimension, as the molar bands and occlusal acrylic will prohibit vertical eruption to correct deep bites.

FUNCTIONAL ORTHOPEDICS

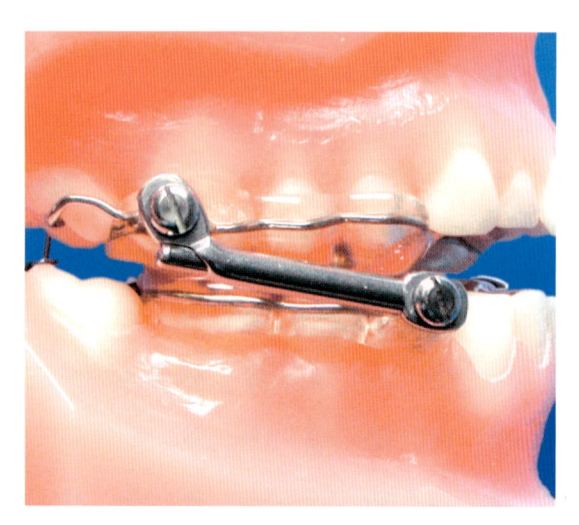

2443 Herbst Appliance

The Herbst is a two-piece fixed appliance used in the treatment of skeletal class II malocclusions. In this design, the mandible is held forward with sliding tubes attached buccal to the upper six year molars and the lower first bicuspids.

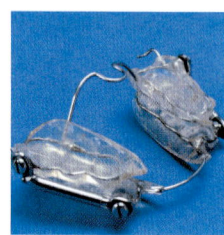

In this example, the Herbst is bonded into place. Retention, however, may be accomplished through banding, bonding or a combination of both, depending upon the situation. The Herbst is suggested for patients who do not readily cooperate with removable functional appliance therapy.

2443C Cantilevered Herbst

This appliance is excellent for correction of skeletal Class II malocclusions, especially if patient compliance is an issue. The effectiveness of this appliance, as with all Herbst designs, is enhanced if the transverse deficiencies are addressed first. However, many of the Herbst appliances in use today include additions to the basic design in order to simultaneously correct multiple factors that may have contributed to the malocclusion.

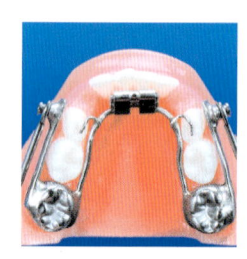

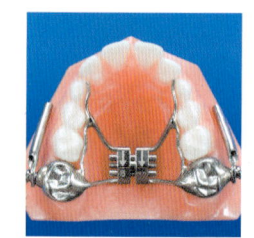

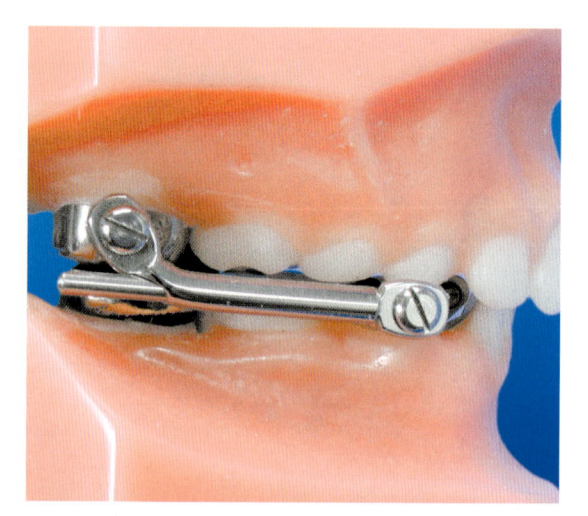

Expansion screws to widen the arches, arch wire tubes to combine fixed appliances, and other modifications extend the treatment effects of the Herbst beyond mere Class II correction. Once expansion of either, or both, arches is accomplished, the Class II correction will occur more rapidly via a combination of dental and skeletal changes, with the end result being a predictable Class I occlusion.

The use of stainless steel crowns, as illustrated in this appliance, are quite popular due to excellent patient acceptance and the ease of clinical application and removal when compared to the acrylic bonded Herbst designs.

FUNCTIONAL ORTHOPEDICS

2708 MARA

The MARA (Mandibular Anterior Repositioning Appliance) is attached to stainless steel crowns on the first molars. Crowns are preferred over bands in that they are needed to help withstand the tremendous leverage forces generated by the appliance. It was developed to overcome the complaints that patients expressed when wearing a Herbst appliance, particularly the bulk in the lower bicuspid area. In addition to the normal rectangular arch wire tube, the upper first molar has a large .062 square tube, which accepts an adjustable .060 square "elbow" that hangs vertically as illustrated.

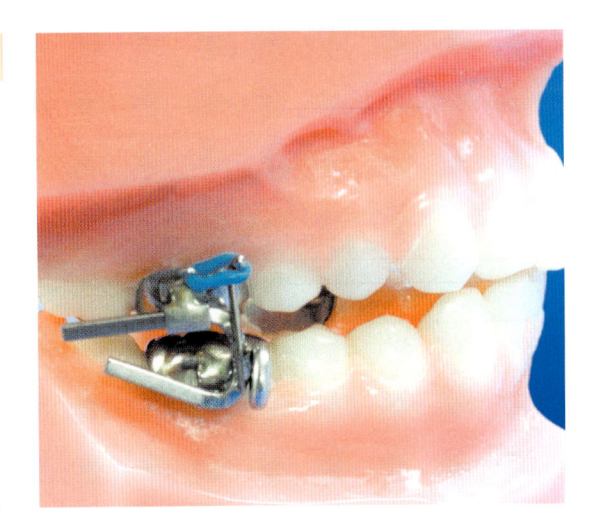

The lower first molar has the normal rectangular tube as well as an .059 round wire "arm" projecting buccally from the mesial. The upper elbow hits the lower arm and prevents the teeth from occlusion unless the patient holds the lower jaw forward so that the lower arm is in front of the elbow. Typically, the lower crowns or bands are stabilized by either a lingual arch or lower braces to prevent unwanted mesiolingual rotation of the lower molars resulting from the resting pressure of the elbows. Additional mandibular advancement is achieved by periodically placing shims on the elbows. The elbows are held in place with either elastics or ligature wire.

Most skeletal Class II cases, with normally positioned maxillas and retrognathic mandibles, have constricted maxillary arches. In these situations, a Hyrax screw is typically used to help develop the narrow maxillary arch. It is usually soldered to the lingual of the crowns and incorporates occlusal rests on the first bicuspids, which may be bonded with composite for additional retention. If the maxillary arch is normal in width, a transpalatal arch is typically used to aid in anchoring the molars and help to properly distribute the forces generated by the appliance.

Design Notes:

FUNCTIONAL ORTHOPEDICS

The Frankel Appliance

The Frankel appliances are composed of a system of oral screens that lie in the vestibule of the mouth, free of direct contact with the dento-alveolar systems. The action of the appliance, as described by Dr. Frankel, is to influence arch development by changing the pressure created by the surrounding soft tissue. For example, lateral development of the arch is encouraged by the buccal shields in two ways. The pressure of the cheeks is eliminated allowing the tongue to exert a molding effect on the dentition, and the continuous stretching of the connective tissue fibers in the vestibular fold stimulates bone formation.

There are basically four different types of Frankel appliances. The FR I is designed to treat Class I and Class II Division 1 malocclusions; the FR II treats the Class II Division 2 malocclusion; the FR III is for the treatment of Class III problems and the FR IV is used for open bites and bi-maxillary protrusions.

Because of the importance of growth to the success of the Frankel technique, best results are obtained before the permanent bicuspids and cuspids come into position. Young patients seem to tolerate the appliance very well allowing treatment to be started at a very early age.

Crucial to the proper construction of the Frankel appliance is the taking of proper impressions. The laboratory must receive models that accurately reproduce the vestibules of both upper and lower arches. Care must be taken so pouring and trimming procedures allow as much soft tissue to be shown as possible. This point cannot be emphasized too strongly. In addition, the anterior sulcus in the upper and lower arches of Class I or Class II patients must be accurately represented for proper lip pad placement. In the Frankel appliance, the soft tissues are as important as the teeth!

Taking a proper wax bite is also important.

> For a Class I case with crowding or a Class II malocclusion where the overjet is not in excess of 5 mm, the bite must be taken with the anteriors in an edge-to-edge relationship and a vertical opening of 2-3 mm. In a Class I or II with an anterior open bite, only a minimum bite opening is needed.

> When a Class II is severe do not take your bite in an edge-to-edge position. Correction of the overjet with this appliance may require repositioning of the mandible in stages.

> The Class III bite is taken with the mandible retruded as far back as comfortable and the bite open only enough to allow for correction of an anterior crossbite.

> Regardless of the type of malocclusion you are treating, when taking a bite registration it is essential to align the skeletal and not the dental midlines. An error here could cause the completed appliance to be constructed with the mandible shifted to one side.

Although the Frankel appliance is ultimately worn full time, except when eating, it is advisable to start treatment slowly to allow the soft tissues time to adjust to the appliance. Wearing it one or two hours per day is usually recommended for the first two weeks gradually increasing to full-time wear.

During treatment, few adjustments in the Frankel are necessary. Adjustments that are required usually involve tightening up the wires after movement has been accomplished or repositioning the anterior lip pads.

As with any orthodontic treatment and perhaps even more so with the Frankel appliance, important pre-conditions are necessary for successful treatment. The patients must be carefully selected with the right attitude for treatment. The appliance must be introduced to the patient in a manner that complete cooperation and compliance of the patient is assured.

FUNCTIONAL ORTHOPEDICS

The Frankel III (FR-3) appliance is composed of a system of oral screens which lie in the vestibule of the mouth, free of direct contact with the dentoalveolar systems. The action of the appliance, as described by Dr. Frankel, is to influence arch development by changing the pressure created by surrounding soft tissue. It has proven effective as a primary treatment appliance in Class III patients with mild, moderate, or severe dentoalveolar, skeletal, and/or neuromuscular imbalances. It affects the skeletal, the dentoalveolar, and the soft tissue components simultaneously.

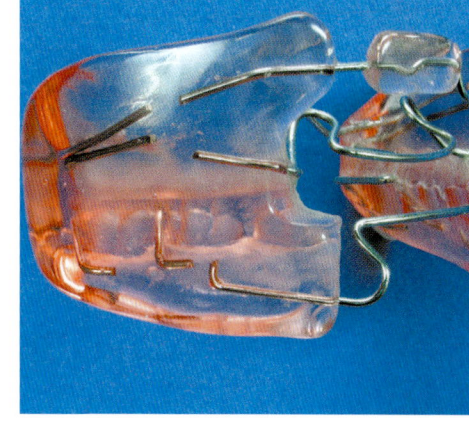

Patient compliance with the Frankel III is typically quite high as it improves the soft tissue profile of the patient with maxillary skeletal retrusion. The purpose of the vestibular shields and upper labial pads are to counteract the forces of the surrounding musculature that tend to restrict forward maxillary skeletal development and cause a retrusion of the maxillary anteriors. The vestibular shields need to be positioned away from the alveolar process of the maxilla, but they must fit closely to the tissue of the mandible. This results in stimulation of maxillary alveolar development and restricting mandibular alveolar development.

Because of the importance of growth to the success of the Frankel technique, best results are obtained before the permanent bicuspids and cuspids come into position. Young patients seem to tolerate the appliance very well, allowing treatment to be started at a very early age.

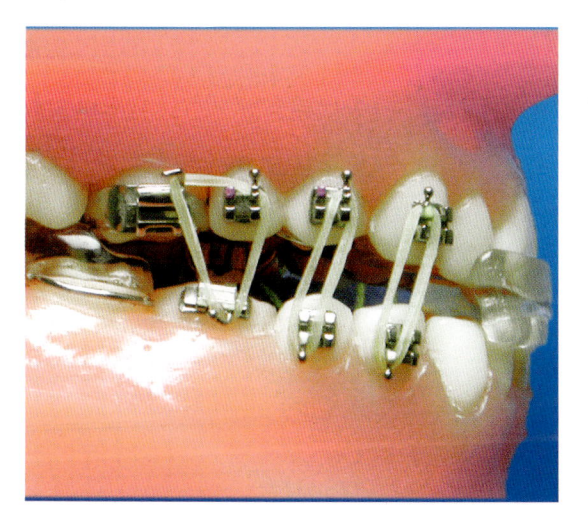

3701 Spahl Split Vertical

The Spahl Split Vertical Appliance is very effective at closing posterior open bites after the mandible has been properly and thoroughly advanced by a functional appliance (such as a Bionator, an Orthopedic Corrector, the Clark Twin Block, the Levandoski Mandibular Stabilization appliance, etc.).

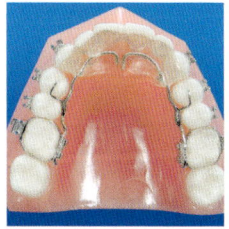

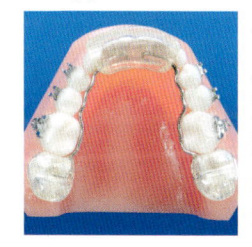

This appliance consists of separate upper and lower devices. The upper has a simple bite plane that is designed to hold the arches at the ideal vertical relationship. This bite plane is placed on a lingual wire that is attached to the first molar bands via a vertical removable bracket assembly. Because it is to be worn 24 hours per day, the bite plane should be kept to a minimum to allow for comfort and ease of speech. The lower part of the appliance is a wire-bodied appliance composed of an anterior bite block that covers the four lower anteriors and a pair of posterior bite blocks that cover the last molar on each side of the arch.

Bonded hooks, buttons, or brackets are placed on the upper and lower cuspids, bicuspids, and first molars. When the lower appliance is in place, vertical elastics are used to initiate eruption of these teeth. By wearing this device a minimum of 12 hours a day (i.e evenings and during sleep) eruption will occur much faster than it could through passive eruption alone.

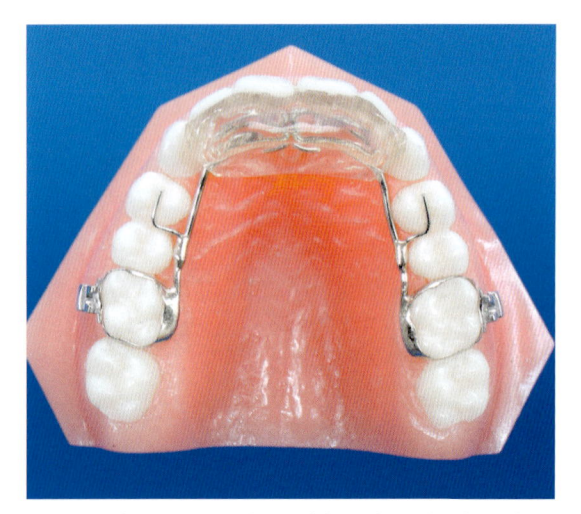

FUNCTIONAL ORTHOPEDICS

2705   Rick-A-Nator

This appliance, designed by Dr. Rick Gallaher, was developed to treat patients who are non-compliant or who have difficulty wearing removable functional appliances. It can be used effectively to treat Class II skeletal malocclusions with normal maxillas, retrognathic mandibles, and deep overbites where the AP correction needed is 4mm or less. The appliance consists of a maxillary anterior inclined plane placed on a lingual wire that is attached to molar bands.

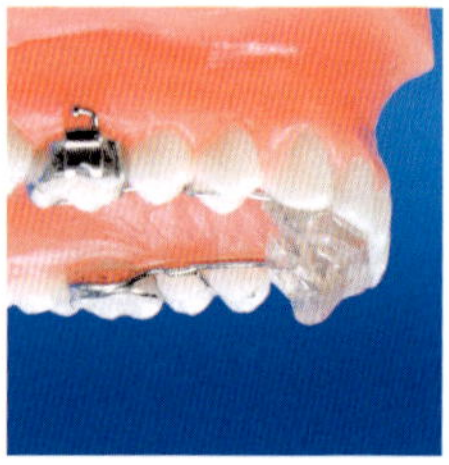

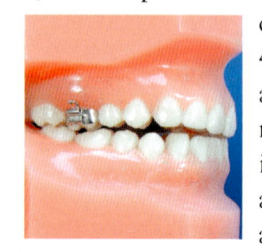

The arch wire can be soldered to the bands, or attached with vertical brackets so that it can be easily removed for cleaning. The incline is made to hold the mandible in the exact AP position desired, but if the overjet is greater than 4mm, it can be stepped forward in segments as treatment progresses. Ideally, cases presenting with Division 2 anteriors should be pre-treated, however, when patient compliance is a problem, lap springs can be added to correct the retroclined incisors as the mandible is being translated. Similar to the Spahl appliance, vertical elastics can be used to reduce treatment time when the patient has an excessively closed vertical relationship. (See Appliance #2706 Rick-A-Nator 2 for the correct design.)

The advantages of this appliance over the removable functional approaches are that patient compliance is not an issue, the appliance is virtually undetectable from an esthetic point of view and it can be worn during active straight wire therapy. The Rick-A-Nator has minimum affect on speech and can be worn 24 hours per day, therefore treatment time is typically reduced. Finally, it can be used as a TMJ appliance as it provides for mandibular advancement and vertical opening. (See Appliance #2706 Rick-A-Nator 2 for the correct design.)

Note - The incline incisal ramp must be partially tooth-born and tissue-born to provide for proper support without causing sensitivity to the teeth or the soft tissues. This appliance can be fabricated with a flat plane so that the inclined portion can be generated chairside, or if a construction bite is provided, the lab, will complete the appliance in every detail.

Design Notes:

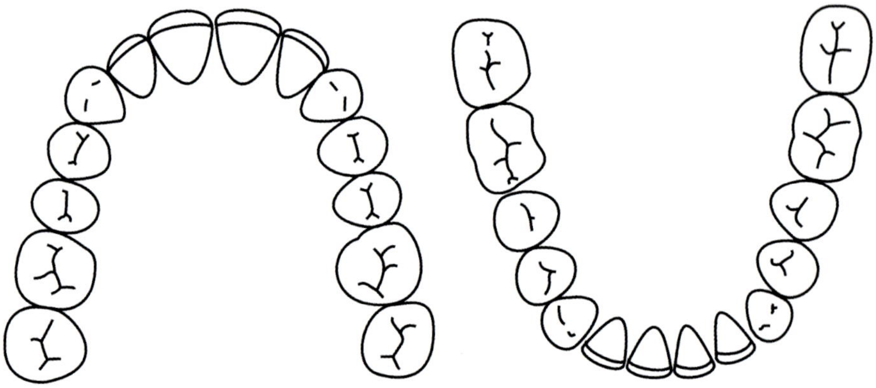

9.16

FUNCTIONAL ORTHOPEDICS

2706 Rick-A-Nator 2

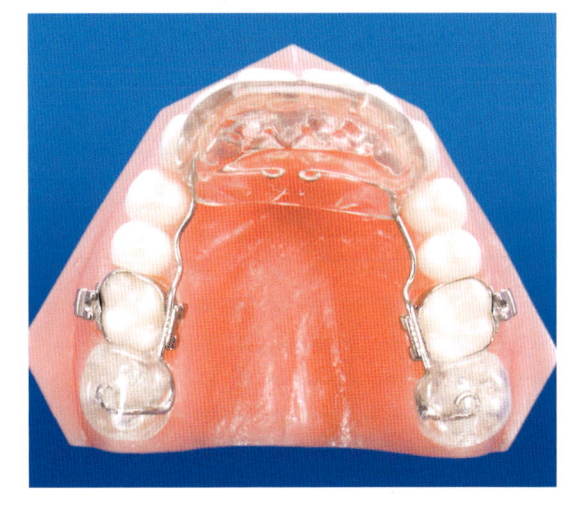

The Rick-A-Nator 2 can be used effectively to treat Class II skeletal malocclusions with normal maxillas, retrognathic mandibles, and deep overbites where the AP correction needed is 4mm or less. It has distal extensions to support acrylic pads that cover the occlusal surface of the maxillary second molars. The purpose of these pads is to provide a tripod effect so that when the mandibular anteriors are contacting the incisal ramp, the lower second molars are also contacting the posterior acrylic pads.

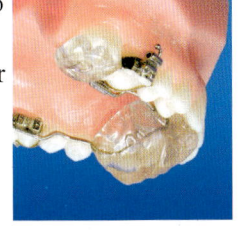

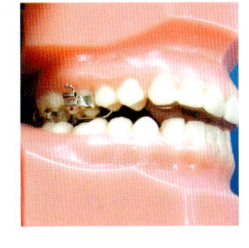

This feature is extremely important, especially if the patient has signs and symptoms of TMJ dysfunction. The tripod effect creates the posterior support needed to prevent the condyles from moving superiorly and causing the discs to become displaced. These pads also allow for the addition of posterior-vertical mechanics with inter-arch elastics without the worry of rotating the condyle superiorly and posteriorly.

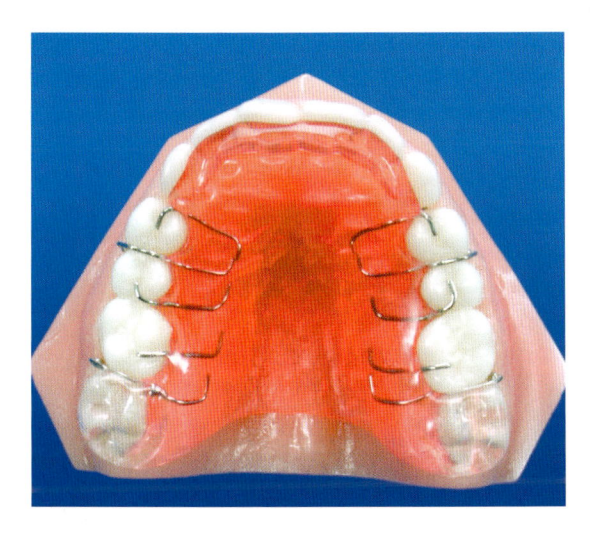

1706 Removable Rick-A-Nator 2

After a Class II has been corrected, this appliance is commonly used as a Support Phase appliance during fixed mechanics, when you plan to use posterior forced eruption mechanics to settle in the occlusion. One of the benefits of this design is that the appliance can be removed for social functions, but obviously it needs to be worn as much as possible, especially during the application of vertical mechanics. This appliance provides the same condylar support function as the Fixed Rick-A-Nator 2 (appliance #2706).

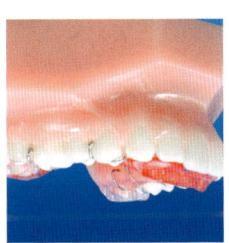

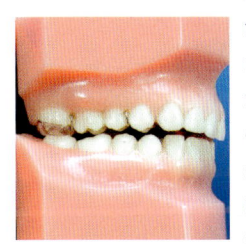

Note - Because it is removable, this design is not recommended for TMD patients who need continual condylar support.

FUNCTIONAL ORTHOPEDICS

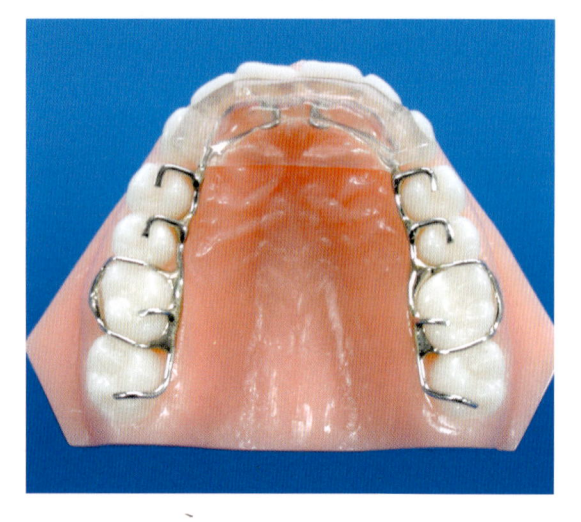

3706 Modified Rick-A-Nator

The Modified Rick-A-Nator can be used when patient compliance is not an issue and you are looking for a repositioning appliance where bands do not need to be placed and the palate needs to be kept free of acrylic. Its design is similar to the upper part of the Spahl appliance with the exception that Crozat Clasps are used on the molars instead of molar bands.

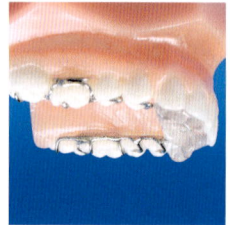

Typically, it is used as a maintenance appliance once functional repositioning has occurred and passive settling of the posteriors is desired. However, it can be used for any procedure where you would use a Rick-A-Nator. For example, by simply adding posterior pads, it can be used with inter-arch elastics to actively erupt the lower posteriors.

1141 Incline Plane

The anterior incline plane has been used for many years to aid in repositioning the mandible forward for patients with a Class II tendency. Since the advent of modern functional appliances, such as the Twin Blocks, Bionators and Ortho Correctors, to name a few, this appliance has been relegated to the position of a maintenance appliance.

After the patient's Class II skeletal relationship has been corrected, this appliance is used as a "reminder" to help the patient function in the forward position during initial retention.

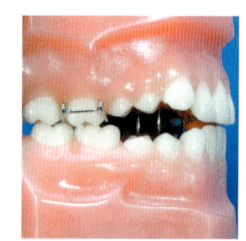

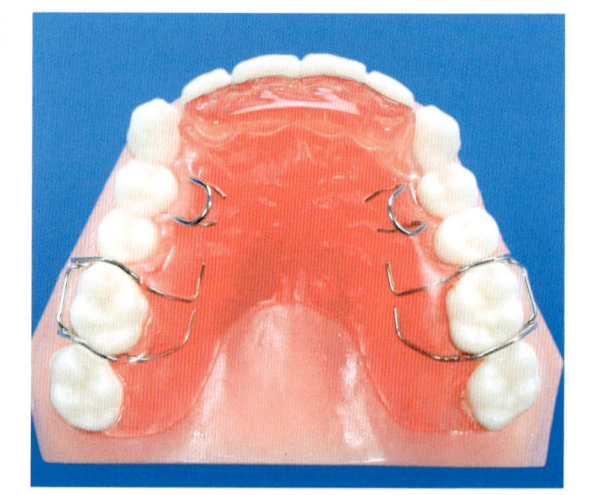

In this example, lingual loops have been added to keep the tongue from inhibiting bite closure in the bicuspid region.

Design Notes:

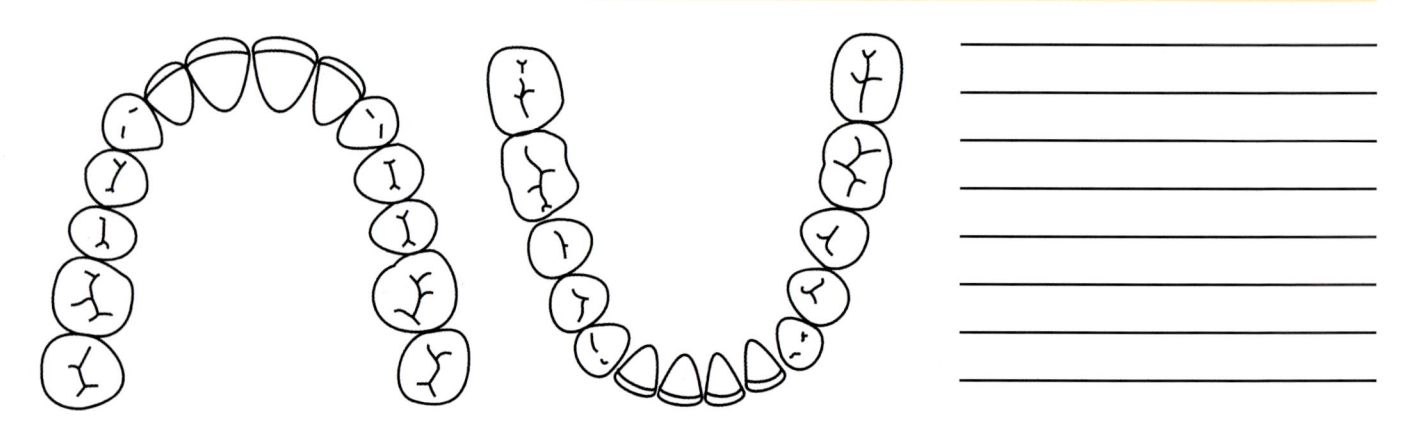

9.18

FUNCTIONAL ORTHOPEDICS

2444 Inter-Oral Face Mask Appliance

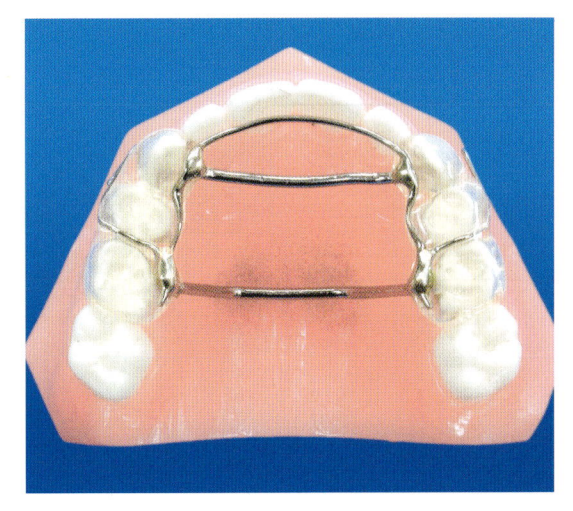

This utility appliance is designed to be used in conjunction with a facemask as described by Henri Petit. Mask therapy can provide effective treatment for mid-face insufficiency, mandibular prognathism, maxillary hypoplasia, clefts, and tongue problems.

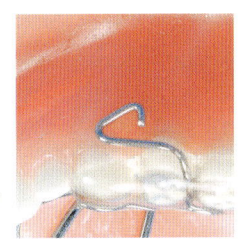

The appliance consists of occlusal onlays to free the bite and hooks buccal to the cuspids for the attachment of the elastics to the facemask. This force can then be used to affect the forward movement of the maxilla as a whole, the rotation of the maxillary pyramid or the "dental drawer" movement of both arches.

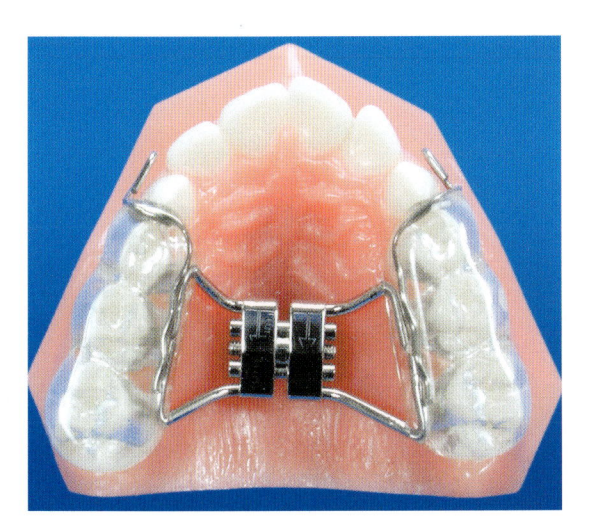

2444E Bonded Maxillary Face Mask/ Expansion Appliance

Face Mask therapy can be used to treat patients who have a mid-face insufficiency, mandibular prognathism, maxillary hypoplasia, clefts, and tongue problems. Although the Bonded Maxillary Face Mask/Expansion Appliance shown here is very similar to a bonded rapid maxillary expansion appliance, within the context of facial mask therapy, the expansion effect of this appliance is quite different. Simply put, it disrupts the maxillary sutural system and enhances the effect of the orthopedic facial mask by making sutural adjustments occur more readily. Midfacial orthopedic expansion has also been shown to be beneficial in the treatment of Class III malocclusions, as rapid palatal expansion can produce a forward movement of Point A with a slightly downward and forward movement of the maxilla.

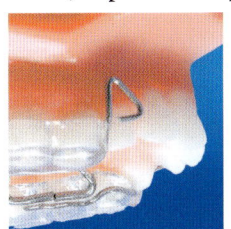

In the mixed detention, the bonded occlusal part of this appliance usually covers the first and second deciduous molars and the permanent first molars. The hooks for the elastics are placed in the anterior aspect of the appliance in the region of the upper first deciduous molars. In cases where only the deciduous detention is present, the splint usually covers the cuspids as well as the deciduous molars. In this instance, the hooks for the elastics are placed adjacent to the upper cuspids.

In late mixed or early permanent dentition cases, the occlusal coverage portion of the appliance may require the following modifications. If permanent second molars are erupted, it is necessary to place occlusal rests against these teeth to prevent them from erupting during appliance wear. The framework itself does not extend to the second molars because of the danger of opening the bite due to placement of acrylic on the occlusal surface of the upper second molars.

In all cases the occlusal acrylic can be finished with either a flat occlusal surface or with light general indexing of the lower posteriors. Many doctors prefer the light indexing, as it is believed to make mastication easier. Please indicate your preference when ordering the appliance.

Design Notes

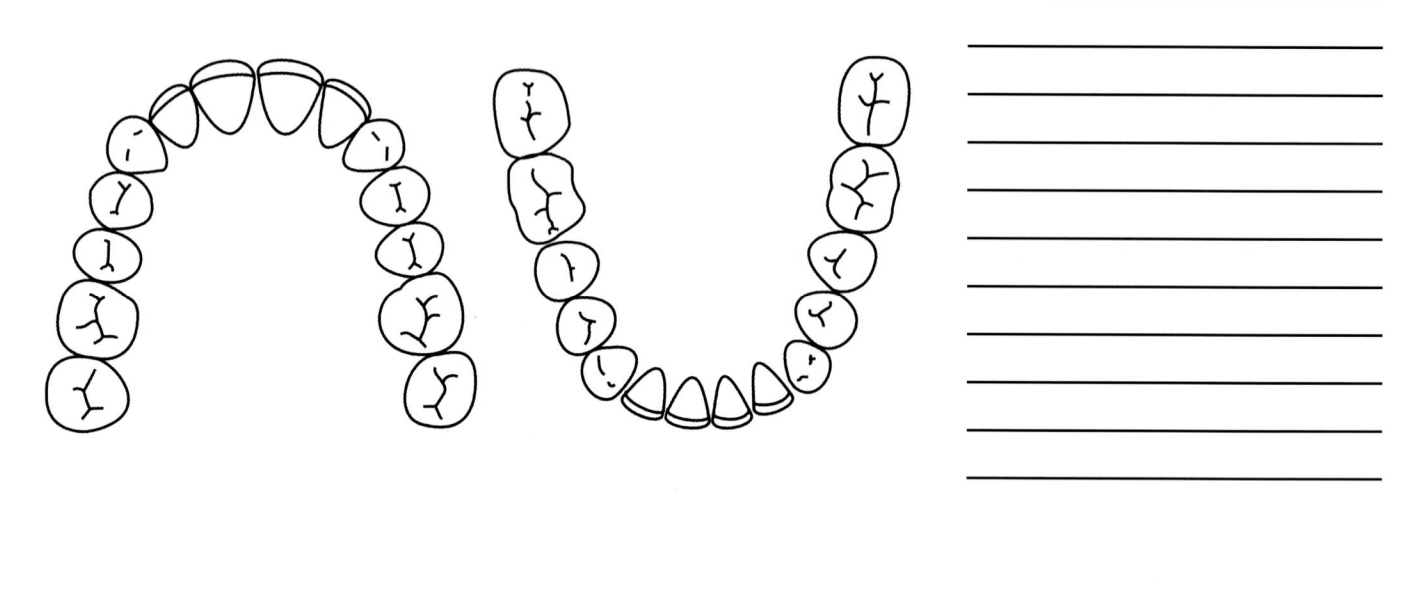

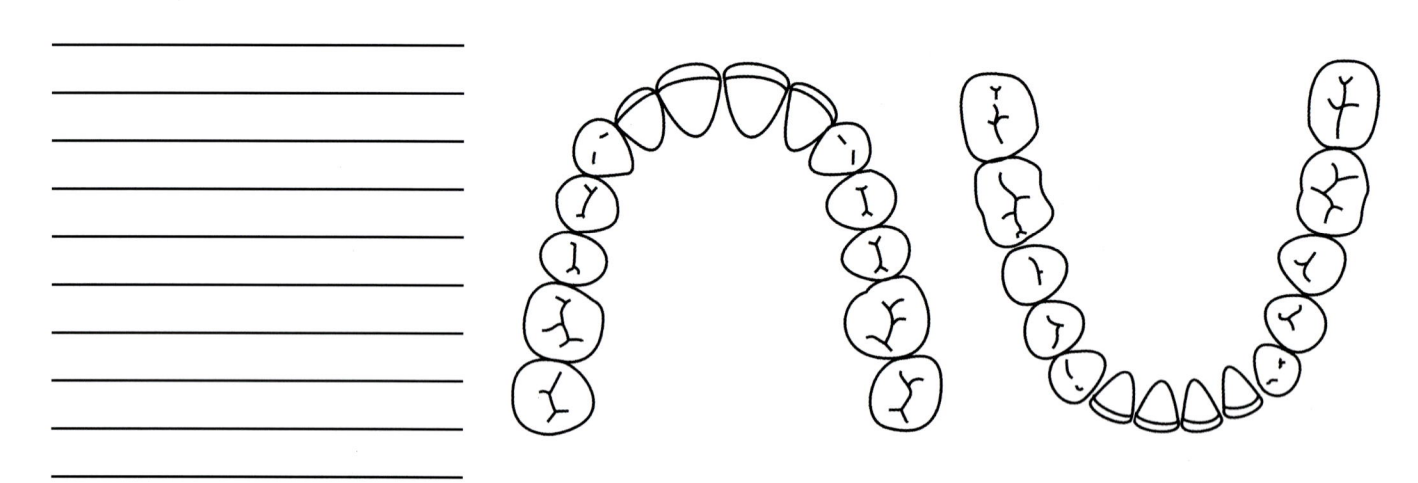

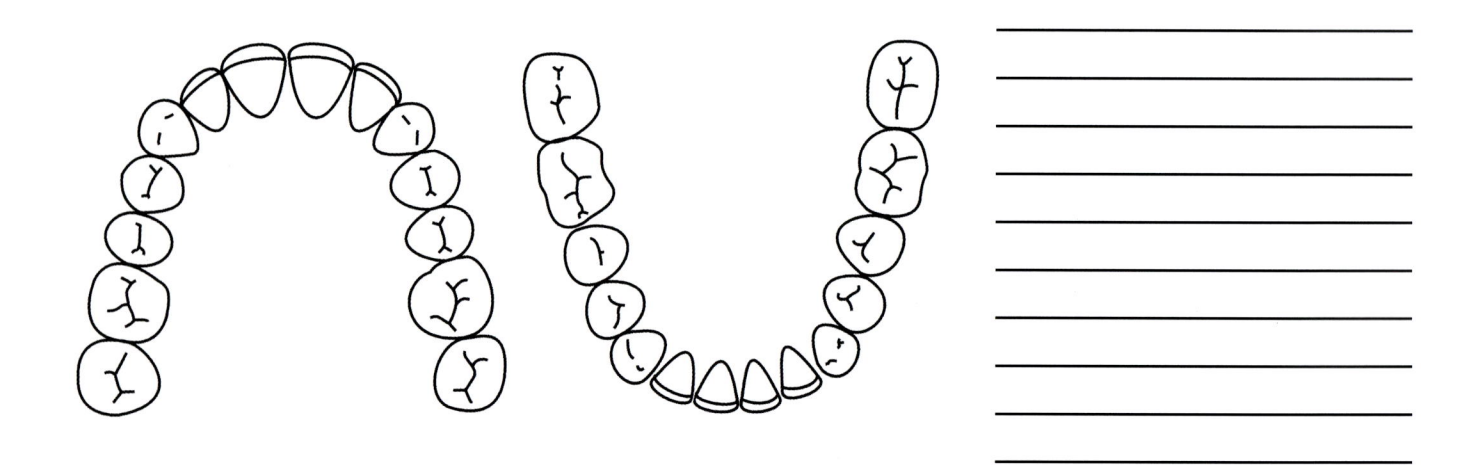

ORTHODONTICS

an overview: ORTHODONTICS

Chapter 10

Whenever the desired objective of your treatment plan requires bodily tooth movements, significant tooth rotations, root torquing or leveling, aligning, and rotating of entire arches, it is necessary to utilize full arch fixed mechanics.

When observing a well-aligned dental arch, it is apparent that the ideal position of each tooth is defined by three parameters: the "in-out" position, the crown angulation or "tip," and the crown inclination, or "torque".

For many years, orthodontic brackets were the same for all teeth making it necessary for the clinician to incorporate into the main arch wire, three bends for each tooth in order to place the tooth in its ideal position. This was a rather complicated and arduous task that required a great deal of skill, effort, and multiple readjustments of the arch wires throughout treatment.

As a result of extensive studies conducted in the early 1960s, Dr. Lawrence F. Andrews introduced pre-adjusted "Straight Wire" type brackets. These brackets are specific for each tooth in that they have the necessary torque, tip, and in-out position built into the individual brackets.

Provided that the bracket is positioned ideally on each tooth in the middle of the clinical crown, parallel to the incisal edge, and along the long axis, the Straight Wire appliance has the capability of finishing treatment with little or no bends in the arch wire. The only wire bending usually necessary involves small compensating bends in the arch at the end of treatment for final detailing.

To further streamline and simplify treatment with fixed appliances, Drs. William and Robert Wilson developed the 3D® Modular System. As shown in the following pages, the Wilson 3D® System involves the use of various components that are attached to the molar bands via vertical brackets. The components are removable for ease of adjustment and are used primarily to enhance treatment. Their use can reduce overall treatment time, provide greater control of reciprocal forces, and allow for precise control of lateral as well as sagittal development.

Every year, new wires and bracket systems are introduced by the various orthodontic companies in an attempt to make treatment easier and faster. Most of these products are excellent. However, as with all orthodontic therapy, there is usually a learning curve associated with using these new tools. We highly recommend that you take a class in the use of any new product before you use them.

Your laboratory can provide you with stainless steel or esthetic ceramic brackets, molar bands with buccal tubes, the series of arch wires of your choice and any Wilson 3D® components necessary for you to completely treat your patient with pre-adjusted appliances. Technical assistance in choosing the right system for your patient is only a phone call away.

In addition to supplying a complete kit of all of the necessary straight-wire brackets, arch wires, and accessories on a per patient basis, your laboratory can do the actual set-up, as well. Each bracket is placed in the correct position on the patient's model as per your instructions and a plastic matrix material is vacuum formed over the brackets. This creates a tray that holds the brackets for transfer to the patient.

ORTHODONTICS

The Wilson 3D® Modular Orthodontic System

The Wilson 3D® system utilizes a series of precision modules (lingual arch wire assemblies) that are designed to enhance the efficiency of most fixed appliances. These snap-in modules fit into double lingual tubes that are attached to molar bands. Used properly, the modules can produce a variety of rapid, supplementary movements, with positive control of reciprocal forces and without interfering with other appliances. The various modules can be used individually or selected in a number of combinations and sets.

Rapid results from using the Wilson 3D® system are possible due to the twenty-four hour per day wearing time. A full spectrum of modules are available for both the mixed and adult detention without the need to alter any full-banded/bracketed system that you may already be using. Treatment time and cost savings with this system are truly significant.

The modular concept does not replace or limit the force systems of present orthodontic appliances. Instead it gives added control and predictable results. The system provides more than one hundred additional appliance functions. Four of the most popular modular units are shown below.

We highly recommend that anyone using this system should have a good working knowledge of it. The use of the Wilson appliances, including the adjustments and the directional movements possible, are superbly described and illustrated in the "Enhanced Orthodontics Mechanotherapy Manual" available from RMO.

Note - Wilson 3D® Modular Orthodontics is a registered trademark of Rocky Mountain International Associates Inc (RMO).

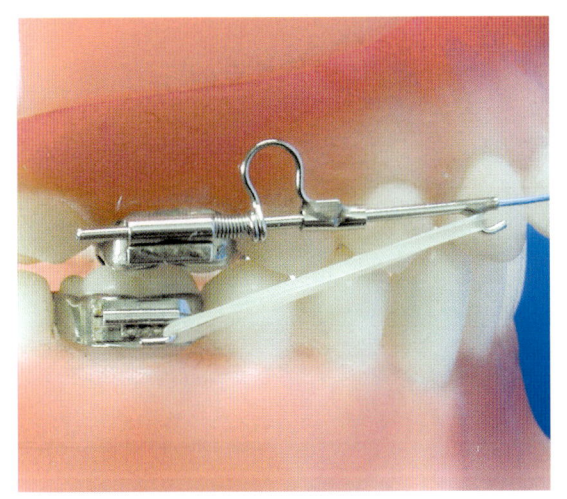

2501 3D® Maxillary Bimetric Distalizing Arch   U

This appliance produces rapid, bilateral or unilateral, friction-free distalization of the maxillary molars without the need for headgear (a real plus when treating young, appearance-sensitive patients). The appliance is composed of maxillary and mandibular components. The maxillary components consist of a labial arch wire with an omega loop and a hook, anterior brackets, compressed coil spring and molar bands.

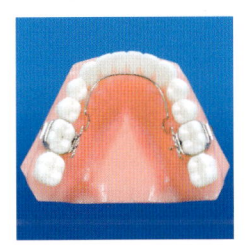

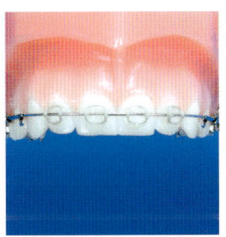

The set-up is as follows: The arch wire is ligated to the anterior brackets. Compressed coil spring is then placed on the labial wire between the adjustable omega stop and the buccal tube. The labial arch wire is then run through the buccal tubes of the molar bands. This set-up allows the coil spring to apply distal pressure on the molar while the omega stop allows for periodic reactivation of the spring as treatment progresses. The mandibular component is a fixed lingual arch wire running from molar to molar (appliance #2502 on page 10.2). It acts as an anchorage unit. It is extremely important to connect the maxillary arch wire to the lower anchorage unit so that the maxillary anteriors remain passive while the molars are distalized. This is easily done by attaching an elastic from the hook on the maxillary arch wire to the hook on the mandibular molar band. The elastics should remain in place at all times during active therapy.

10.1

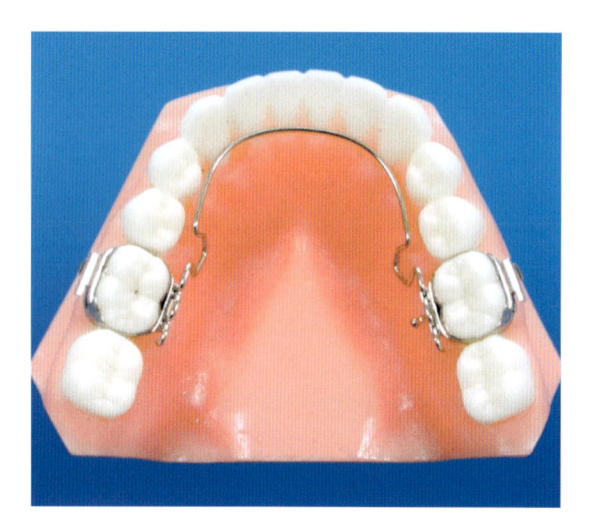

ORTHODONTICS

2502 3D® Lingual Arch   L

The 3D® Lingual Arch is a very versatile modular component. The adjustment loops in the wire (referred to as "Activators") make this lingual arch much more than just an arch length space maintaining device. The Activator is a diamond shaped loop that is easily adjusted with a flat-on-round Light Wire Plier. Proper adjustment of the Activator loops can provide a number of different movements such as: Anterior-Posterior arch length increase, buccal expansion, distal molar movement, molar torque or tip, and molar rotation. The fact that this arch wire is removable from the bands makes adjustment quite easy. The adjustments, and the directional movements possible, are superbly described and illustrated in the "Enhanced Orthodontics Mechanotherapy Manual" available from RMO.

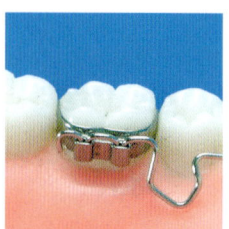

2507 3D® Nance   U

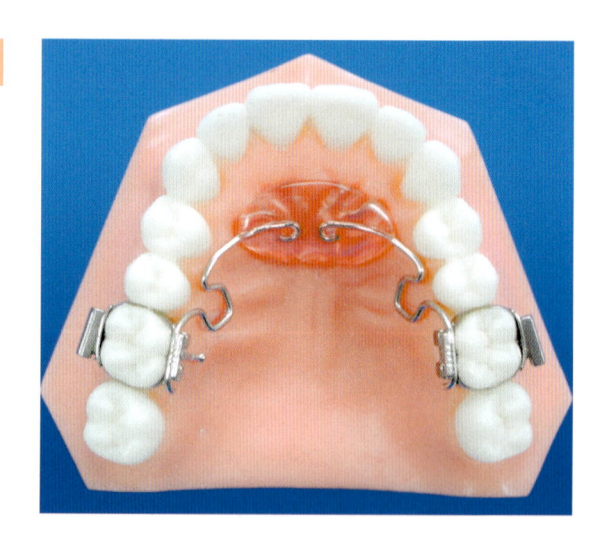

The 3D® Nance appliance is used (1) to maintain molar position during the mixed dentition and (2) to create an anchorage unit and prevent mesial molar drag when using fixed mechanics to torque the incisor roots lingually.

The advantage of placing the Nance button with Wilson 3D® lingual attachments is its ease of removal for both hygiene purposes and adjustments. Once the significant orthodontic movements are completed, the Nance button can be easily removed without having to cut solder joints or remove bands.

Note - This appliance must be monitored carefully as the acrylic pad can act as a food trap. Left unresolved the pad could actually become embedded in the tissue. This can easily be controlled with the use of an oral irrigator.

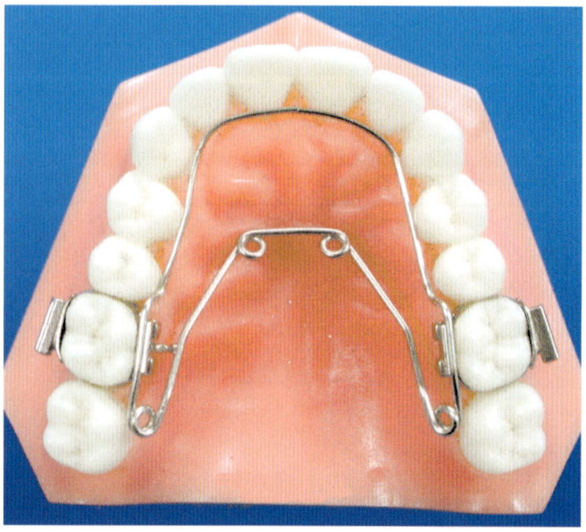

2503 3D® Quad-Helix   U

The 3D® Quad-Helix Appliance is a multi-purpose maxillary arch development appliance. The appliance plugs into the 3D Lingual Tube and the twin posts produce a tight friction-lock, with no free play. The .036 Tru-Chrome™ (RMO) stainless steel construction assures both stability and flexibility.

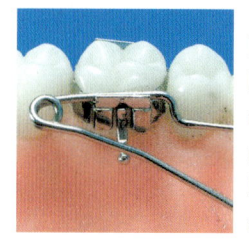

In addition to being used for the traditional lateral arch development, this appliance can be used for unilateral expansion, molar rotation, molar buccal or lingual tip, molar buccal or lingual torquing, as well as anterior advancement.

ORTHODONTICS

2504 3D® Quad-Action Mandibular Appliance   L

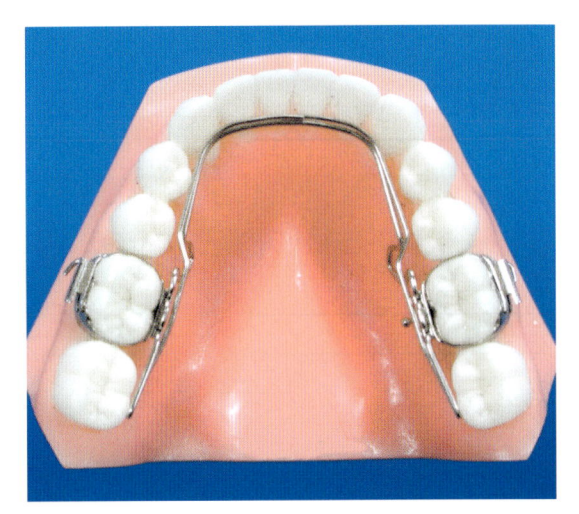

The 3D® Quad-Action Mandibular Appliance offers simple, inexpensive alternatives to more than 20 different sagittal and transverse removable appliances. This versatile appliance can produce unilateral or bilateral rapid arch expansion or contraction; can expand or contract bicuspid position; can advance or retract incisors; and can rotate, tip, or torque the molars. The adjustments necessary to accomplish these movements are easily made since the arch wire is simple to remove from the molar bands.

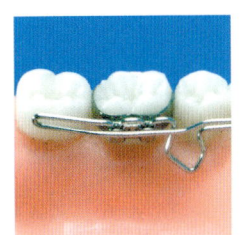

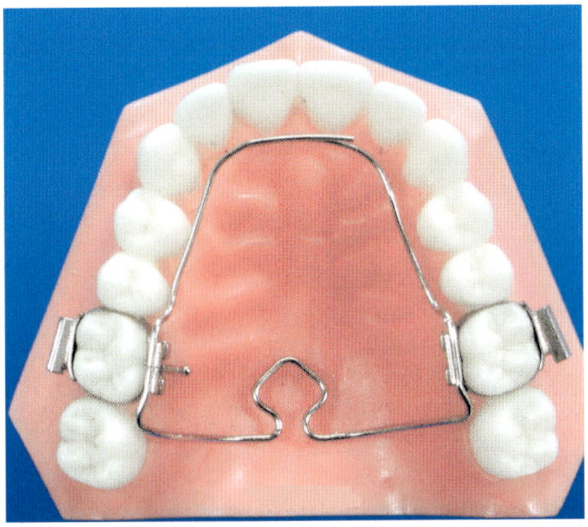

2505 3D® Multi-Action Palatal Appliance   U

The 3D® Multi-Action Palatal Appliance offers an alternative to using the Quad-Helix appliance. It, too, offers a simple, inexpensive alternative to numerous sagittal and transverse removable appliances. Often used in conjunction with the Quad-Action Mandibular appliance, this appliance produces rapid arch expansion or contraction, unilaterally or bilaterally; expansion or contraction of the bicuspids; advancement or retraction of the incisors; and tip, torque, and rotation of the molars. Buttons placed on the cuspids are used to keep the lingual wires (termed "extenders" in the 3D® system) functioning in a horizontal plane and not riding up the lingual incline when activated.

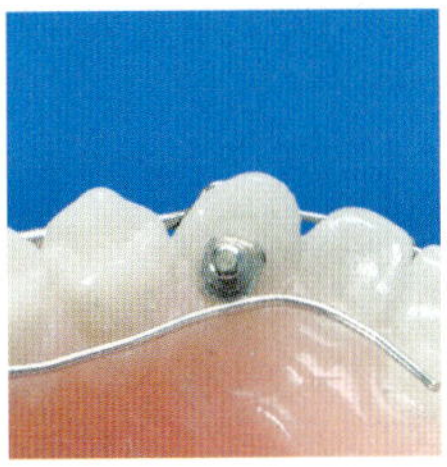

2511 Clark Trombone   U/L

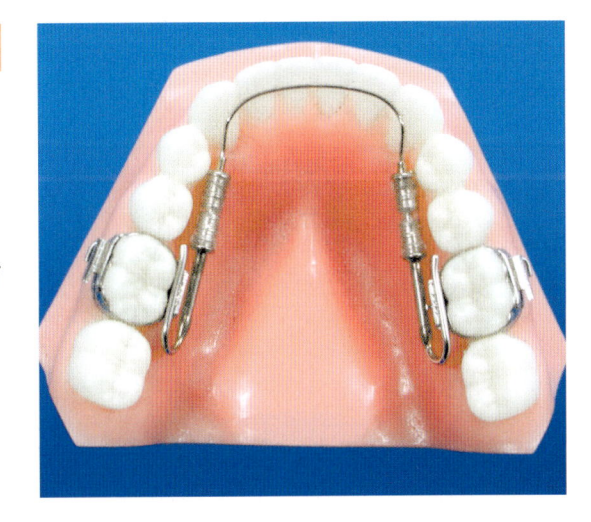

The principal goal of this appliance is to manage a loss in arch length by using a pre-activated system. The original design of this appliance used coil springs to provide the necessary force, and chain elastic attached to mesial and distal hooks to control the force. In the new design shown here, the AP force is provided through a unique Compression Tube Activator that is comprised of fine bore silicone tubing. Replacing the springs and hooks with this new material has greatly improved the stability and safety of the appliance.

The advantages of this appliance are that it is removable from the bands giving the doctor complete control, it is virtually invisible, and it can be used in conjunction with any conventional fixed appliance technique.

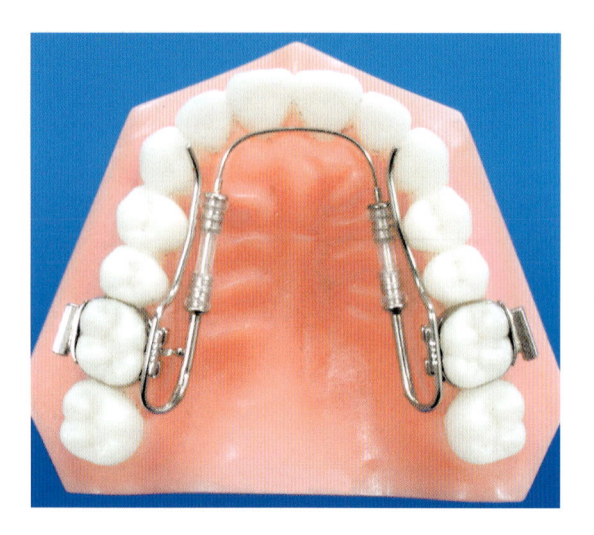

ORTHODONTICS

2521 Clark Trombone and Lingual Arch Developer U/L

This version of the Clark Trombone/LAD has mesial extensions which serve to apply additional buccal and labial force. These extensions are occasionally required to apply buccal pressure to align a palatally displaced bicuspid. Bayonet bends are placed mesial to the molar tubes to expand the arch transversely in the bicuspid region and match the expansion of the molars.

As with the #2511 appliance outlined previously, the Trombone/LAD appliance is often used in conjunction with conventional fixed orthodontic therapy to provide more positive and controllable AP and lateral forces. As a result, treatment times are typically reduced when using this technique.

2443C Cantilevered Herbst

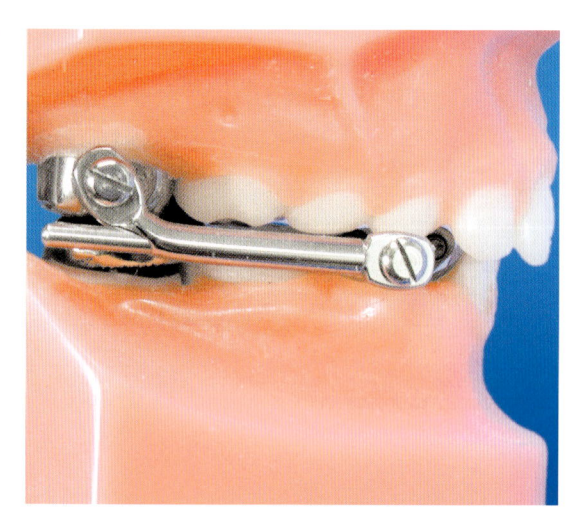

Herbst appliances are excellent for the correction of skeletal Class II malocclusions, especially if patient compliance is an issue. When primary molars are missing or cannot be used for retention and a bonded approach is contraindicated, the Cantilevered Herbst shown here is a good choice. In fact, the use of stainless steel crowns as a method of retention is quite popular because they are easy to place and remove. This is especially true when compared to the acrylic bonded Herbst designs. Patient acceptance of this appliance is also excellent.

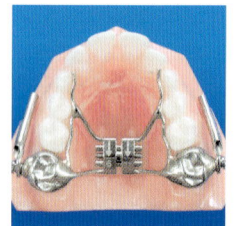

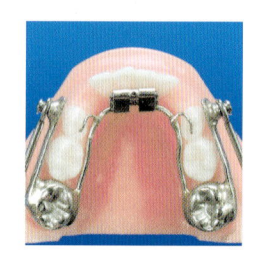

The effectiveness of all Herbst designs are enhanced if transverse deficiencies are addressed first. Once expansion of either, or both, arches is accomplished, the Class II correction will occur more readily via a combination of dental and skeletal changes. Today, however, many of the Herbst appliances include additions to the basic design that allow the practitioner to simultaneously correct multiple factors that may be contributing to a malocclusion. Expansion screws to widen the arches, arch wire tubes as part of a straight wire set-up, and other modifications, extend the treatment effects of the Herbst far beyond the mere correction of a Class II malocclusion.

ORTHODONTICS

5511 The Positioner

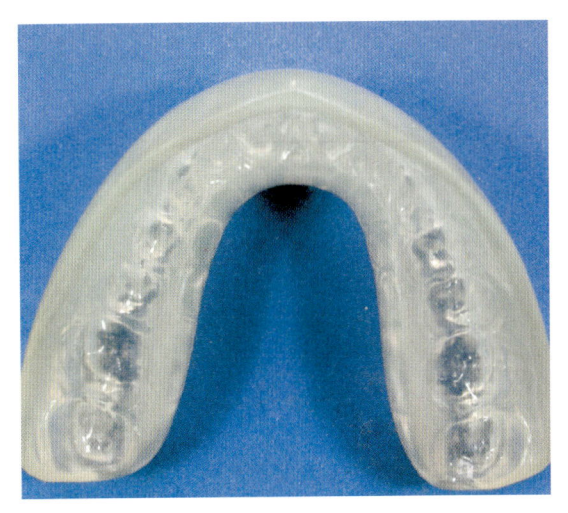

The Positioner is mainly used to help settle in the occlusion at the end of a full fixed bracket and band case. This retaining appliance is fabricated from flexible plastic (silicone or rubber) and is typically made into a slightly over-treated Class I relationship.

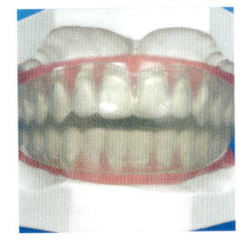

The appliance is fabricated after the individual teeth are cut from a current set of models and reset into an ideal relationship. Impressions for this appliance can be taken with brackets still in place. This will allow you to deliver the appliance immediately on the same day that you plan to remove your bands and brackets. Upon delivery, the patient is instructed to clench into the Positioner on a scheduled basis. This action not only allows for a gentle settling-in of the individual teeth into their correct positions, but it also has a functional element of establishing a correct interarch relationship. Various colors, as well as the standard clear material, are available for this appliance.

Note - A specific "Set-up and Positioner Prescription" form is available upon request.

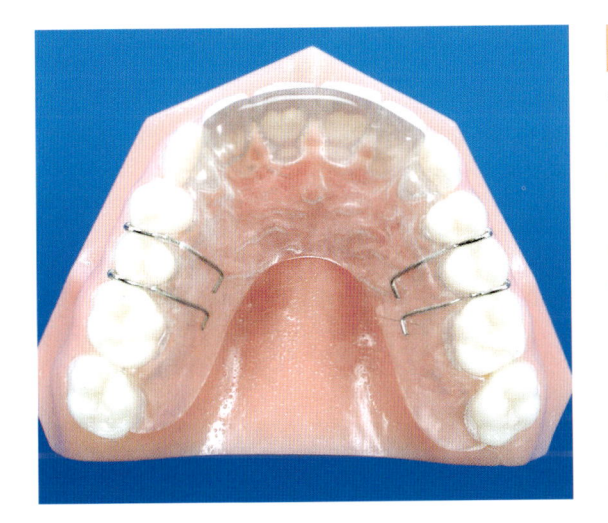

1163 Fixed Therapy Removable Bite Plane

This removable anterior bite plane appliance can be used in conjunction with full arch fixed mechanics when an increase in vertical dimension is needed. By using ball clasps for retention, it is possible to remove and replace the appliance without disturbing the fixed components. This design is easy to adjust during treatment and more hygienic than most fixed approaches.

Note - If the loss of vertical dimension is over-closed to the point that the lower anteriors cannot be properly bracketed, this removable approach is contraindicated. Instead, consider using a fixed bite plane.

10.5

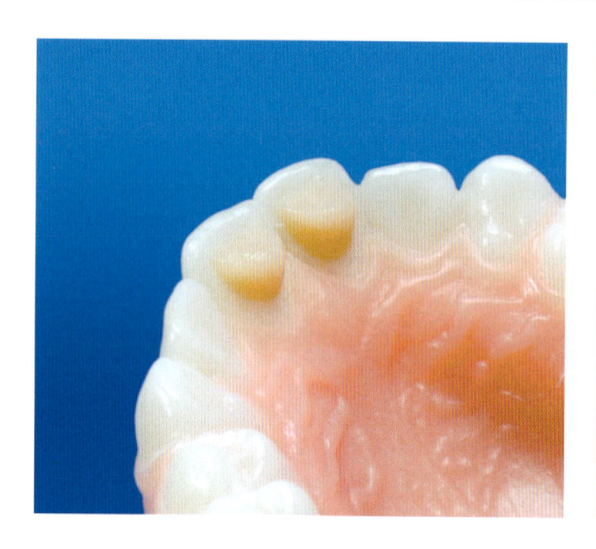

ORTHODONTICS

1400 Incisal Blocks

Lingual Bonded Incisal Blocks are regularly used during full fixed appliance therapy and can be employed to perform several functions. One of the most common uses is to expedite therapy in cases where an excessively deep bite prohibits bracketing of the lower incisors. By placing incisal blocks, the clearance needed to allow for mandibular bracketing at the beginning of treatment can easily be accomplished. This allows you to begin aligning the lower arch and improving the vertical dimension immediately, while protecting the lower brackets from being sheared off by the upper anteriors.

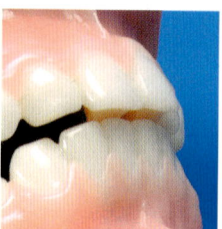

After the incisal blocks are bonded, speech can be slightly affected for a day and mastication for a week—sometimes longer for adults. Molar contact will be re-established after three to four months in children and four to six months in adults, but the blocks should not be removed until an effective occlusion with normal incisor relationships is established.

The incisal blocks can be fabricated chairside from composite, can be lab-made out of acrylic and delivered with or without a transfer tray, or purchased from several orthodontic supply companies (which typically supply "stainless steel" incisal blocks).

Note - The Incisal Blocks in the accompanying photo are fabricated from a darker tooth shade for visibility purposes. In fact, some suggest following this procedure when placing incisal blocks on your patient. A contrasting tooth shade makes it easier to remove all residue when de-bonding the blocks.

Note - When using Incisal Blocks, vertical dimension changes occur because changes in occlusal forces create intrusion of maxillary incisors and canines, intrusion of mandibular incisors and canines, extrusion of maxillary molars and extrusion of mandibular molars. Care must be taken to control these forces to achieve an ideal outcome.

Design Notes:

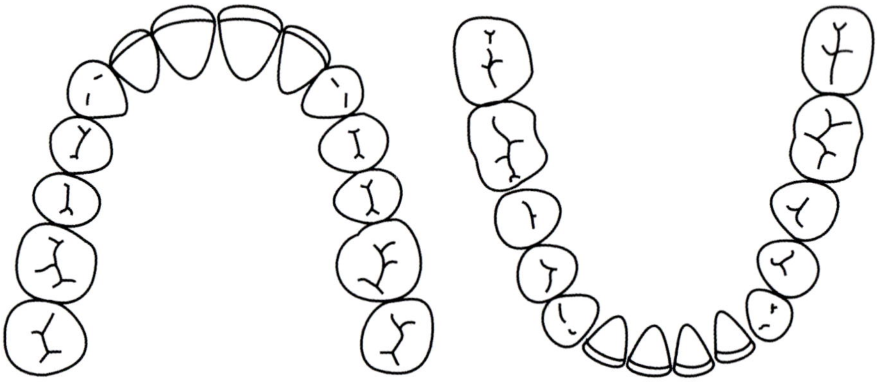

ORTHODONTICS

Indirect Banding and Bonding Service

Many clinicians find it convenient and economical to have your laboratory prepare their full band cases in an indirect set-up. Upon receipt of clean accurate models, custom bands are fitted to individual dies made for each tooth that needs to be banded. Appropriate brackets and arch wires are selected and your complete appliance is returned in a special compartmentalized box, pre-sterilized, and ready for cementation. If you prefer, brackets can be accurately placed on the model and a custom matrix made to assist you in seating them.

A variety of brackets are available in metal, plastic, and tooth shade ceramics for most fixed appliance techniques. They can be purchased individually or in complete sets. These sets can include molar brackets; however, conventional molar bands are still preferred by most practitioners. It is recommended that at least five sets of upper and lower brackets be kept on hand for emergencies or to replace a bracket that comes off.

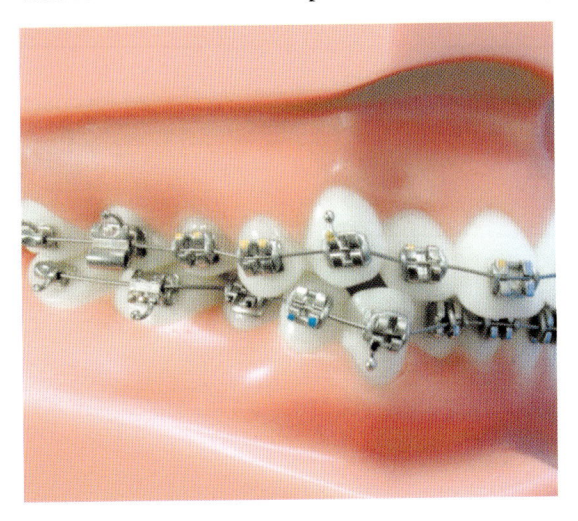

2152 The Straight-Wire Technique

The standard straight-wire appliance is designed to move teeth to their desired location in the arch form by using straight wire brackets in conjunction with a series of preformed arch wires. Straight wire brackets have the ideal tip, torque, angulation and in/out position built into each individual bracket for each tooth.

Once the bands and brackets are cemented and bonded in their ideal position, the doctor simply flexes the first arch wire to fit into the bracket slots and ligates it into place. As the arch wire attempts to return to its original shape, it will place a corresponding force on the individual teeth until the wire lies passive within the brackets. The arch wires are then progressively changed until a normal occlusion is achieved. Some of the advantages of this system are: limited or no arch wire bending, shorter overall treatment time and consistent quality of the end results. Since the ideal tooth position is built into the brackets, once they are placed correctly, less chair time is required as treatment progresses.

Bands

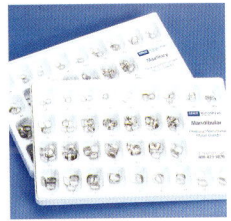

Bands are usually made for molars and bicuspids and are cemented in place with a band cement. These bands are used to provide a means to attach a wire, bracket, or other auxiliary device to that tooth for anchorage or active tooth movement.

Excellent custom bands can be fabricated for your fixed appliances, or you can choose to use pre-formed bands. Please see Chapter 1, page 1.21 for more detailed information. To use pre-formed bands, you must purchase a kit of bands with a selection of at least five sizes for each tooth to be banded. A band is then selected and pre-fit directly on the patient, being sure to adapt it accurately and tightly.

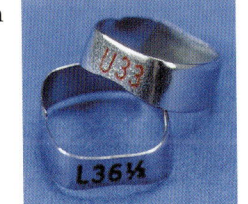

Once this is accomplished, the band, or bands should be removed, appropriately identified and placed in a protective box or envelope prior to taking the impression. The impression should then be taken, poured immediately, allowed to set up completely, checked for accuracy, and then sent to the lab along with the Rx slip and bands.

DO NOT pour up the bands in place. If there is even the slightest movement, it is extremely hard to detect and difficult to correct in the laboratory. This will cause the appliance to not fit and you'll need to start over with new impressions.

10.7

ORTHODONTICS

2619 Transfer Trays

In addition to supplying a complete kit of all of the necessary straight-wire brackets, arch wires, and accessories on a per patient basis, Space Maintainers can do the actual set-up as well. Each bracket is placed in the correct position on the patient's model as per your instructions and a plastic matrix material is vacuum formed over the brackets. This creates a tray that holds the brackets for transfer to the patient.

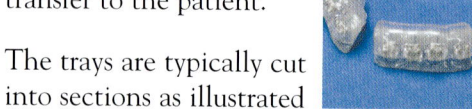

The trays are typically cut into sections as illustrated here and are flexible enough that it is easy to fit them over the patient's teeth. This makes the bonding procedure cleaner and more predictable. The tray material is also transparent so light-cured cements can be used if desired.

Some clinicians prefer a dual tray system. With this system, a second hard tray is designed to fit over the flexible tray that holds the brackets. Immediately after placing the soft tray, the hard tray is placed directly over it. Then a cotton roll is placed over the top of the hard tray and the patient is instructed to close carefully but firmly. This pressure holds the brackets firmly in place until the bonding process is complete.

Note - When using a transfer tray technique, please specify the type of brackets, where you would like them placed, and which tray system you prefer.

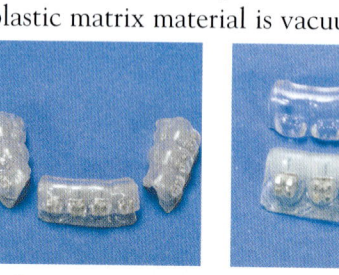

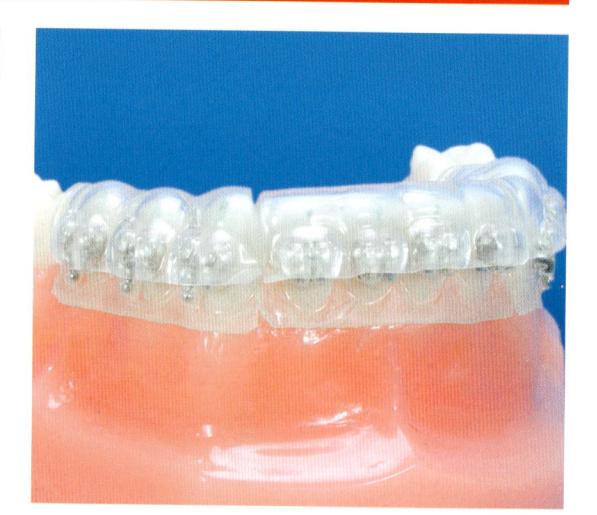

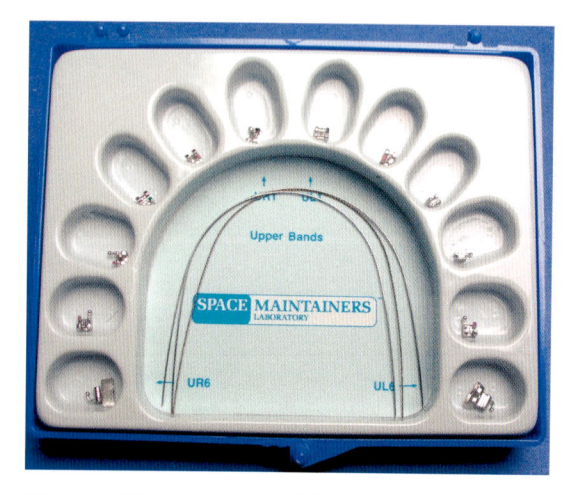

Trauma Kits courtesy of Space Maintainers Laboratory®

Trauma Kits

Unfortunately, in our modern, active society, oral facial trauma occurs all the time. Whether it is due to an auto accident, sports injury, fall, or some other incident, the dental practice needs to be able to effectively treat these injuries on an emergency basis. Every dental office should be prepared for these accidents by having a trauma kit in reserve. This kit consists of all the brackets, wires, and ligature ties necessary to quickly stabilize and immobilize injured teeth.

FINISHING / MAINTAINING

an overview: FINISHING/MAINTAINING

Chapter 11

After completing orthodontic therapy it is not uncommon to still need a little fine tuning to settle-in the occlusion or align a tooth that still has a slight rotation. This is particularly true in patients who have undergone extensive orthodontic therapy and are simply "burned out". Numerous appliances have been designed that will allow you to finish these cases through a combination of minor orthodontic corrections and the use of a patient's normal function.

Once tooth movement is completed, the final step in most orthodontic procedures is to use some method of retention until the soft tissue and bony changes have stabilized and are able to support the teeth in their new location.

To be effective, a retaining appliance should meet certain objectives. It should securely retain each tooth in its new position and prevent the tendency toward relapse. It should permit as much functional activity as possible allowing the teeth to respond in a normal physiological manner. Finally, the devices should be comfortable, easy to maintain, and as inconspicuous as possible.

Choosing the best approach will be different for each patient. Some of the factors that must enter into your decision process are:

1. the type of orthodontic treatment performed.

2. length of retention expected.

3. the age of the patient.

4. the ability of the patient to maintain his or her oral hygiene.

5. the periodontal condition.

6. the patient's future restorative needs.

Although the most common combination of retention appliances seems to be a removable upper retainer and a simple fixed lower retainer, this would clearly be an inappropriate choice for a patient who cannot use a floss threader to maintain the oral hygiene of his or her lower anteriors. For this type of patient a removable appliance would be a better selection.

Choosing the right appliance after aligning the upper anteriors and placing veneers is another example where you must take some time to select the best method of retention. Here, the metal labial used in a Hawley retainer could cause damage to the facial surface of the veneers. A better selection would be a thermoplastic Talon™ splint. This appliance will not only retain your orthodontic corrections but it will protect the veneers against abnormal forces and control the damage that can occur from bruxing at night.

an overview: FINISHING/MAINTAINING

Chapter 11

Where full-fixed orthodontic therapy has been used, impressions for removable final retainers may be taken while the bands and brackets are still in place. The laboratory will then carefully carve the bands and brackets off the models and complete the necessary appliances. If you have a specific lingual and/or palatal finish line in mind, please use a standard lead pencil to mark your desired finish line directly on the model.

When a patient does not wear the final retainers prescribed, relapse will usually occur, especially the return of crowding in their upper or lower incisors. When this happens, patients often prefer to have this corrected without having to wear brackets again. If the relapse is caught early enough, a removable finishing appliance is often sufficient to correct the problem.

Note - It is also possible to add a variety of patient-pleasing touches to the acrylic portion of the appliance. Different colors (including glow-in-the-dark colors), decals and even have the patient's name added to the plastic. An appliance color selection chart is included in the back of this book and is a great way to encourage patient compliance through their involvement in the selection process.

Design Notes

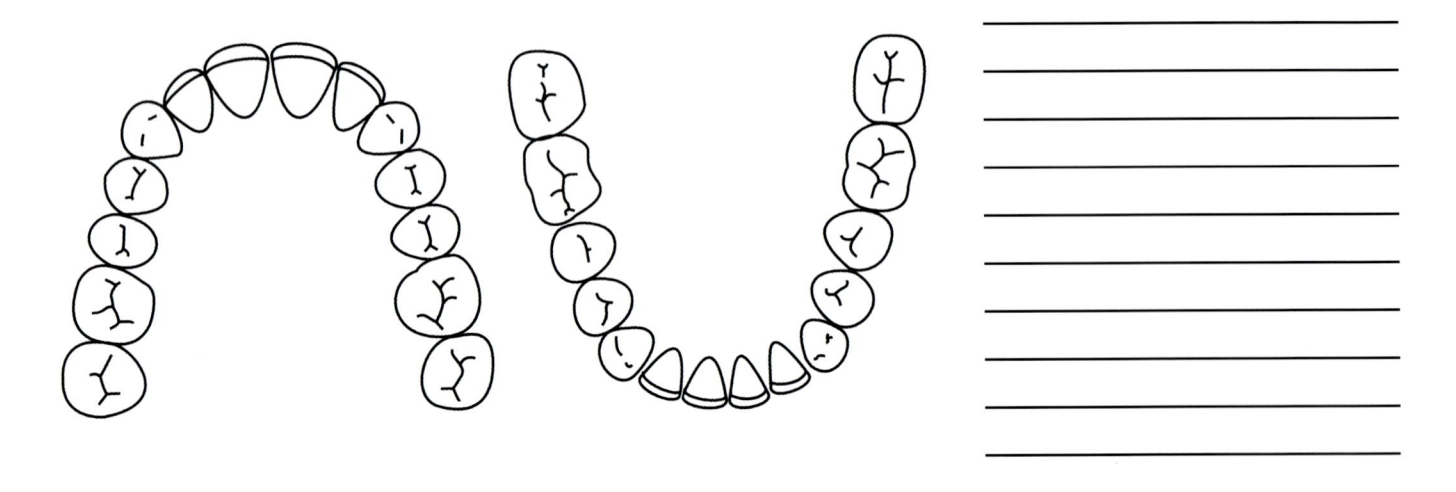

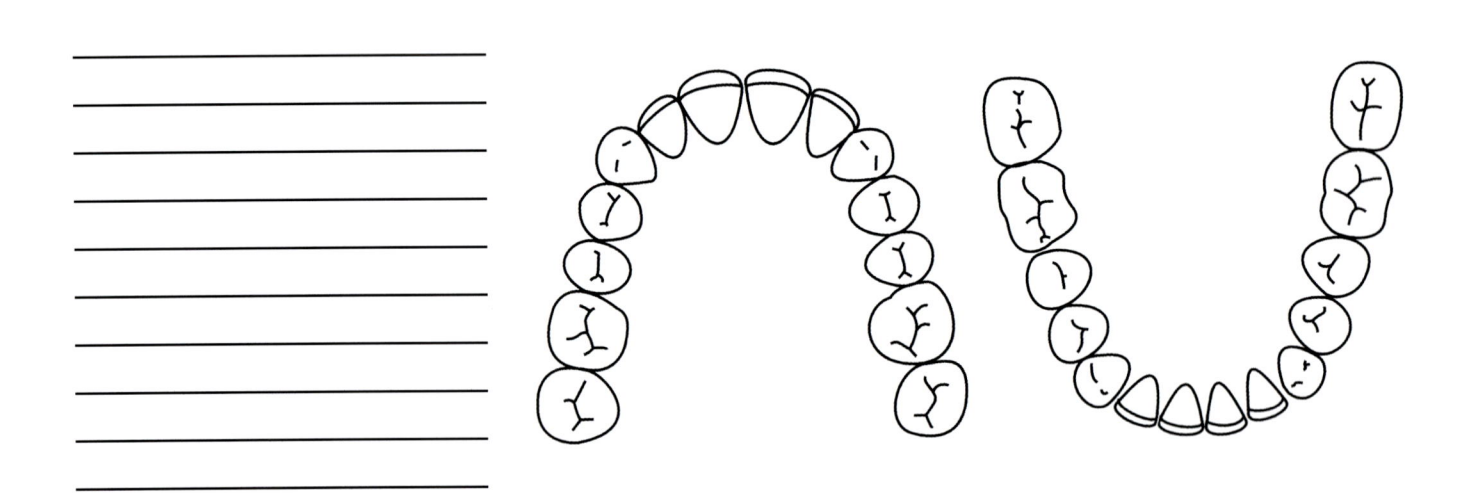

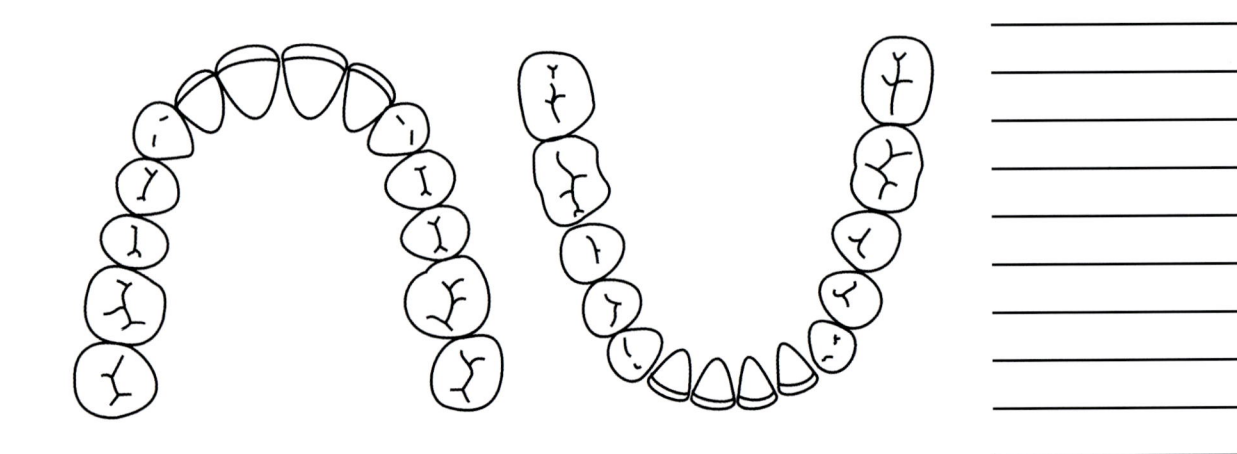

FINISHING/MAINTAINING

1115 Open Palate Retainer   U

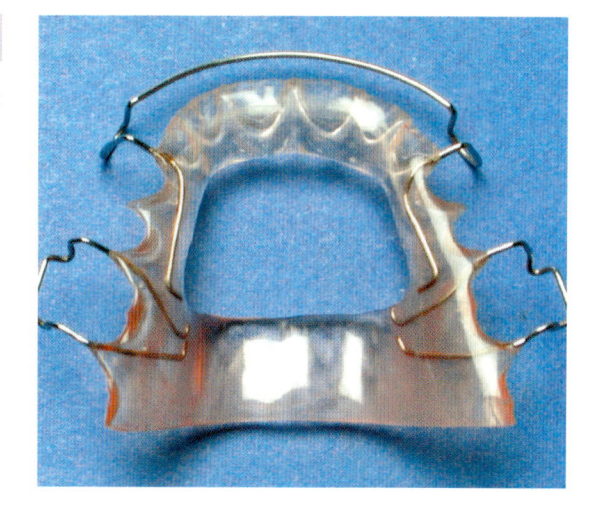

This appliance is designed primarily as a final retainer to be used at the completion of any orthodontic therapy. The area over the hard palate has been left free of acrylic. Speech is left virtually unaffected and there is no danger of the patient developing a deviate swallowing pattern as the tongue never loses its natural contact with the hard palate. The ribbon of acrylic that is contacting the lingual of the anteriors is reinforced with Kevlar in order to reduce the possibility of fracture. Adams clasps are used because they stay retentive over time. Both the clasps and the labial bow must be designed to stay out of occlusion to prevent any unwanted tooth movement.

Note - Always send the lab both upper and lower casts along with a bite relationship for fabrication of this appliance.

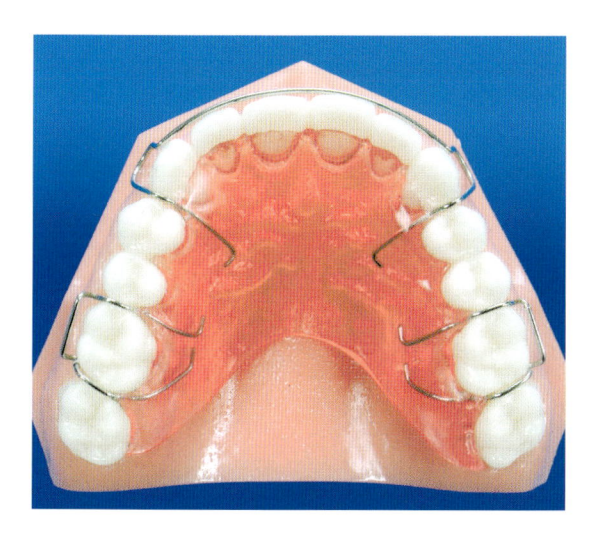

1161 Maxillary Final Retainer   U

Whether you are actively doing orthodontics or not, every dentist at one time in his or her career has had to replace a patient's retainer. There are many different appliance designs and variations but this is the basic retaining appliance. It features Adams clasps on the first molars and a standard, tightly adapted "Hawley" type labial arch wire running from the distal of both cuspids. The acrylic should be well adapted to the palate and the lingual aspect of the teeth. Every effort should also be made to keep it thin for comfort.

Note - Always send the lab both upper and lower casts along with a bite relationship for fabrication of this appliance.

1162 Simple Mandibular Retainer   L

Shown here is a basic lower appliance with a standard "Hawley" type labial arch wire. Rests are placed on the molars for posterior stability and to keep the appliance from over-seating into the tissue. Clasps are optional; the most commonly requested clasps are Adams Clasps as illustrated in the insert photo. Please be very specific as to your design preferences when requesting this appliance.

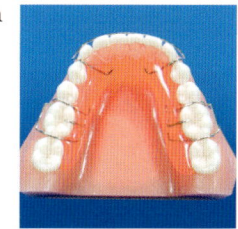

Note - Always send the lab both upper and lower casts along with a bite relationship for fabrication of this appliance.

11.1

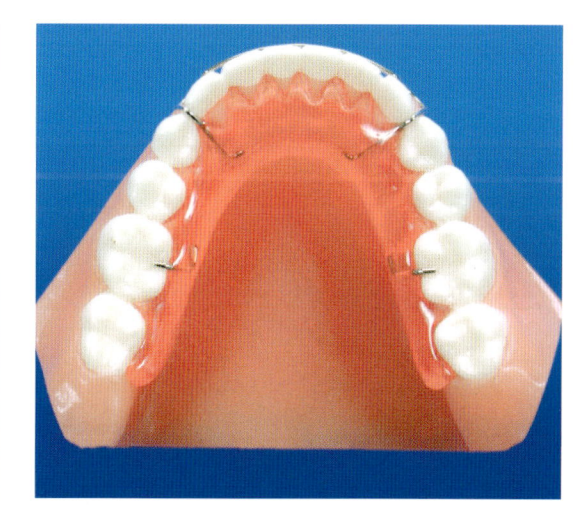

FINISHING/MAINTAINING

Labial Arch Wire Options

Several different designs are available for the labial wire portion of these retainers. Detailed description and applications of the most common ones are listed here and are described in greater detail in Chapter 1.

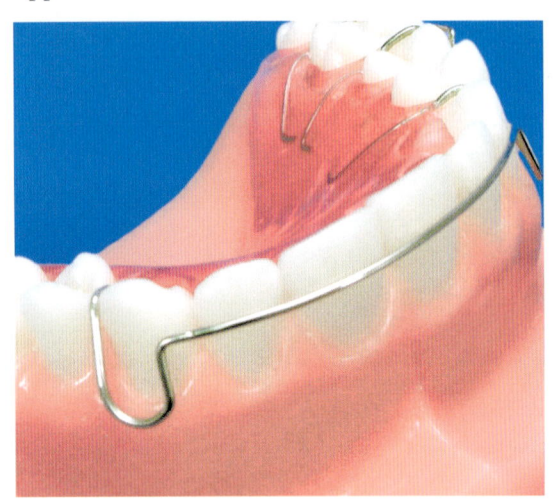

Standard

The most common arch wire design is shown here. The labial bow will generally embrace the six anterior teeth and join the acrylic between the canine and the first premolar. However, the labial portion may be restricted to any part of the anterior region, or extended as far distally as the first molar.

Round Contoured

A Round Contoured arch wire is bent to closely fit against the labial surface of the anteriors. It is used to securely hold the teeth in their final position after active treatment is completed.

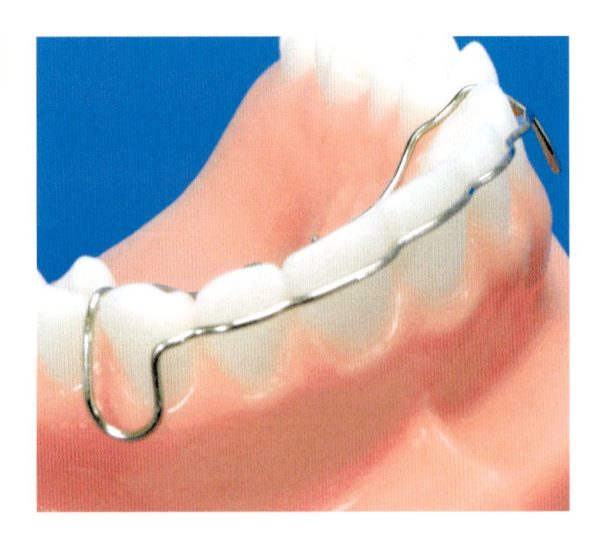

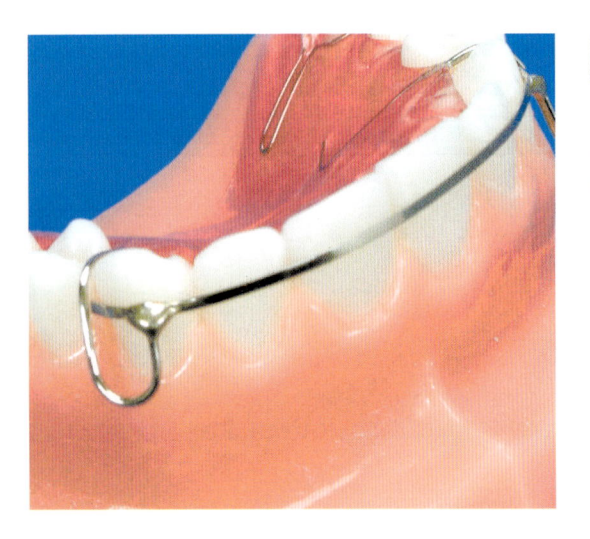

Flat Hawley

A flat wire is used to contact the labial surface of the anterior teeth and is soldered to the adjustment loops at the cuspids. The flat wire is carried back to the distal of the cuspids and affords added retention to stabilize the cuspids after movement.

FINISHING/MAINTAINING

Flat Contoured Hawley

Similar to the Flat Hawley, this wire is individually contoured to the entire labial and interproximal surfaces of the incisors.

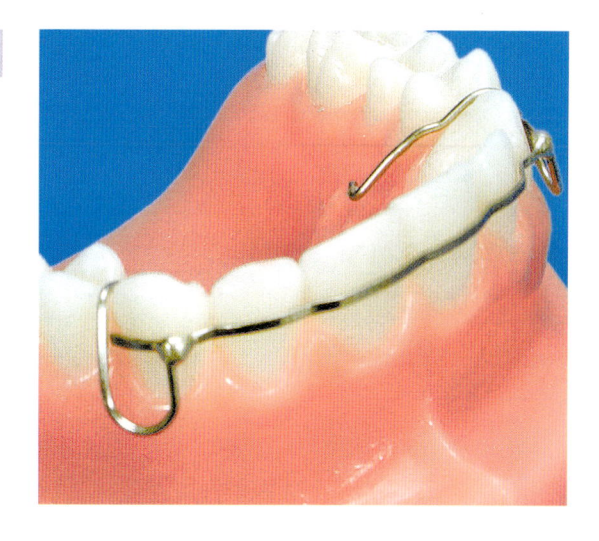

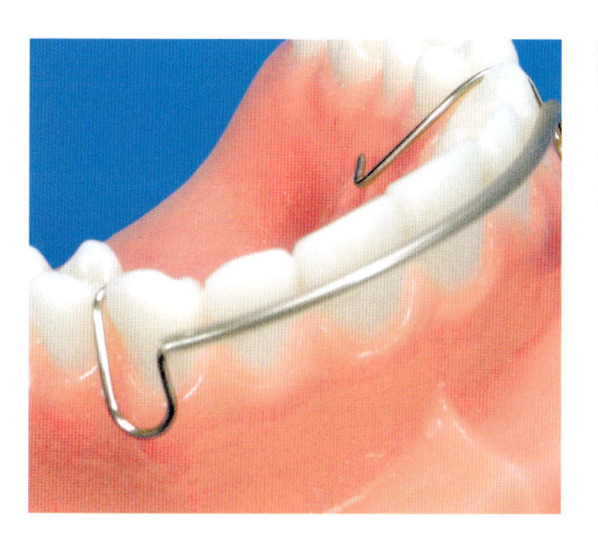

Plastic Coated Hawley

This Labial wire is preferred on retainers when the anterior teeth are restored with veneers. The Plastic coating protects the porcelain surfaces from possible abrasion from the wire.

Acrylic Arch Wire

This wire gains superior anterior retention through the use of clear acrylic that tightly conforms to the labial and interproximal surfaces of the incisors. This prohibits movement, and particularly rotation, of the incisors and is often used on "Wrap Around" labial wires to aid stability.

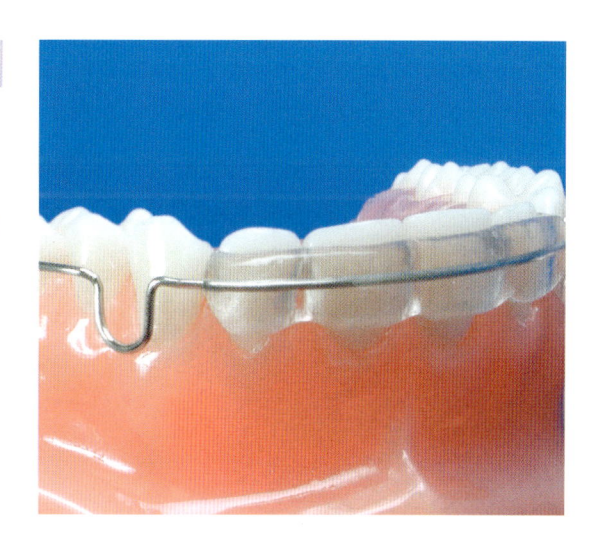

FINISHING/MAINTAINING

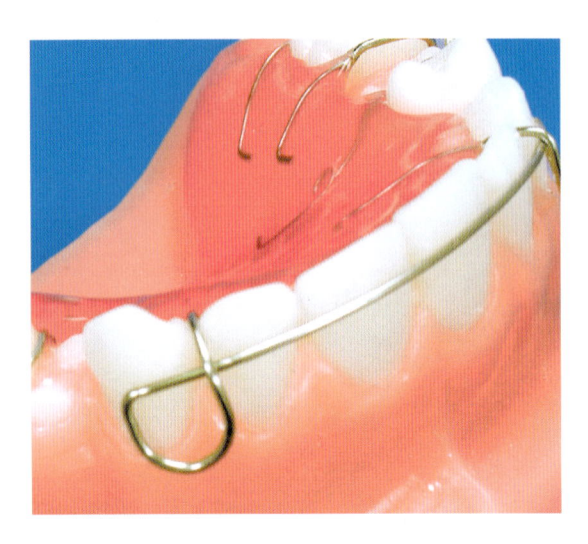

Reverse Hawley

The Reverse Hawley is fabricated with the labial wire crossing between the cuspid and lateral with the adjustment loop running from the distal to the mesial. This labial wire is excellent when you do not want any wire coming over the distal of the cuspids. A typical scenario requiring this design is when positive cuspid control is needed, particularly if the cuspid has been rotated significantly during orthodontic therapy.

Ricketts Arch Wire

The Ricketts arch wire, like the Reverse Hawley, crosses the dentition through the embrasures interproximal to the laterals and cuspids. The "U" Loops are placed on the laterals and the distal recurved arms are contoured to the cuspids. These distal recurves can be used to increase retention as well as help stabilize cuspids that may have required rotation during active treatment. If carefully activated, they can be used to affect minor lingual rotation of the cuspids, unilaterally or bilaterally.

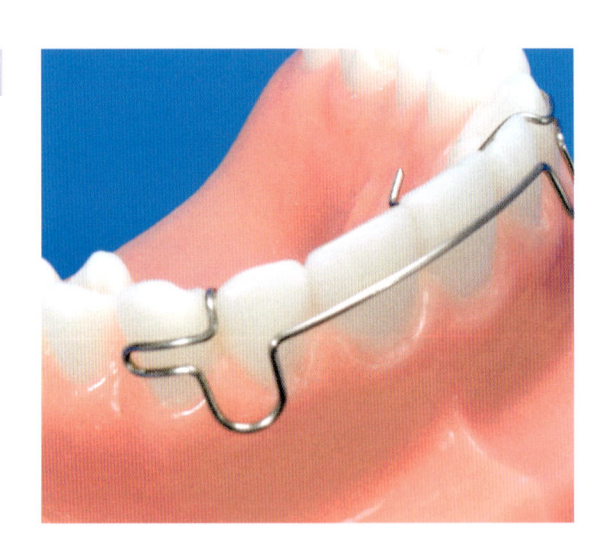

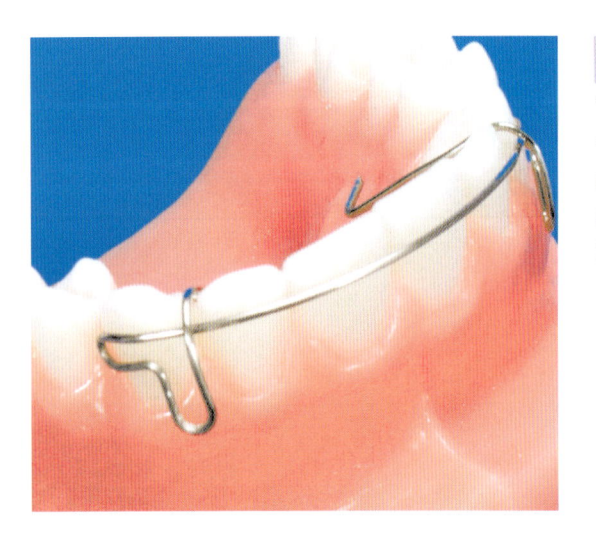

Witzig Double Loop

This design is a modification of the Ricketts arch using a narrow vertical loop. It is excellent for final stability of the anterior segment but only allows for very minor adjustments during retention. It is typically used only when a removable final retainer is preferred after completion of orthodontic therapy.

FINISHING/MAINTAINING

Apron Spring Labial (Roberts Retraction Arch)

The Apron spring is an active labial arch wire that is primarily used to retract severely flared anteriors. It features two spring coils for light, continuous, lingual movement and is easily activated with finger pressure.

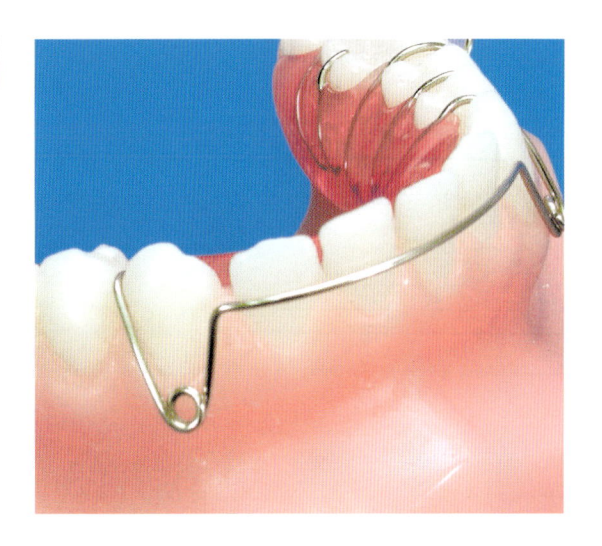

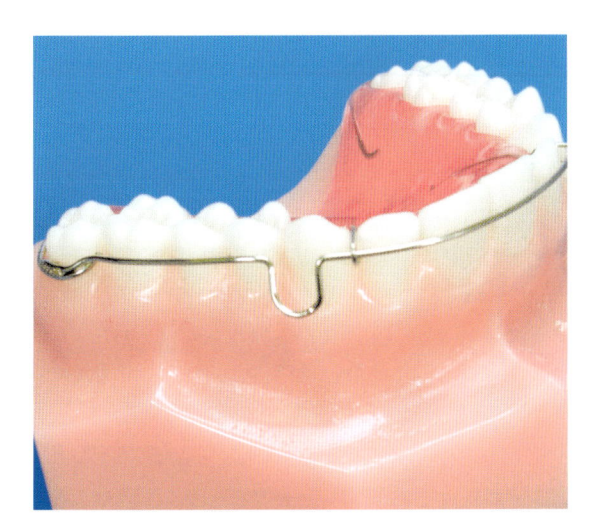

Wrap Around

The Wrap Around labial is excellent for final retention. It is usually soldered to the buccal bar of the Adams clasp or to "C" clasps. Wrapping around in this manner eliminates the possibility of occlusal interferences or opening interproximal contacts.

Design Notes:

FINISHING/MAINTAINING

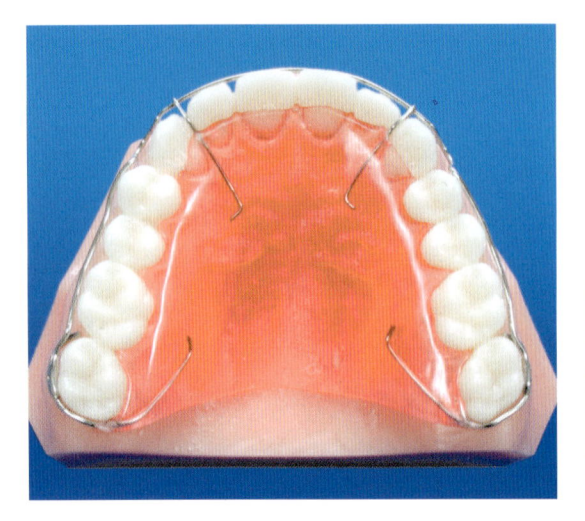

1165 The San Antonio Retainer   U/L

Named for the Texas Study Club that first described it, this retainer has many special features worthy of consideration. The labial arch wire extends from molar to molar for excellent retention and control of the entire arch. Since it does not pass over the occlusal surface, there is no occlusal interference to prevent proper function.

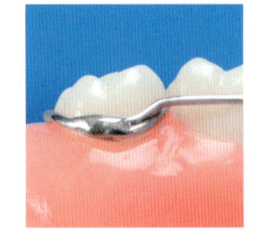

To stabilize the labial, two small interproximal support wires pass from the acrylic and wrap around the arch wire between the cuspids and the laterals. (Also note the extended arms to the cuspids to provide support and prevent rotation.)

Usually "C" clasps are used distal of the twelve-year molar for retention of the appliance. These are preferred in order to prevent any occlusal interference. If retention is a problem, it is advisable to place a small composite ledge on the molars to create a retentive undercut for the clasp.

Finally, a thin, heat-cured acrylic base is used for strength and comfort. During finishing, extra care must be taken to be sure that the acrylic is in contact with the entire lingual surface of each tooth.

Note - Always send the lab both upper and lower casts along with a bite relationship for fabrication of this appliance.

1169A Wrap Around Retainer   U/L
with Labial Acrylic Support

Often, due to the long span of the labial arch wire in the "wrap-around" design, the labial wire has a great deal of flex and can come out of adjustment if the appliance is handled roughly. To help alleviate this problem, and to add stability and retention to the anteriors, clear acrylic is processed tightly against the labial surface of the incisors as illustrated. This feature adds superior retention to the overall appliance and eliminates the need for a small interproximal support wire distal to the lateral incisors as seen in the San Antonio design.

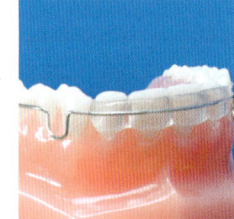

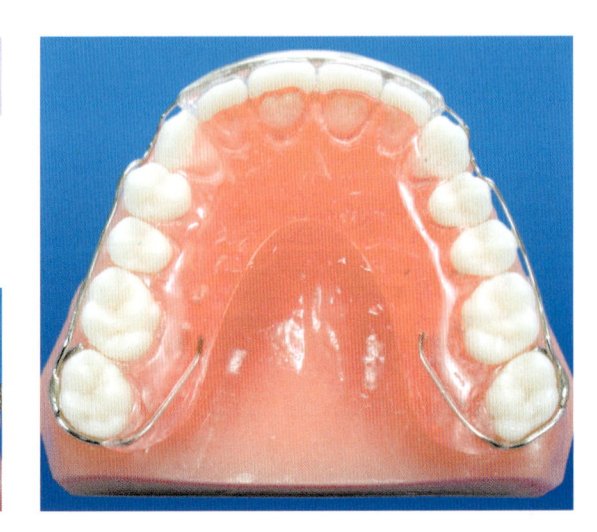

11.6

FINISHING/MAINTAINING

1065 The Spring Hawley Retainer   U/L

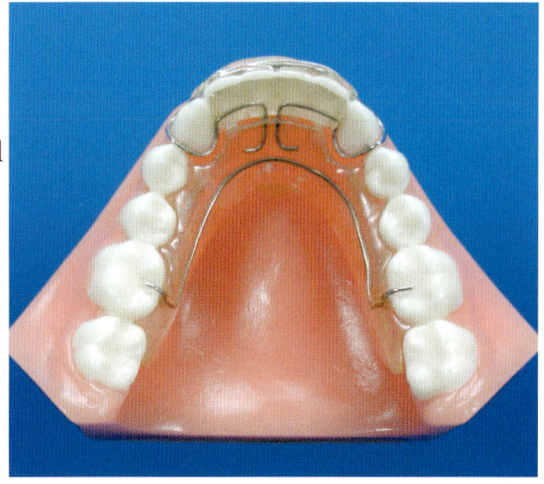

This appliance is useful in correcting minor rotations and crowding up to 1-1/2mm from cuspid to cuspid in the anteriors. The space necessary to correct this crowding is gained by judicious interproximal recontouring in the anterior region only, as the appliance is NOT designed to gain any arch width or length.

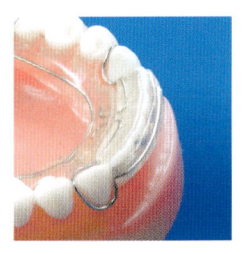

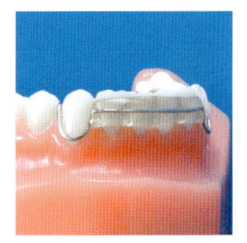

Before fabricating the appliance, the lab will separate the rotated and crowded anteriors from the stone cast and reset them in an ideal alignment. The appliance is then fabricated to this corrected anterior position and sent back to you for delivery. On the day of delivery, complete the necessary interproximal recontouring, then place the appliance. When worn, the spring action of the cuspid wires will direct a light labial-lingual force to align the teeth. Since this appliance has been constructed to the "ideal" setting, it may not seat well in the patient's mouth until the teeth adapt to their new position. Once the teeth are straight, the appliance can continue to be worn as a final retainer.

Note - Since tooth movement is in a labial-lingual direction, adequate vertical dimension is essential. If the patient has a closed vertical and the upper and lower anteriors are already in contact, tooth movement will not occur.

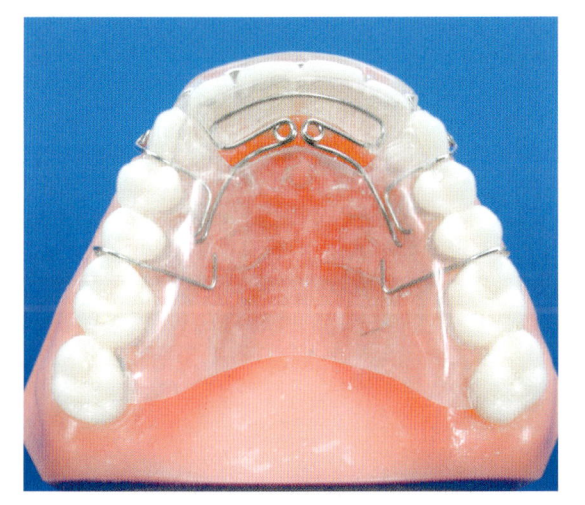

1333 Modified Spring Retainer   U/L

This design is useful for correcting minor rotations of the upper anterior teeth. The teeth are set-up in the corrected position on the model and then the appliance is constructed. The dentist completes the necessary interproximal recontouring on the day of delivery. When in place, the resulting labial-lingual force will align the teeth.

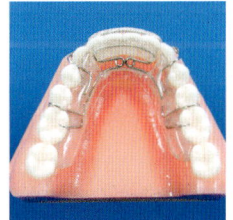

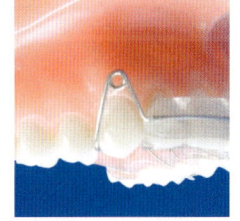

The helical coil in the labial wire portion, and the "mushroom" helical coil spring design of the active lingual component, make this appliance very effective for quickly aligning the incisors.

Adequate space for alignment of the anteriors is essential and this design will NOT gain arch width or length. The appliance may also be used as a final positioning retainer but is not recommended for closing spaces.

FINISHING/MAINTAINING

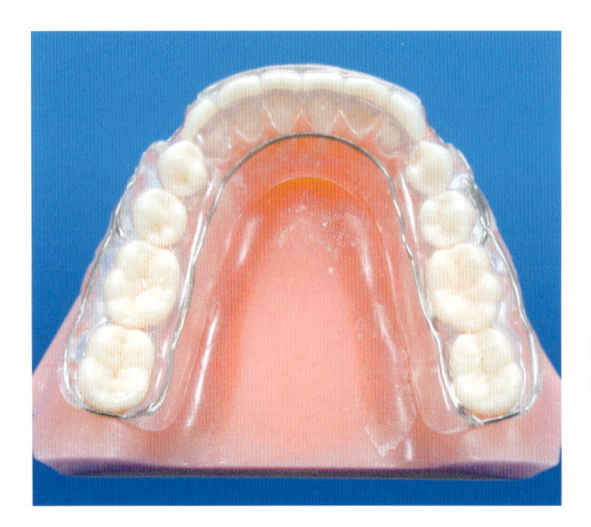

1332 Modified Adaptor™   U/L

The Modified Adaptor™ appliance is used for minor tooth rotations and alignments of both the posterior and anterior teeth. It works like the spring retainer in that the teeth on the working model are carefully placed in their ideal position prior to fabricating the appliance.

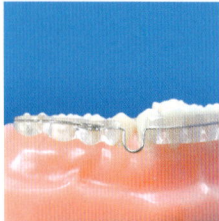

This unique design features a solid lingual acrylic base that is tightly contoured to all of the lingual surfaces. The buccal posterior segments are joined to the lingual via stainless steel wires, and the labial portion covering the six anterior teeth is joined to the posterior segments via stainless steel Omega Loops in the cuspid/bicuspid region.

Once seated, this highly flexible appliance gently settles the teeth in the correct alignment. Since the Modified Adaptor™ allows for full occlusal contact of the posterior teeth, natural function aids in a rapid and secure settling in of the buccal segments. Unlike a Positioner, it is extremely comfortable, virtually undetectable, and can be worn full time, except while eating.

Please note, however, that it is essentially a finishing retainer and no significant rotations or mesial/distal movements should be attempted with this design.

1164 RAM Retainer
designed by Dr. Robert A. Meese   U/L

The RAM final retainer adds a twist to the wrap around designs seen in other final retainers. First, there are no clasps or support wires crossing the occlusion. Then by using a sliding labial bow, a small amount of space closure and retraction can be accomplished. The sliding labial consists of a .010 X .022 wire that runs through tubes placed buccal to the first bicuspid region. Bilateral elastics are then placed from hooks at the distal end of the labial wire to hooks in the molar region that are on the distal support wires.

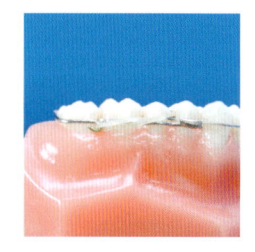

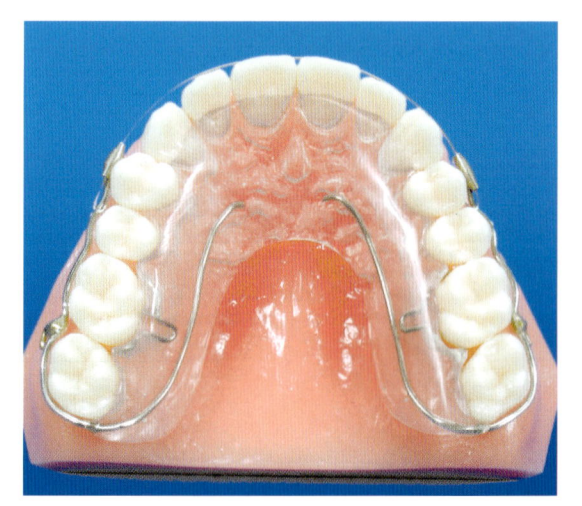

Note - A positive overjet is necessary if lingual retraction is required for the space closure.

FINISHING/MAINTAINING

1076F Bloore Aligner   U/L

After completing orthodontic therapy, it is not uncommon for patients to experience a small amount of relapse crowding in their upper or lower incisors. This is especially true when they have not been diligent in wearing their final retainers. When this happens, patients often prefer to have this corrected without having to wear brackets again. The Bloore Aligner is excellent for this purpose.

Springs, called eyelet arms, are placed lingual to each incisor and individually activated to move the teeth into alignment. As needed, interproximal reductions and incisal re-contouring are utilized to gain room and provide an esthetic result.

Note - When used on the lower arch, it is important to make sure that the incisors are not coupling with the lingual of the uppers prior to initiating treatment, as vertical and AP clearance are required in order to successfully correct the lower anteriors. Once the anteriors are re-aligned, it is recommended to consider using a fixed lingual retainer for final retention.

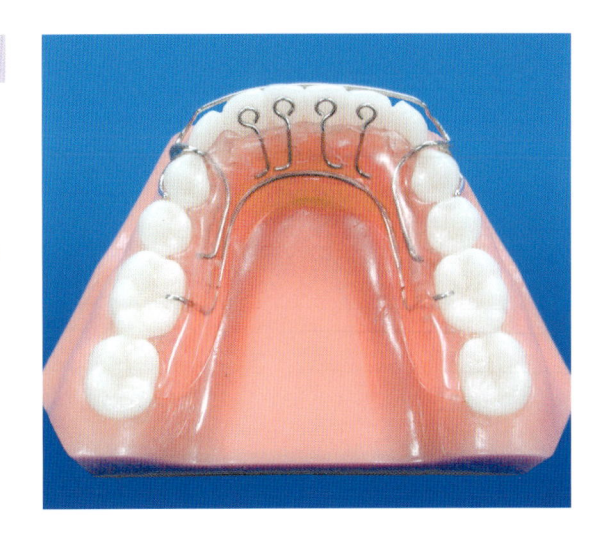

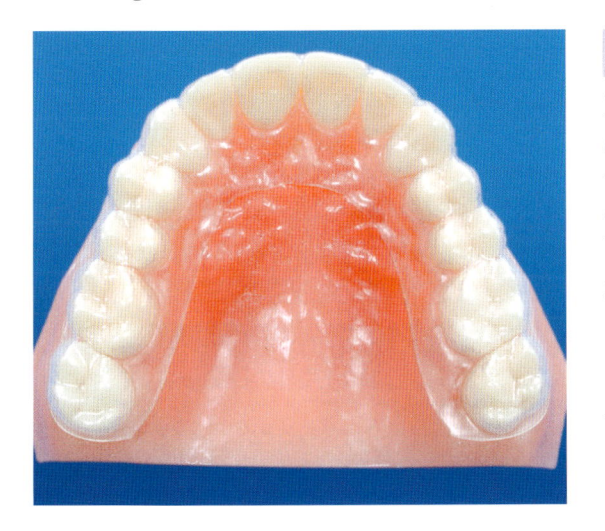

1116 The "Invisible" Retainer   U/L

Here is a popular retainer design for the extremely appearance conscious patient. It is fabricated from a thin sheet of clear acrylic that is vacuum-formed to the occlusal and incisal surfaces of the entire arch. The completed appliance typically extends over the buccal and labial surfaces, and is typically finished just short of the gingival margins on the labial and buccal surfaces. On the upper appliance, the palate is horseshoe shaped for patient comfort.

Note - These retainers are quite thin and are contraindicated for anyone who bruxes their teeth. Also, the patient needs to be instructed on the gentle care required for this appliance.

Design Notes:

FINISHING/MAINTAINING

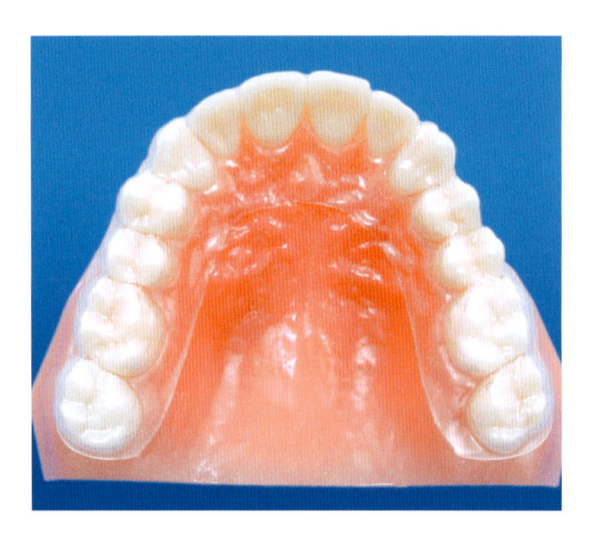

1116E - Essix U/L

The Essix retainer is a popular retainer for the extremely appearance-conscious patient. It is fabricated by thermoforming a thin sheet of Essix material over the entire arch. Essix material is made of a clear acrylic that is tough, stain and abrasive resistant and has the light-reflecting properties to make the teeth appear brilliant when the retainer is in place. The appliance, as illustrated here, covers the buccal, labial, and lingual surfaces and extends onto the gingival tissue.

Note - Please provide a detailed description when ordering this appliance if you have a specific finish line in mind.

2164 Three-to-Three Fixed Banded Retainer

Shown here is a cuspid-to-cuspid banded lingual retainer which can be made either from your preformed bands or from our own custom fit bands. The lingual wire is carefully adapted to be in direct contact with the lingual surfaces of each anterior tooth and is typically placed 2mm below the incisal edge.

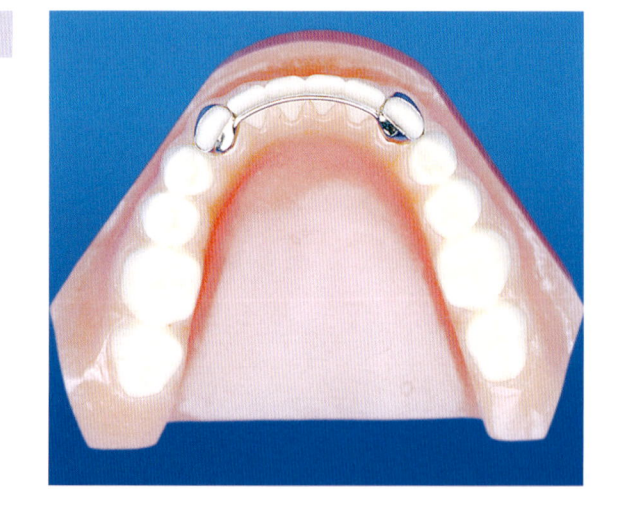

Note - Recent research shows that it is necessary to bond each tooth individually to maintain them in their corrected position. Individual anterior teeth can be secured to the lingual wire by simply adding composite over the lingual wire.

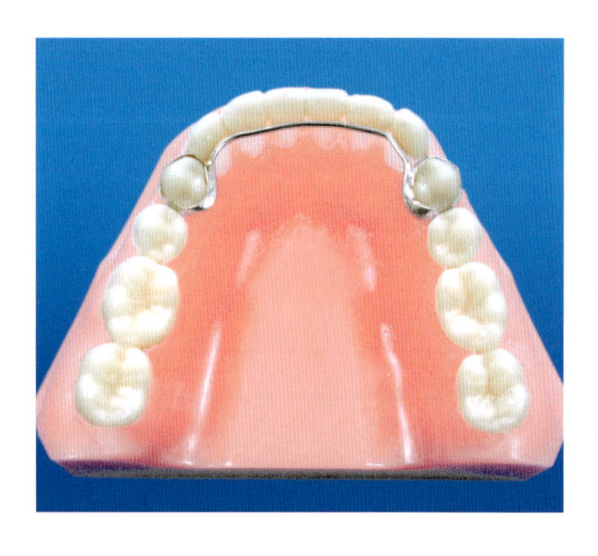

2166 Banded 4x4 Retainer U/L

Many clinicians recommend including the first bicuspids in all fixed retainers. This is especially true when significant orthodontic movements have been necessary to achieve the desired final results. The lingual wire is carefully adapted to be in direct contact with the lingual surfaces of each anterior tooth and is typically placed 2mm below the incisal edge.

Note - Recent research shows that it is necessary to bond each tooth individually to maintain them in their corrected position. Individual anterior teeth can be secured to the lingual wire by simply adding composite over the lingual wire.

FINISHING/MAINTAINING

2165 Direct Bond Fixed Retainer

This appliance is bonded to the lingual of the cuspids by the use of custom contoured, direct bond pads. These pads have a metal-mesh backing for superior retention. The lingual wire is carefully contoured and routinely placed 2mm below the incisal edges unless prescribed otherwise. Additionally, many choose to add the first bicuspids into the retentive unit as illustrated in the inserted photo.

Note - Recent research shows that it is necessary to bond each tooth individually to maintain them in their corrected position. Individual anterior teeth can be secured to the lingual wire by simply adding composite over the lingual wire.

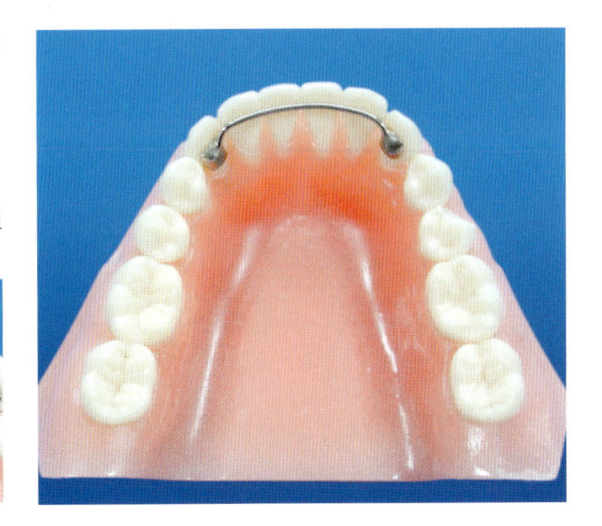

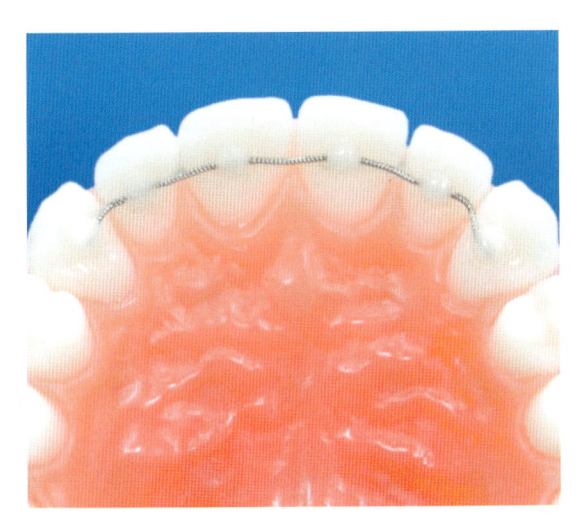

2212 E-Z Bond Lingual Retainer   U/L

The E-Z Bond Retainer is a multi-strand, dead-soft wire that is carefully contoured to the lingual of the six anterior teeth and is light-cured with composite to each of the six anterior teeth. The key advantage to this appliance is use of a laboratory fabricated transfer tray that makes correct placement of the wire easy with a minimum of chair time.

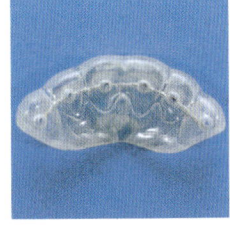

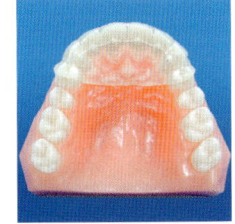

The transfer tray has small reservoirs at each bonding site with an excess material escape channel directly lingual to each of the anterior teeth. This assures a complete wrap of bonding cement around the lingual wire.

To place the appliance, the reservoirs are filled with composite by use of a syringe. The tray is then gently seated by finger pressure, allowing any excess composite to flow out of the escape channels. Then it is light cured. After curing the material, any excess cement is removed from the tray with a high speed hand piece and a diamond. Then the tray is slowly and carefully lifted off of the teeth. The top of the individual composite buttons can then be polished for patient comfort with a composite diamond or disc. Complete, step-by-step, chairside instructions are provided with your first E-Z Bond Retainer.

Note - When requesting an E-Z Bond Retainer for the maxillary anteriors, it is important to send an opposing model and a wax bite. Sufficient overbite and overjet is essential to provide clearance for the maxillary E-Z Bond Retainer.

FINISHING/MAINTAINING

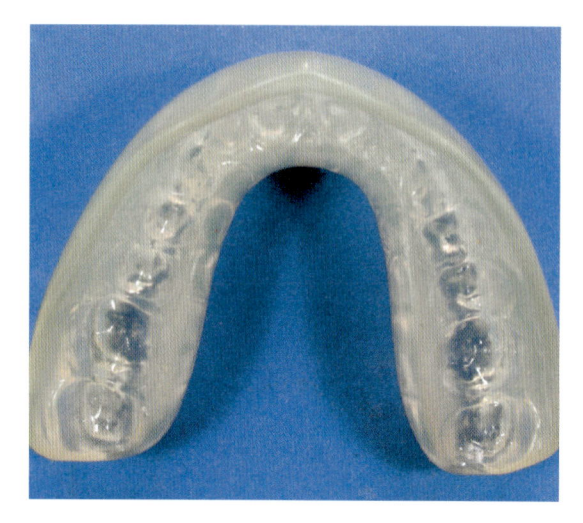

5511 The Positioner

The Positioner is mainly used to help settle in the occlusion at the end of a full fixed bracket and band case. This retaining appliance is fabricated from flexible plastic (silicone or rubber) and is typically made into a slightly over-treated Class I relationship.

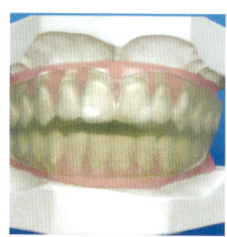

The appliance is fabricated after the individual teeth are cut from a current set of models and reset into an ideal relationship. Impressions for this appliance can be taken with brackets still in place. This will allow you to deliver the appliance immediately on the same day that you plan to remove your bands and brackets.

Upon delivery, the patient is instructed to clench into the Positioner on a scheduled basis. This action not only allows for a gentle settling-in of the individual teeth into their correct positions, but it also has a functional element of establishing a correct interarch relationship. Various colors, as well as the standard clear material, are available for this appliance.

Note - A specific "Set-up and Positioner Prescription" form is available upon request.

2166M Direct Bond Fixed Retainer   U/L

Long-term, post-orthodontic treatment studies suggest that some degree of relapse is inevitable. The most recent research shows that it is necessary to bond each tooth individually to maintain them in their corrected position. This is hard to accomplish without making it more difficult for the patient to maintain hygiene. Typically patients who have lingual bonded retainers have to use floss threaders to clean interproximally.

The lingual bonded retainer, shown here, is designed to allow the patients to floss normally making it much easier for them to maintain a healthy oral condition. Using Australian wire, loops are placed between all the teeth except in the lower incisor region where the interproximal distances are too close. These loops avoid the interproximal areas allowing patients to floss. A floss threader is recommended for use between the lower incisors.

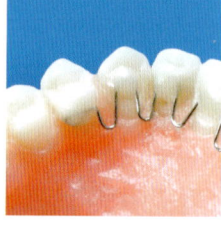

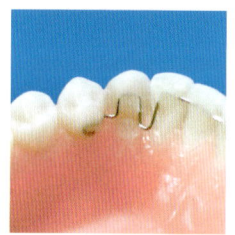

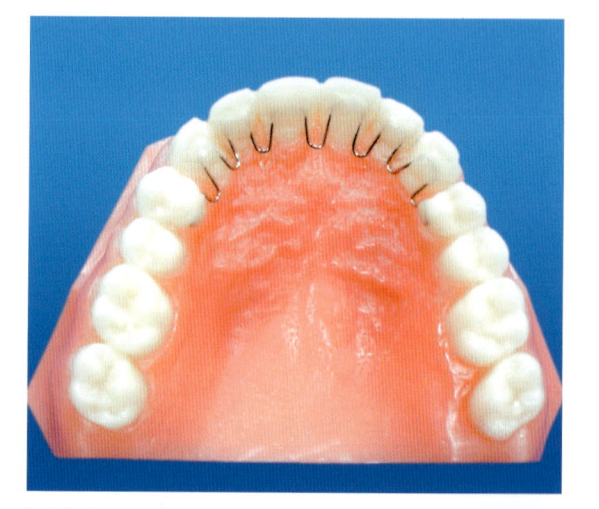

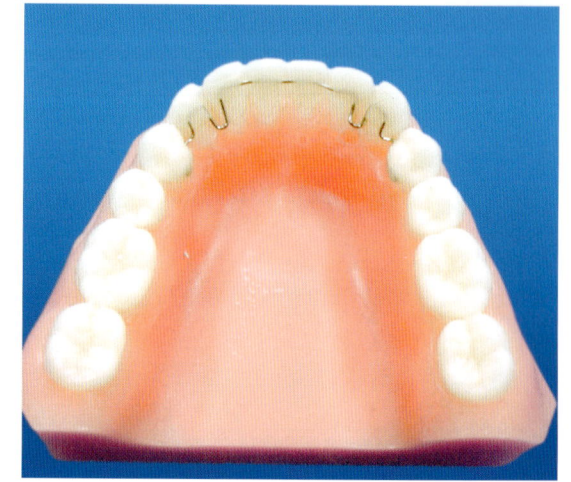

11.12

MOUTHGUARDS

an overview: MOUTHGUARDS

Chapter 12

Adults and Children

Most people wear a mouthguard during sports in an effort to prevent any damage to their teeth. The new generation of mouthguards has been shown to reduce forces that not only protect the teeth but also can prevent concussions, neck injuries, jaw fractures, cerebral hemorrhage and even death. This is accomplished by separating the jaws, to prevent the condyles from being displaced upward and backward against the wall of the glenoid fossa. The proper use of a mouthguard can reduce the incidence and severity of injuries during sports and athletic activities of any type.

Every person in your practice, who is involved in any athletic activity where contact can be made or a fall can occur, should be using an athletic mouthguard. Some examples are baseball, basketball, boxing, rugby, hockey, squash, soccer, racquetball, tennis, lacrosse, karate, judo, volleyball, touch and contact football, bicycling and skating. Therefore it is recommended that patients be routinely asked if they are involved in any sports.

To get patients to wear a mouthguard on a regular basis, it must be comfortable, not impair breathing and allow for normal speech. The mouthguards shown in this text have these characteristics and are custom formed for the individual patient. The ready-made, store-bought tooth protectors and thermoplastic mouthguards usually fall short in one or more of these important features and therefore should not be recommended.

Mouthguards are most commonly made for the maxillary arch. For the athlete with a prognathic mandible, it is recommended that a custom mouthguard be made to cover the mandibular arch as well.

Prior to delivering the mouthguard, you will need to accomplish the following:

1. An oral exam should be completed to ensure that the patient is in good dental health.

2. All new or recurrent caries should be treated prior to the fabrication of a mouthguard.

3. Special care needs to be taken when designing mouthguards for the edentulous patient. Please consult with the lab for specific information.

4. Removable prosthodontic devices (appliances) should be removed prior to taking impressions for the mouthguard. The patient must be instructed to remove these appliances while wearing the mouthguard.

5. The most frequent site of mandibular fracture is in the area of unerupted third molars. Serious athletes in a contact sport may want to have their third molars evaluated for possible extraction.

6. Any area where teeth will be erupting should be blocked out on the model prior to appliance fabrication.

7. Mouthguards should be modified to allow for the anticipated changes over a 3-month period. Patients in fixed appliances should be wearing either separate mouthguards on both the upper and the lower arches, or bi-maxillary mouthguards to prevent the possibility of severe soft tissue trauma.

an overview: MOUTHGUARDS

Chapter 12

Upon delivery, take some time to discuss how to wear, clean and store the appliance. The mouthguard should be kept moist to maintain its flexibility and resilience. After use, it should be scrubbed with a toothbrush and placed in a container.

The patient should be aware that exposure to heat or pressure may permanently deform the mouthguard appliance. This may occur if the mouthguard is squashed in the bottom of a player's sports bag, left in a hot car, or out in direct sunlight. Even with excellent care, mouthguards will need to be replaced every two years as they lose their reliance and flexibility. In the growing patient, mouthguards should be replaced at least every year.

Many doctors supply mouthguards for their patients at cost because of their effectiveness as a marketing tool. Some practice-building ideas others have found effective are:

- offer this service to local gyms and sports clubs.

- become a school dentist.

- give talks to community service clubs i.e. P.T.A., Rotary.

- make service available to neighborhood sports teams.

- contact businesses such as martial arts studios, gymnastics schools, sporting goods stores and bike shops.

- cooperative coupons and flyers can be used to promote your mouthguard services to local businesses.

Design Notes

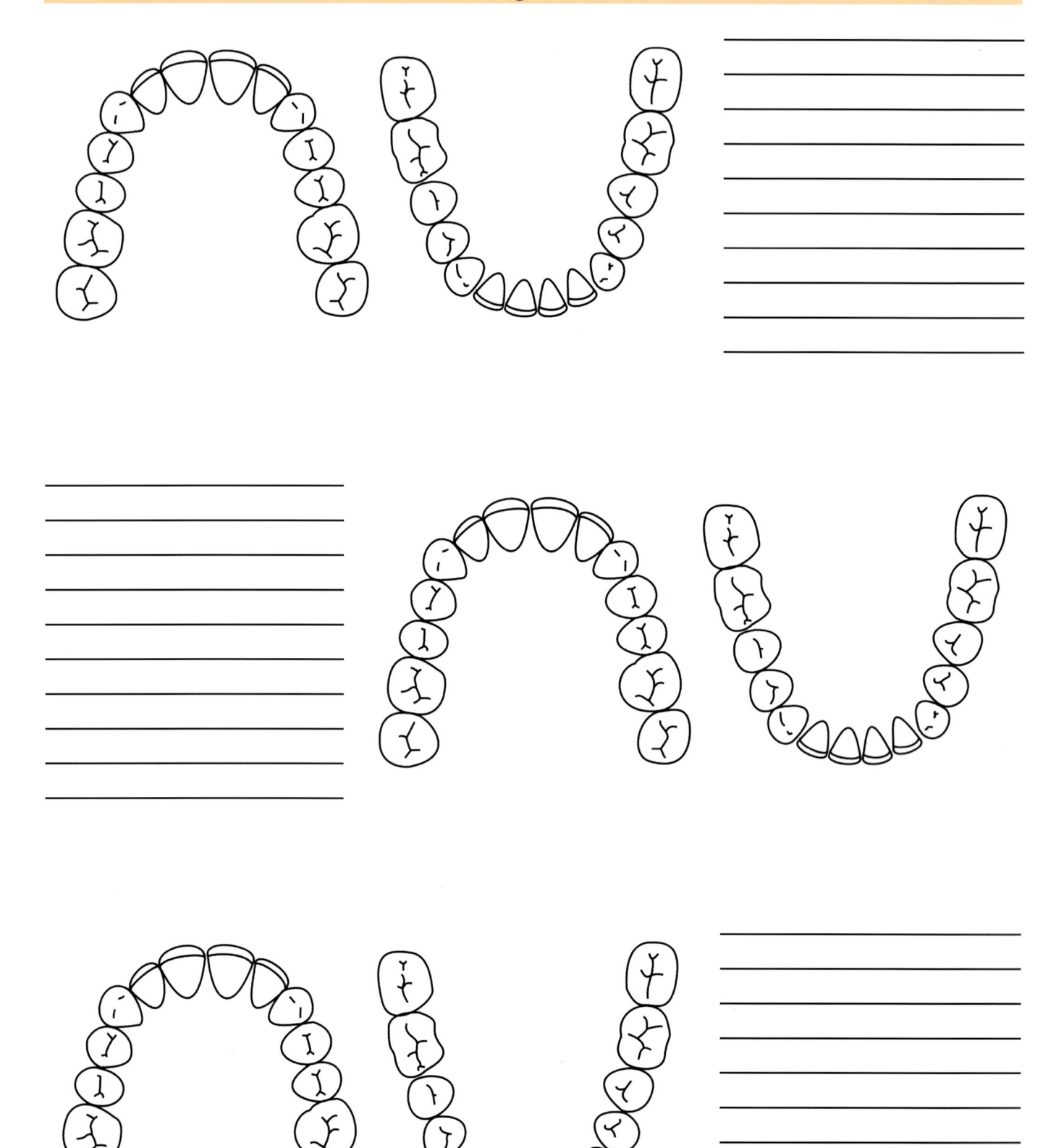

MOUTHGUARDS

The Intact™ All Sports Mouthguard

Heat/Pressure Laminated Thermoformed Mouthguards

This type of mouthguard is constructed on upper and lower models of the patient's teeth within close specifications of material, technique, machinery and design. Each mouthguard is fabricated with a special high heat/pressure-forming machine, under six atmospheres of pressure.

The advantages over all other mouthguards, including the vacuum-formed type, are:

- precise adaptation due to the increased pressure.

- negligible deformation when worn for prolonged periods of time. (There is no elastic memory when high-heat is combined with high pressure during fabrication.)

- ability to thicken any area as required because of the laminated ability of the machinery used.

- ability to customize for each sport, age and level of competition, orthodontics, mixed dentition, clefts, missing teeth, anatomical variations of occlusal Class I, II, III.

- ability to insert a hard polycarbonate layer between the soft ethyl vinyl acetate layers for additional protection against high velocity impact sports such as hockey and football.

- ability to achieve constant occlusal separation and proper occlusal balance necessary for concussion prevention.

- no interference with breathing and speech.

- individually designed to specifications predetermined through consultation of dentists, technicians, and sports professionals.

These multi-laminated mouthguards are now the treatment of choice for the ultimate in oral/facial athletic protection. During impact, this mouthguard will deliver the intended protection expected by the athlete. Shock absorption will occur and there will be an equal distribution and transfer of the impact forces throughout the mouthguard. Due to the correct occlusal coverage and thickness, bony structures of the head and neck, like the condyle, fossa and vertebrae, are protected, thereby minimizing the chance for concussion and other serious injuries.

Selecting the Correct Intact™ Mouthguard

All Intact™ Mouthguards are finished on articulated models to a balanced occlusion, creating the best protection for the joint and dentition.

Intact™ All Sports Mouthguards have four different designs, which are based on the parameters specified above. These designs follow immediately.

MOUTHGUARDS

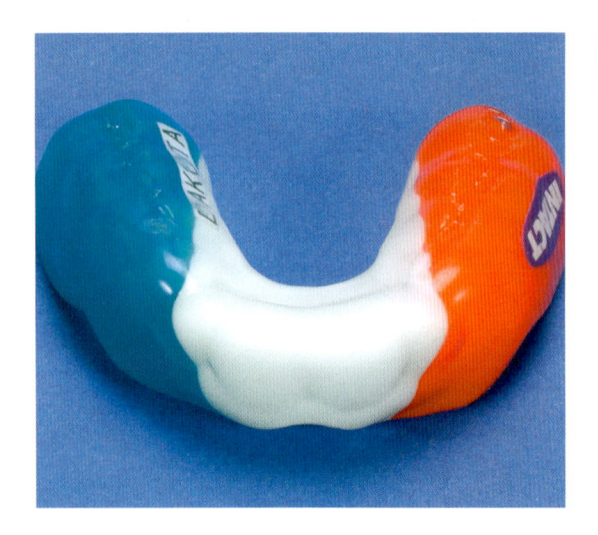

61401 The Intact™ Youth Mouthguard

The Intact Youth Mouthguard is recommended for athletes who are in primary and mixed dentition. Given all the pertinent information (i.e. sequence of exfoliation, type of orthodontic movement being accomplished) the mouthguards can be modified to allow for these changes.

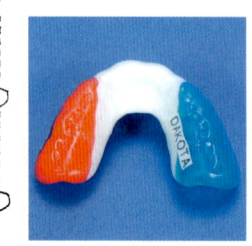

Because children's arches continue to change, it is necessary to have a guard that will provide an adequate amount of retention and protection, yet is inexpensive enough to be replaced throughout growth. This guard is usually 3-4 mm in thickness.

61402 The Intact™ Adult Mouthguard

The adult mouthguard is recommended for the majority of athletes with an adult dentition who are involved in recreational sports. This mouthguard is made to last. It is composed of 2-3 laminated sheets making it a thicker and stronger than the youthguard.

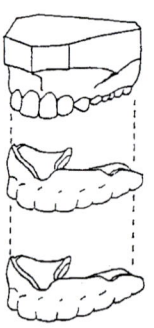

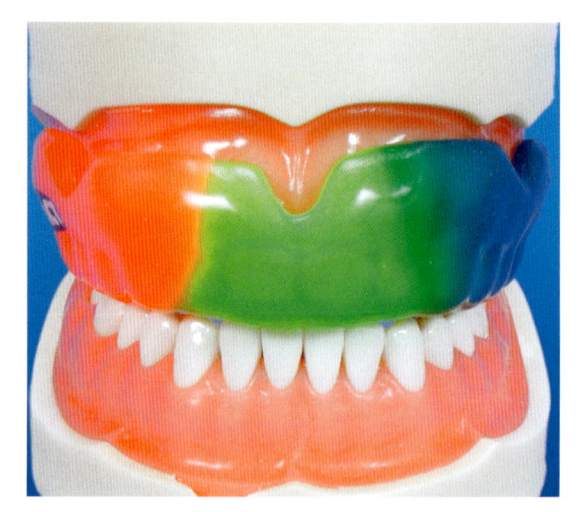

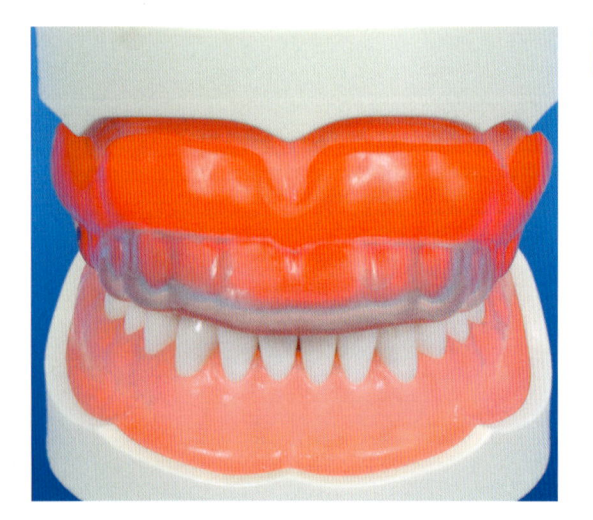

61403 The Intact™ Professional Mouthguard

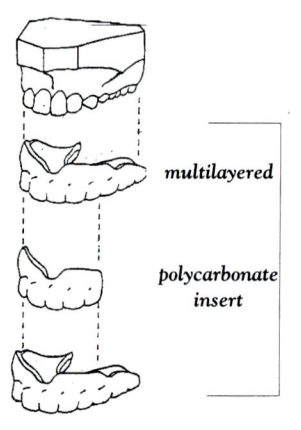

multilayered

polycarbonate insert

This guard is recommended for professional athletes and for anyone involved in a sport where hard impacts to the face and jaw are to be expected. Some examples are hockey, football, rugby and most racquet sports. These guards are multi-layered with a thin polycarbonate insert on the labial and buccal surfaces of the teeth. This extra protection is also needed for anyone who has a history of trauma.

MOUTHGUARDS

61404 The Intact Martial Arts Mouthguard

This guard is recommended for someone involved in any of the martial arts or boxing. Because these athletes often receive strong impacts to the face and jaw, a mouthguard must protect not only their teeth, but also their temporomandibular joint. With that purpose in mind, the Martial Arts guard is composed of three layers (9mm) to give these athletes the added protection they need.

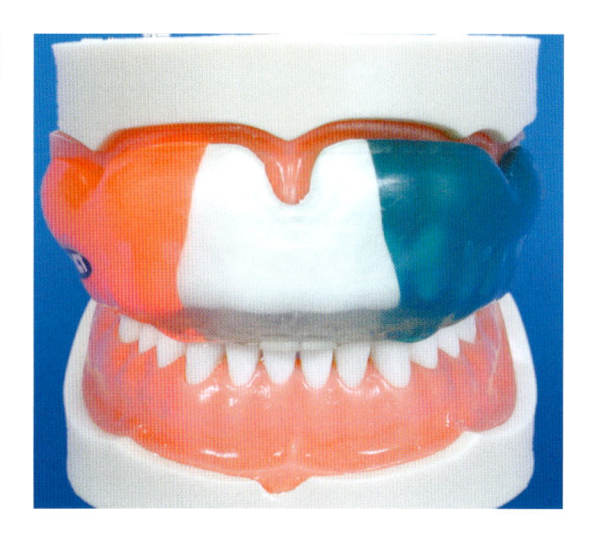

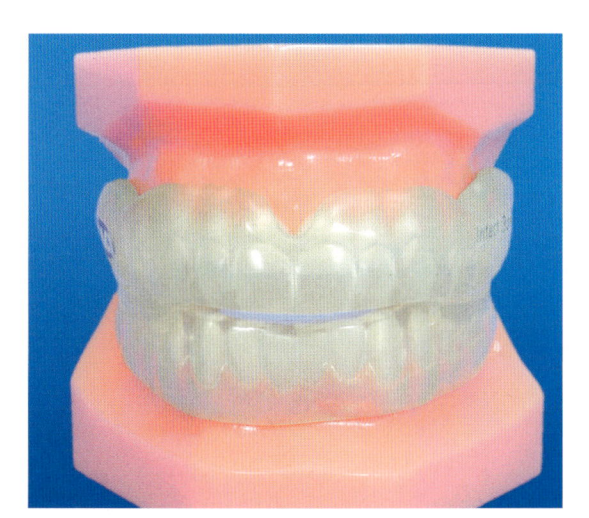

61409 Professional Boxer's Mouthguard

This guard is ideal for any athlete where intentional contact to the head or face is involved, such as boxing and martial arts. It is also recommended for any athlete with a prior history of multiple concussions, mandibular trauma and temporomandibular dysfunction. It is fabricated using two separate mouthguards laminated together at the mandibular relation provided by your properly taken construction bite.

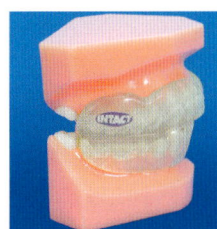

Color Availability

Many sports teams, especially those affiliated with schools, require that mouthguards be clearly visible so that it is obvious when the guard is being worn.

Intact Mouthguards are available in clear, yellow, blue, red, black, fluorescent orange, purple, fluorescent yellow, fluorescent green, white and pink.

Multi-color mouthguards (example: red, white & blue) are also available.

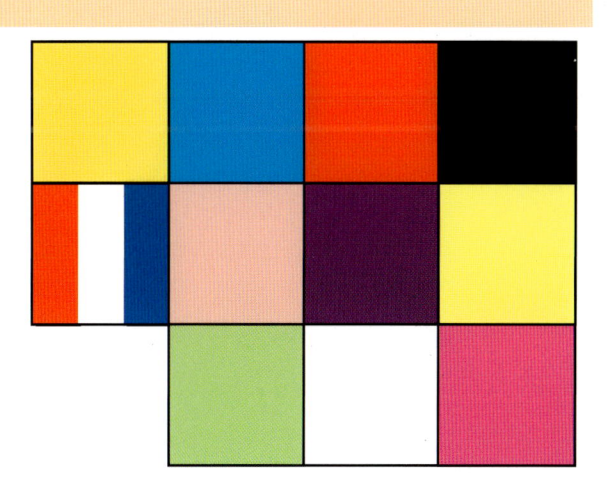

MOUTHGUARDS

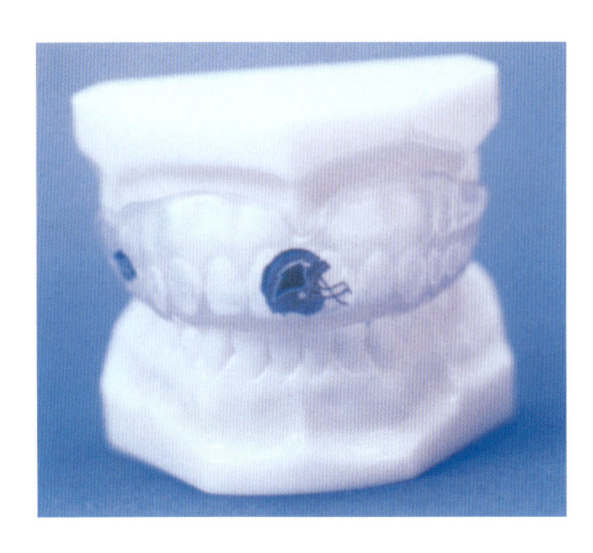

Team Logos & Helmet Straps

A team logo as shown here, patient name and even doctor's name and phone number are often added to these mouthguards.

Helmet Straps - Helmet straps are an unfortunate result of the poor fit inherent with "boil and bite" type mouthguards. Intact's superior, custom fit make the use of helmet straps unnecessary. Intact Mouthguards are so comfortable the athletes will be able to keep the mouthguards in place the entire game. However, should the use of a helmet strap be required by your sports organization, we'll be happy to add a breakaway strap to your Intact Mouthguard.

MOUTHGUARDS

62020 Pro-Form™ Mouthguard

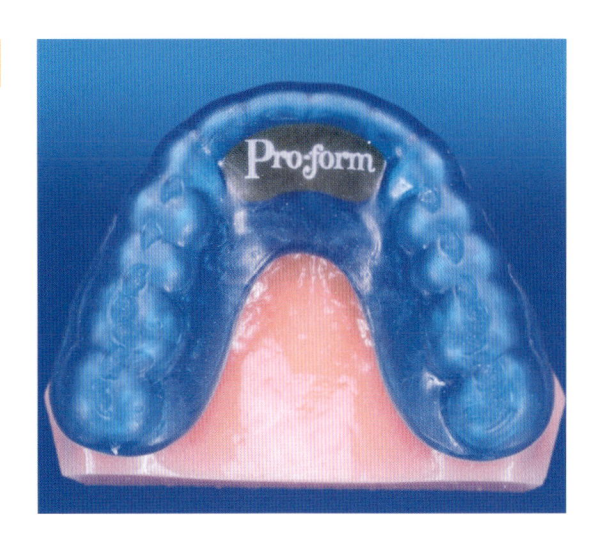

The Pro-Form™ laminated mouthguard is constructed of bonded sheets of injection molded, cross-woven vinyl, which provide strength and resistance to distortion. A palatal brace of hardened plastic is incorporated into the material behind the upper anterior teeth for added support and to transmit the shock of shear forces away from the area.

Increased resiliency helps minimize condylar fractures and/or possible concussion.

Pro-Form™ mouthguards may be ordered in clear, red, blue, green, orange, purple, black, and red/white/blue. Please call for a current selection.

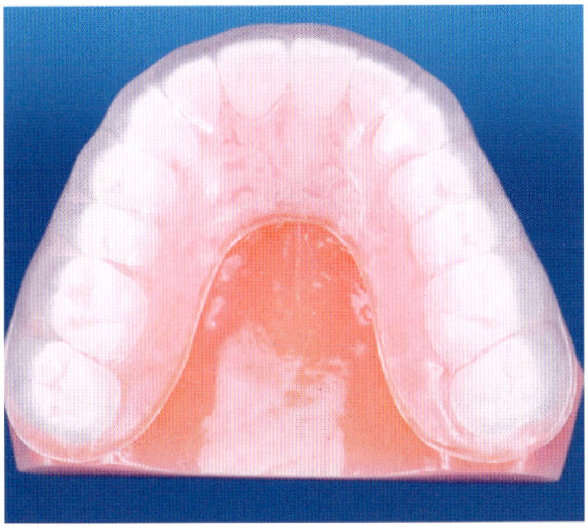

62010 Standard Mouthguard

Constructed of a soft polyethylene material, this appliance is usually custom molded to the maxillary arch to prevent oral trauma during contact sports. Other uses for this device include use as a tissue conditioning appliance for treating hyperplasia and as an excellent fluoride tray. It can also be used by bruxism patients when the usual hard acrylic splint cannot be tolerated.

62023 Pro-Form™ Mouthguard with Helmet Strap

The perfect fit of a custom mouthguard generally makes it so comfortable that patients typically do not find the need to remove it until the competition is over. However, when desired, the Pro-Form mouthguard and the standard #6201 mouthguard can be made with a helmet strap for fastening to a football helmet face guard bar. These straps have a built-in safety feature that allows them to break away under 12 pounds of strain. The straps come in the same colors as shown in #6202.

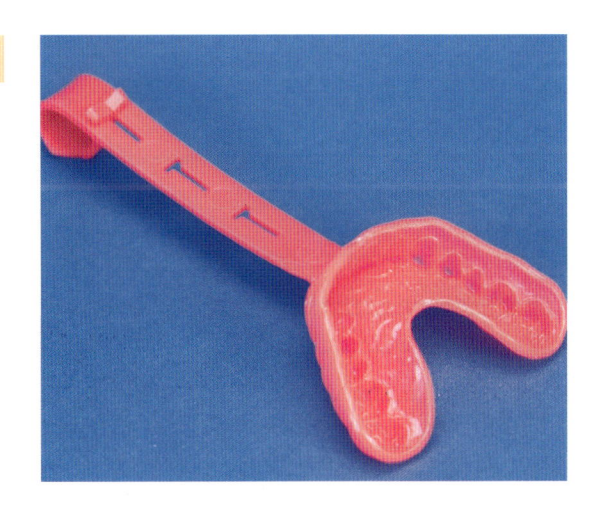

12.5

MOUTHGUARDS

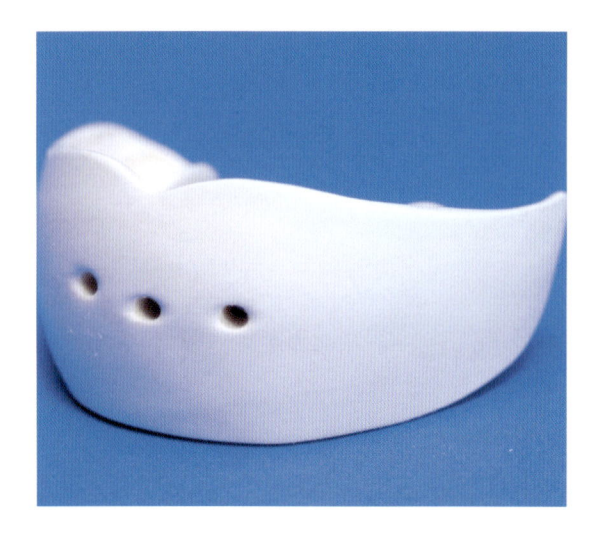

62080 Boxer's Mouthguard

This Mouthguard is designed as a single unit and covers both the upper and lower dentition. As the name implies, it is used primarily by boxers or any other direct contact sport. The anterior breathing holes are made as large as possible without reducing the protection to the anterior teeth.

Since this appliance is designed to protect the TMJ as well as the teeth, it is essential to provide a construction bite along with the models. The construction bite should not only open the vertical sufficiently to allow for breathing holes, it should also translate the lower arch forward slightly to compensate for mandibular flexion. If the bite is only opened vertically and the mandible is not adjusted slightly forward, it could possibly create a "glass jaw" syndrome for the Boxer.

Design Notes:

SPLINTS

an overview: SPLINTS

Chapter 13

Occlusal splints are removable appliances that are usually made of hard acrylic and fit over the occlusal surface of either the maxillary or mandibular dentition to create a precise occlusal relationship with the teeth of the opposing arch. These appliances are some of the most versatile tools used in dentistry. A properly designed splint can:

- break up doodling patterns and cover any facets of wear.
- protect the teeth from abnormal forces that may create a tooth fracture or breakage of restorations.
- protect the bony and soft tissue supportive structures against abnormal forces that would cause their breakdown.
- introduce an optimum occlusal position.
- deprogram the musculature and reorganize neuromuscular reflex activity.
- encourage normal muscle function.
- alleviate any occlusal stresses to the posterior teeth by providing anterior guidance.
- establish a new vertical relationship.
- alleviate occlusal stresses to the anterior teeth by controlling the vertical dimension.
- provide the teeth with protection from diurnal and nocturnal bruxism.
- provide a more stable or functional joint position.

As our society becomes more complex, the incidence of the Bruxism and Temporomandibular Joint Dysfunction seems to be on the increase. Nocturnal Bruxuism may be the most destructive form of bruxism because the patient is not aware of the habit until it is to late. Temporomandibular Joint Dysfunction is an extremely complex problem that effects a large percentage of the population.

Although a wide variety of treatment approaches and appliance designs are available for the treatment of these disorders, the most common appliance is a splint. A splint can protect the patient against the destructive forces of nocturnal bruxism and act as a diagnostic and treatment tool in the management of Temporomandibular Joint Dysfunction. Regardless of the treatment technique, early intervention can prevent many of the severe problems associated with Bruxism and TMJ dysfunction.

Before treating either of these problems, an accurate history and examination is vital to a sound diagnosis as breakdown in the system may occur at the level of the teeth in the form of wear, the periodontium in the form of mobility or the TMJ in the form of muscle spasms or splinting.

This examination should include radiographic information (FMX, Panorex, Cephalogram, Tomograms), a physical exam that includes palpation of the muscles, listening to the joint sounds, watching the mandible during functional movements, and a thorough investigation of the timing and duration of the pain. To do this the clinician must have a thorough understanding of the anatomy of the TMJ, including the muscles of mastication, ligaments, and mandibular movements.

Regardless of whether you are treating a bruxism problem or a joint disorder, splint therapy is almost always your first line of defense. This is because they are generally reversible, non-invasive and very effective at reducing symptoms.

an overview: SPLINTS

Chapter 13

Splints also act as an excellent diagnostic tool, as their very presence can alter some of the etiologic factors of Temporomandibular Joint Dysfunction. For example when a malocclusion is suspected of contributing to joint pain, a splint can quickly and reversibly introduce a more optimum occlusal condition.

There are several varieties of splints. Each design is aimed at eliminating a specific causative factor. To select the right splint, you must first identify the proper factor. Therefore the importance of a thorough history, exam and diagnosis cannot be overemphasized.

Splints are generally classified according to their intended function. The two most common types of splints are the disengaging/occlusal correcting splints, and mandibular or anterior repositioning splints.

The disengaging splints eliminate chronic and acute malocclusion and induce relaxation of the masticatory muscles. This is accomplished by introducing an optimum occlusal position that allows a reorganizing of the neuromuscular reflex activity and a deprogramming of the musculature.

Mandibular repositioning splints are used to prevent the disc-condyle complexes from returning to the fully occluded position, or to set the condyles in a more favorable condyle disc relationship in the fossa so that normal function can be established.

Some techniques require a smooth bite plane, while others call for having the occlusal facets ground into the completed splint. Still, others call for a cuspid rise or anterior guidance inclines.

Design Notes

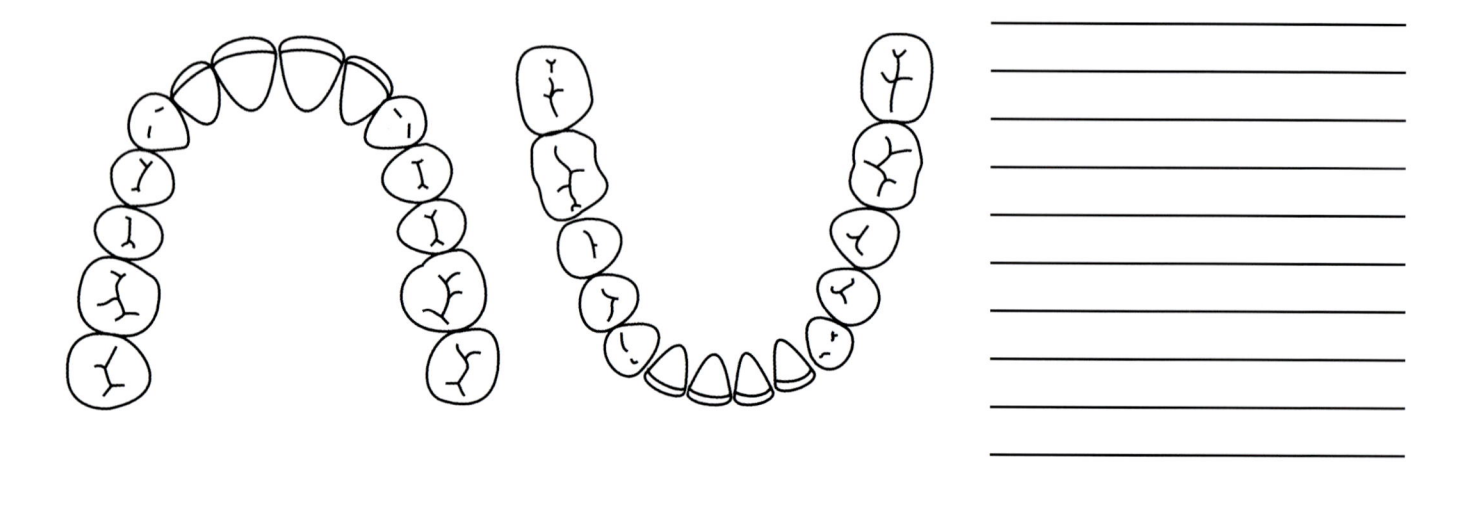

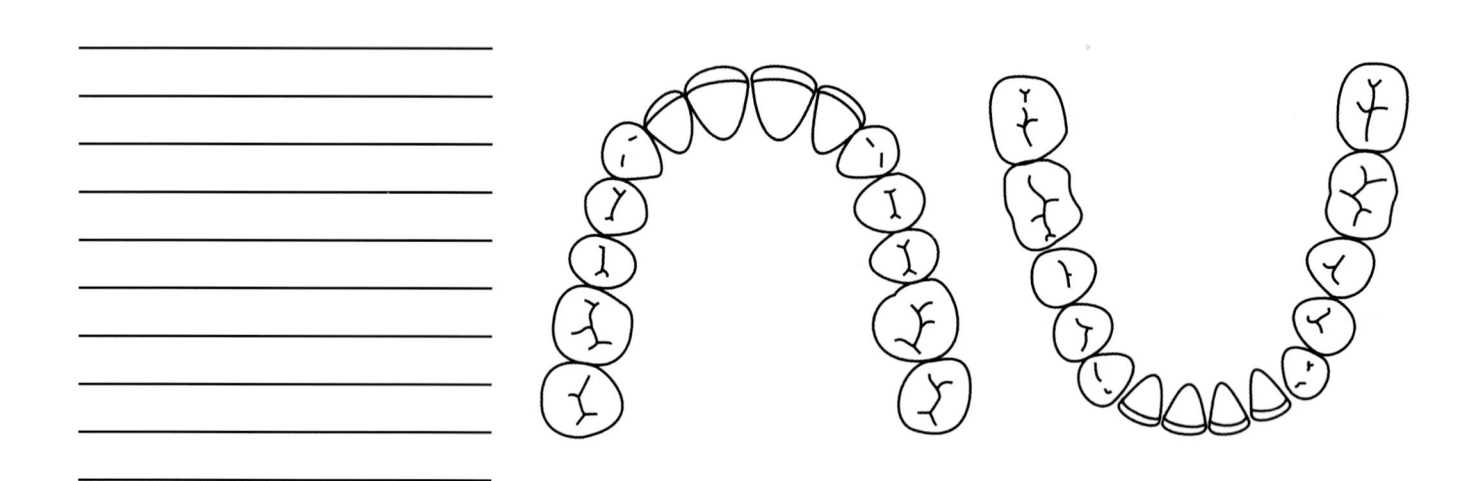

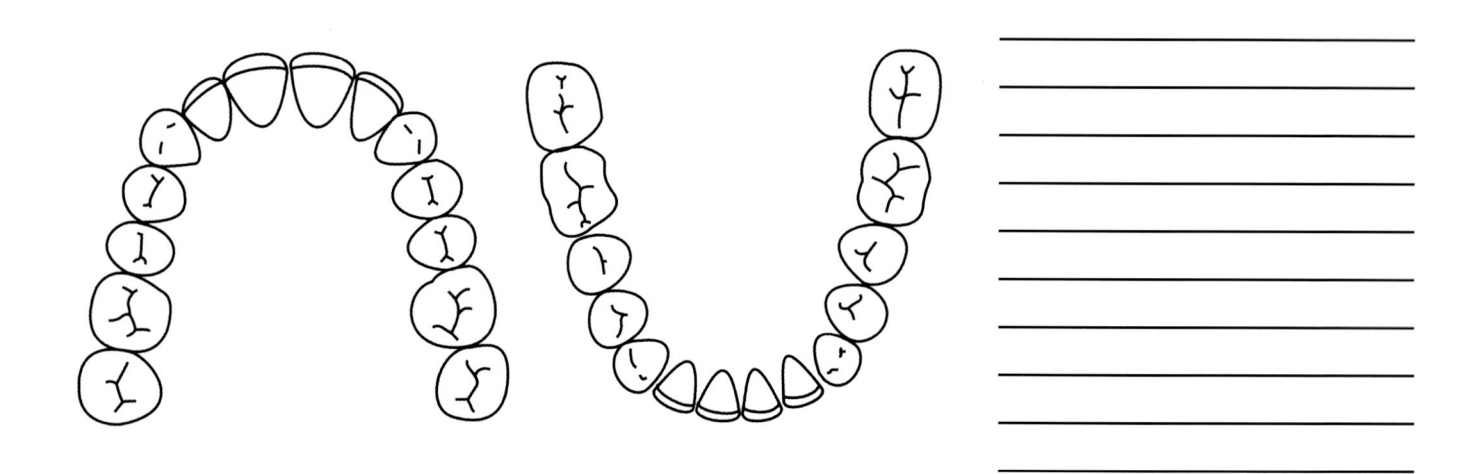

SPLINTS

Disengaging and/or Occlusal Correcting Splints

6191 Full Palate Maxillary Bruxism Splint   U

Splints are valuable tools used to distribute forces, decrease occlusal trauma and protect against excess tooth mobility due to primary or secondary occlusal trauma. Over 80% of the splints made are maxillary splints.

This design has clear acrylic over the entire arch and is finished with full palatal coverage. The palatal coverage provides extra stability when tooth mobility is an issue. The occlusal surface can be finished in whatever manner desired, i.e. smooth with point contact, positive facets for opposing dentition, cuspid rise, and/or anterior guidance to disarticulate the teeth in protrusive movements.

Note - Careful finishing is required so that each opposing tooth will make equal contact with the acrylic biting surface. To avoid unnecessary chair time adjusting a splint, always provide the lab with an accurate set of working casts and a construction bite that precisely represents the vertical and horizontal occlusal relationship that you want in the final product.

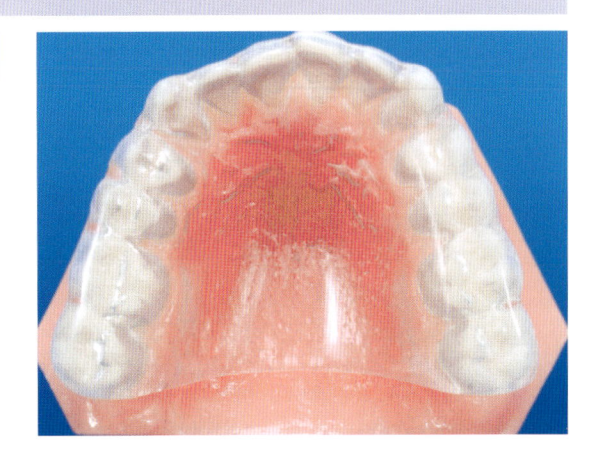

6193 Maxillary Horseshoe Splint   U

This bruxism splint is palate-free. Although it is not as strong as the full palatal appliance, the open palate design is much more comfortable and allows the patient's tongue to sit in its normal rest position.

Simply put, greater patient comfort leads to better compliance. A twisted stainless steel reinforcement wire is carefully placed across the lingual anterior position of the appliance for added strength. The occlusal surface can be finished in whatever manner desired, i.e. smooth with point contact, positive facets for opposing dentition, cuspid rise, and/or anterior guidance to disarticulate the teeth in protrusive movements.

Note - Careful finishing is required so that each opposing tooth will make equal contact with the acrylic biting surface. To avoid unnecessary chair time adjusting a splint, always provide the lab with an accurate set of working casts and a construction bite that precisely represents the vertical and horizontal occlusal relationship that you want in the final product.

13.1

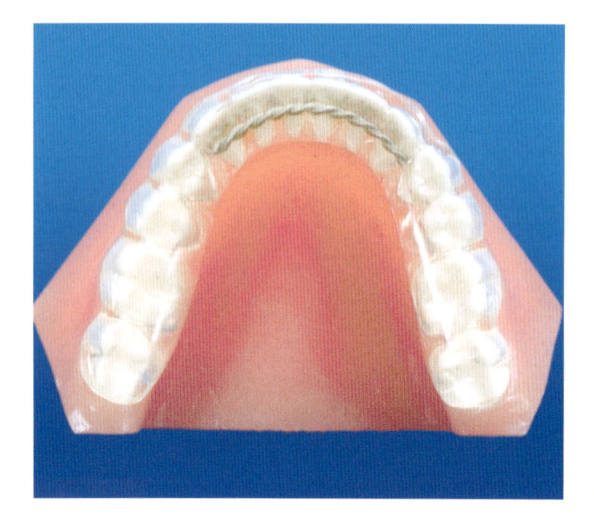

SPLINTS

6192 Mandibular Bruxism Splint   L

The design shown here is a basic mandibular splint typically used for bruxism protection. The occlusal surface is finished smooth with the opposing dentition making equal point contact. Just like a maxillary splint, the occlusal surface can be finished smooth with point contact, with positive facets for opposing dentition, with cuspid rise, and/or anterior guidance to disarticulate the teeth in protrusive movements. A twisted stainless steel wire is placed lingual to the anteriors to add additional strength to the appliance.

Note - Careful finishing is required so that each opposing tooth will make equal contact with the acrylic biting surface. To avoid unnecessary chair time adjusting a splint, always provide the lab with an accurate set of working casts and a construction bite that precisely represents the vertical and horizontal occlusal relationship that you want in the final product.

1163 Oakes Splint   U

The Oakes Splint is specifically designed to stop a patient's clenching or grinding habit. It works by using a maxillary lingual anterior bite plane that is built up so that only the lower incisors contact the acrylic. Placing all of the clenching forces on the anteriors initiates the nociceptive trigeminal inhibition response and inhibits the temporalis muscles from making strong contractions. Leaving the posteriors completely out of occlusion not only protects the dentition from damage due to bruxism, but leads to the reduction or total elimination of the clenching and grinding habit.

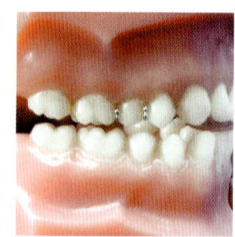

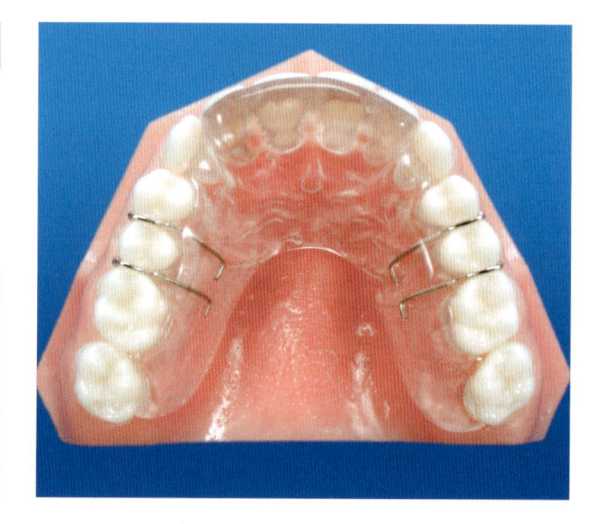

Note - This appliance fits the upper arch like a retainer and is held in place by bilateral ball clasps. The palatal acrylic is finished in a horseshoe shape for patient comfort.

Design Notes:

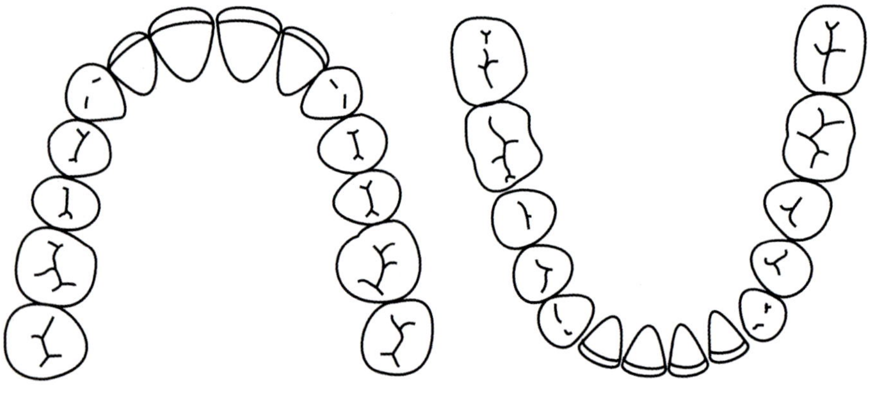

SPLINTS

6191N   Maxillary Anterior Night Splint   U

The design of this appliance is similar in concept to the Oakes Splint. By using Crozat Clasps on the bicuspids, this appliance can be reduced significantly in overall size by eliminating the need for palatal acrylic. Since only the lower incisors contact the acrylic anterior block, the patient will not be able to clench due to the nociceptive trigeminal inhibition response. The anterior portion of this appliance can be left flat or built up at the mid-line so that only the lower centrals initially contact the acrylic.

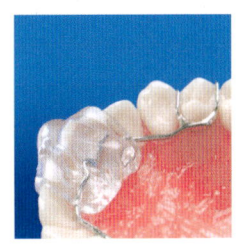

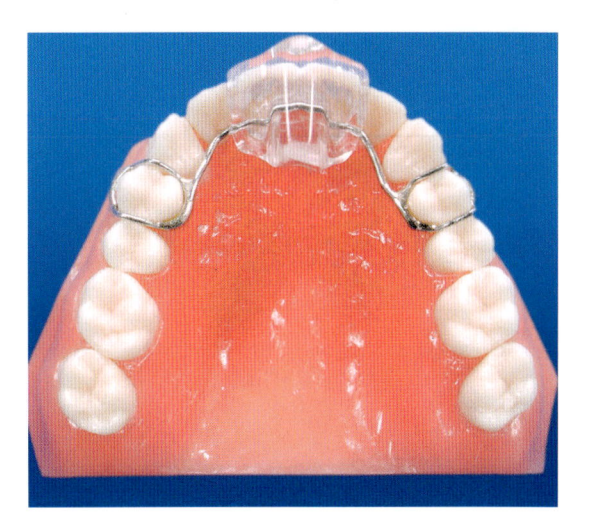

Caution - This appliance is meant for night time wear only.

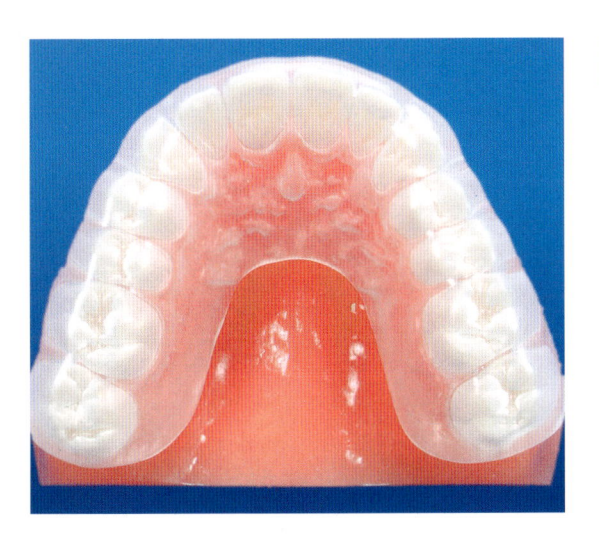

6131 Soft Nightguard   U/L

Soft splints have been advocated for patients who cannot tolerate wearing a hard acrylic splint, but still need some protection. They are believed to be particularly useful when treating those who suffer from repeated or chronic sinusitis that results in extremely sensitive posterior teeth. This soft splint is constructed from bonded sheets of injection-molded, cross-woven vinyl, which provides extra strength and resistance to distortion.

Note - If a parafunctional activity like bruxism is initiated by an occlusal condition, it is unlikely that a soft splint would improve this condition. In fact many clinicians believe that a soft material will only enhance any abnormal frictional forces created during function. Another reason not to use this material as a splint is that it is almost impossible to adjust.

Design Notes:

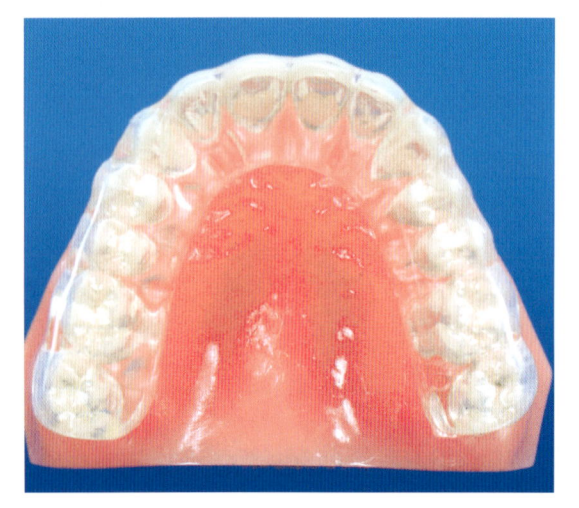

SPLINTS

6196 Talon™ Splint   U/L

Although it often takes numerous appointments to get a hard splint to be comfortable, a soft splint is usually not an acceptable alternative because it cannot be adjusted at all. By choosing a Talon™ splint you can combine the best features of a hard splint and a soft splint while eliminating the inherent disadvantages of either type. The portion of the appliance that covers the buccal, labial, and lingual surfaces is made of a soft, thermoplastic, resilient polymer. At body temperature this material is flexible, but firm. It provides superior retention without creating any forces that can cause the teeth or tissues to become sore. Using this material should also eliminate the need for any internal adjustments.

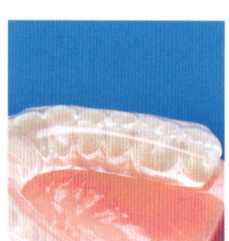

The occlusal surface of the appliance is made of hard acrylic that is chemically bonded to the thermoplastic material. Having a hard acrylic occlusal surface allows the splint to be adjusted as needed. The Talon™ appliance design can be utilized for all splint techniques (i.e., Gelb, MORA, May, etc.).

6194 Protective Splint U/L

The protective splint is a simple, inexpensive, vacuum formed appliance that can be used on either the maxillary or mandibular arch. Because it is vacuum formed, the occlusal facets are automatically duplicated in the appliance.

Due to the thin nature of the material, a minimum bite opening of 1 to 2mm is possible. This is important for those patients who cannot tolerate a significant change in their vertical dimension. However, because it is thin, it will not hold up under excessive bruxing forces.

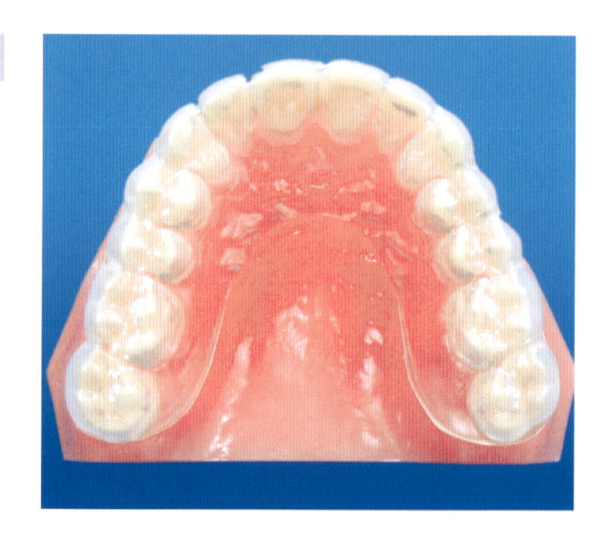

Design Notes:

SPLINTS

T.M.J. Splints - Disengaging

6204 May T.M.J. Splint   L

The May Splint is a mandibular splint that is designed to disengage the patient's habitual occlusal relationship. This splint is usually designed to only allow contact to occur in the first molar region. By using this splint to relieve dental stress, proponents of this technique have been successfully treating a variety of symptoms throughout the body. Advanced study of the technique seems to be a prerequisite to optimum results with this appliance.

The design of this appliance utilizes a lingual acrylic reinforcement with a twisted stainless steel strengthening wire to support the occlusal pads. The lingual anterior acrylic is finished up against the incisors at the level of the cingulum providing added support and increasing the strength of the appliance. Interproximal ball clasps can be added for retention as needed.

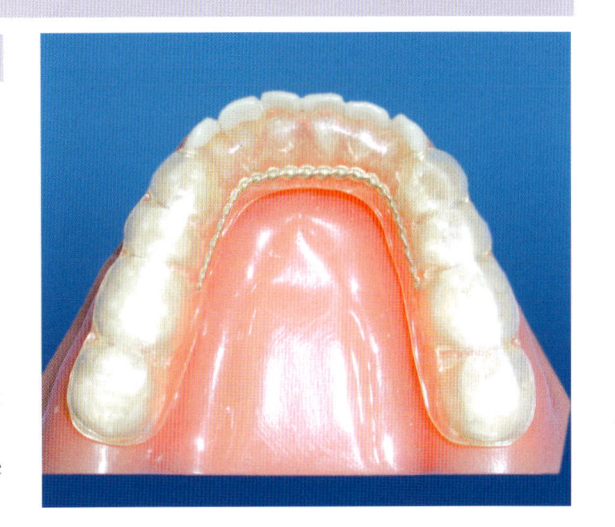

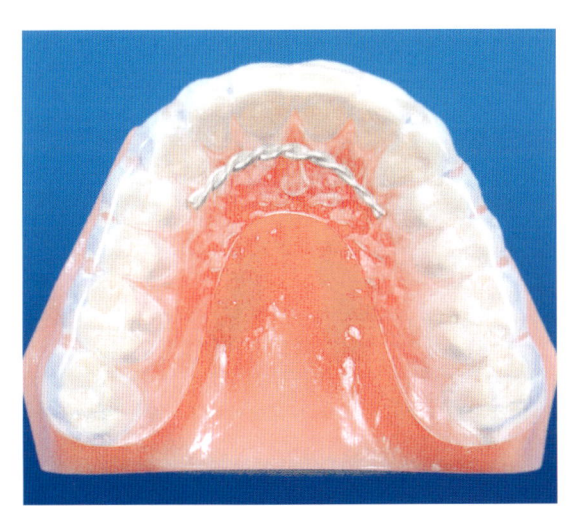

6207 Superior Repositioning Splint   U

This maxillary appliance is a simple disengaging splint that increases the patient's vertical dimension. It provides centric stops for the lower posterior buccal cusp tips and has an anterior ramp that provides incisal guidance and cuspid protection. It is primarily used to treat joint pain in the absence of TMJ clicking.

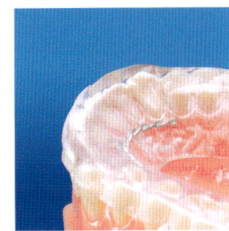

Design Notes:

13.5

SPLINTS

T.M.J. Splints - Repositioning

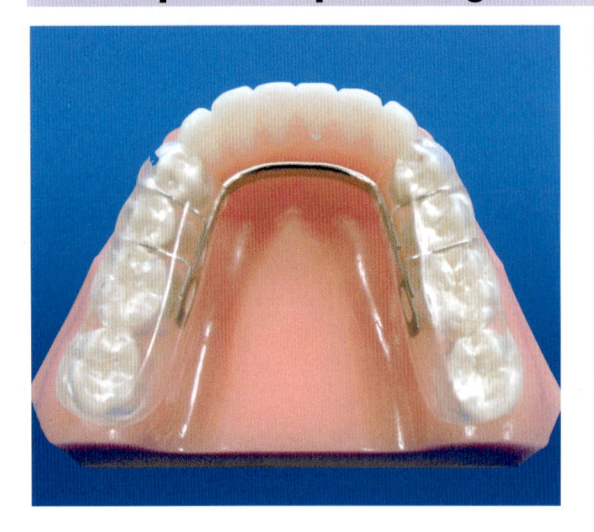

6203 MORA Appliance   L

The MORA appliance, as described by Dr. Gelb, is designed to reposition the mandible to achieve neuromuscular balance and an optimal condylar-fossae relationship. MORA stands for Mandibular Orthopedic Repositioning Appliance. Advanced study in treating temporomandibular joint dysfunction is a prerequisite to achieve optimum results with this appliance.

The appliance itself is simple and elegant. It consists of clear acrylic bite pads covering the molars and bicuspids connected by a heavy, oval lingual bar. Usually the laboratory furnishes the basic appliance with minimal occlusal coverage and the operator establishes the correct neuromuscular and optimal condylar-fossae relationship directly on the patient using cold cure acrylic. Through use of a Verticulator and a very precise wax construction bite, it is possible to complete the entire appliance in the laboratory. (See Appliance #6205)

Note - Besides being used to treat TMJ pain and dysfunction, there has been much interest of late in the use of the repositioning appliance to release or enhance strength in athletes.

6205 MORA/Gelb with Anatomical Occlusion   L

The general design of this appliance is similar to the #6203 MORA appliance with one important difference. Through use of a Verticulator and a very precise wax construction bite that alters the patient's mandibular position, the occlusal surface is finished with a very precise anatomical cusp/fossa contour. The anatomical occlusal finish allows the patient to function normally at the new position. This device is to be worn at all times, even while eating. If desired, the anteriors can also be covered with acrylic.

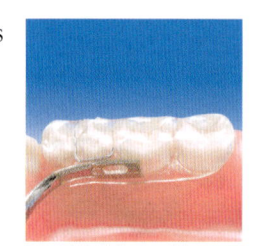

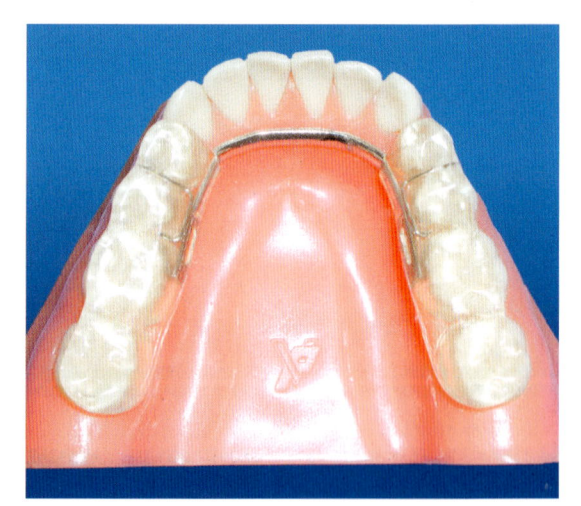

SPLINTS

6206 Anterior Repositioning Splint or Pull Forward Splint   U

This appliance, with an anterior inclined ramp, is typically used when there is a definite clicking in the temporomandibular joint. It is designed to recapture an anteriorly displaced disc. The altered mandibular position is maintained by an upper inclined anterior ramp which rests lingual to the lower anteriors, while the upper occlusal coverage is indexed heavily to accept the lower buccal cusp tips.

An accurate "construction bite" is essential for proper fabrication of this appliance.

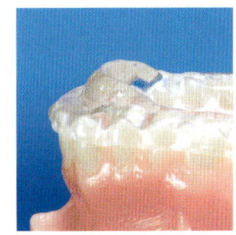

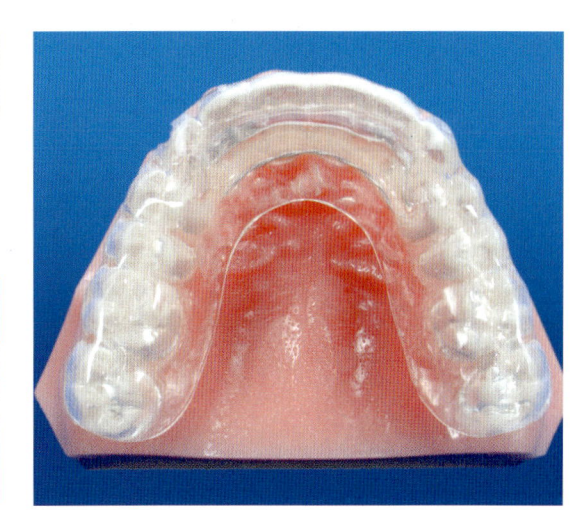

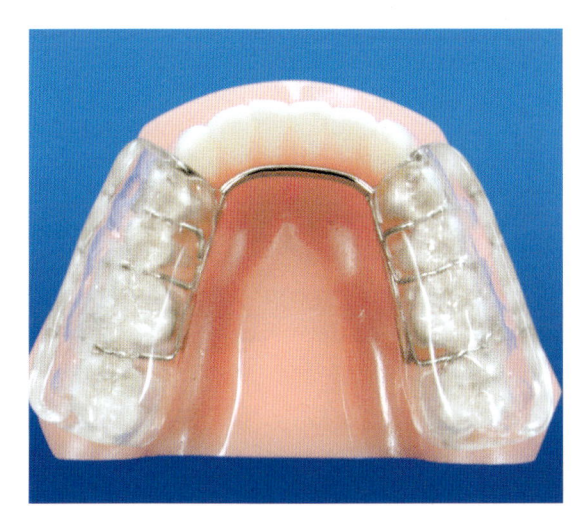

6203F   The FACT Appliance   L

The FACT Appliance is designed to reposition the condyle and decompress the joint space to provide pain relief and allow the battered bilaminar zone and shredded supportive connective tissue of the joint time to heal over a period of months.

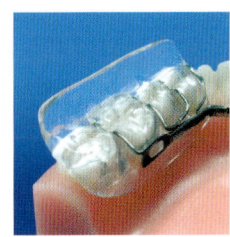

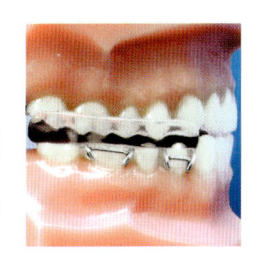

The appliance consists of two acrylic pads with high buccal walls, connected by a Gelb lingual bar. The high buccal walls limit lateral excursive motions of any kind permitting only rotational movement of the mandible.

Since the appliance is intended to be worn at all times, the use of buccal walls to stabilize the mandible is favored over lingual walls because the tongue is then free to move a bolus of food up onto the occlusal table of the splint during chewing.

In order to properly fabricate the FACT appliance, models, along with a construction bite that accurately represents the condyle in its therapeutic decompressed position, must be provided. Radiographic verification of this position should be accomplished prior to appliance fabrication.

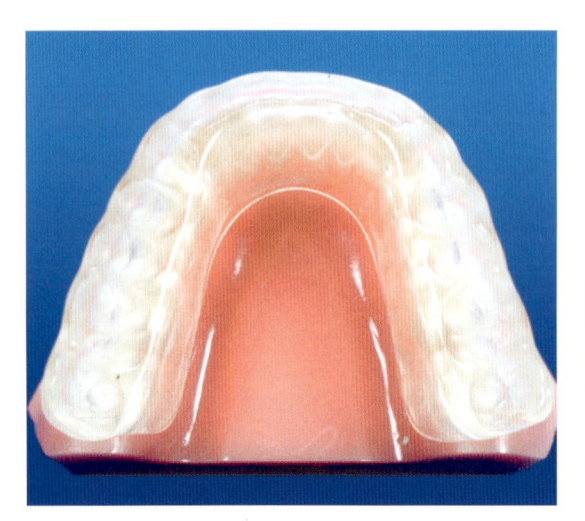

SPLINTS

6209 Levandoski Stabilization Prosthesis   L

The Levandoski Stabilization Prosthesis is a mandibular splint that is designed to precisely position the mandible and hold the condyles in the ideal physiologic position within the fossa. This position is predetermined with the use of precise radiographic records and special equipment.

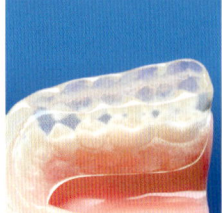

The first step in making this appliance is to mount accurate casts on the Levandowski Articulator. The unique design of this articulator allows for precise adjustments of the X, Y, and Z axes and gives you control of the anterior and posterior vertical dimension. Next, transcranials or tomograms of each joint are taken to precisely determine the position of the condyles in occlusion. Using these radiographs, a vector analysis is completed to determine the ideal physiologic position of the condyles. This information is then transferred to the articulator so that an occlusal record can be generated. Once the occlusal record is generated, new radiographs should be taken of the patient's joint with the occlusal record in place to confirm its accuracy prior to making the appliance.

The appliance itself is designed with high buccal and lingual walls of acrylic and an occlusal surface that is heavily indexed to the upper dentition, including all of the incisors and cuspids. This design assures the stability of the joint even during function as it is meant to be worn 24 hours a day.

6203W Modified Witzig Splint   L

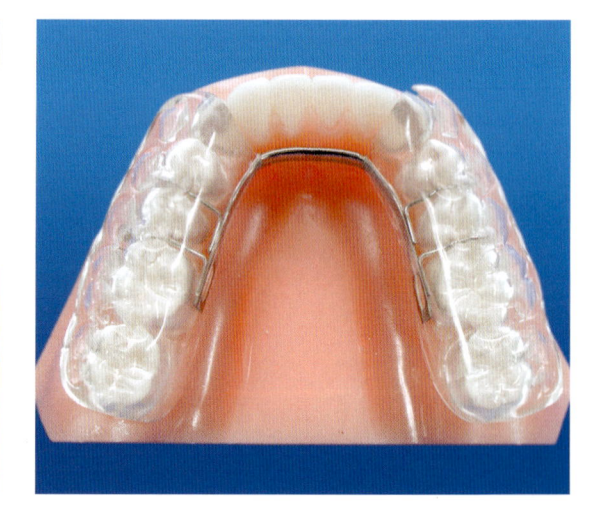

The Witzig Splint is a mandibular splint that is designed to precisely position the mandible and hold the condyles in the ideal physiologic position within the fossa. Like the Levandoski approach, the position is predetermined with the use of precise radiographic records and a unique articulator.

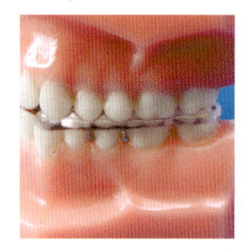

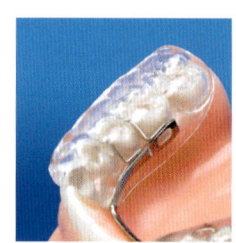

First, the Witzig/Denar articulator and face bow transfer are used to mount accurate casts. Then transcranials or tomograms of each joint are taken to precisely determine the position of the condyles in occlusion. Using these radiographs, a tracing along with measurements of the joint complex are completed to determine the ideal physiologic position of the condyles. This information is then transferred to the articulator so that an occlusal record can be generated at the ideal anterior and posterior vertical dimension. This position should be confirmed radiographically prior to making the appliance.

The actual appliance is a modification of the Mora/Gelb design. The occlusal surface is finished with positive indentations of the upper posteriors, capturing both the buccal and lingual cusps. Once the patient accommodates to the new position, the occlusal indentations can be reduced if desired.

SPLINTS

6205C Chan LVI Neuromuscular Orthotic   L

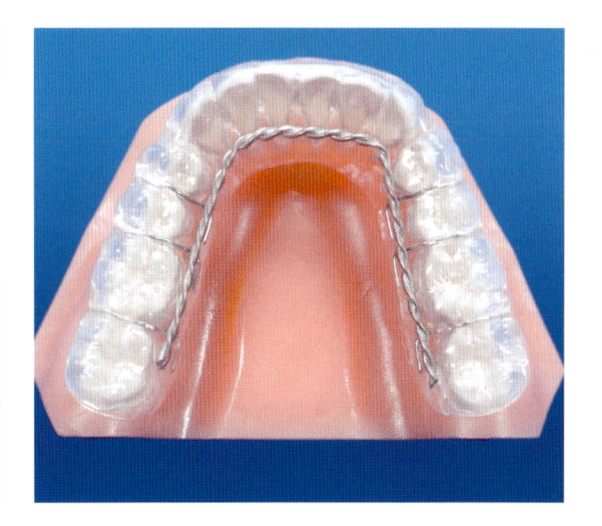

This neuromuscular orthotic is an anatomical mandibular appliance designed to orthopedically realign the mandible to the cranium, stabilizing the temporomandibular joints in six dimensions. This relationship is determined and acquired by the use of ultra low frequency TENS.

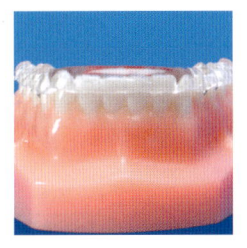

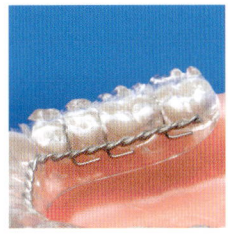

Diagnostic tests are further used to design and construct this appliance by use of accurate and objective data gathered through the use of Myotronic K6-I/K7 instrumentation using computerized mandibular scanning (CMS) and electromyography (EMG) which confirms physiologic resting musculature and mandibular trajectory in harmony with the TM Joints. A reinforcing lingual wire has been placed along with 6 interproximal ball clasps for added retention.

On delivery of this appliance, detailed micro-occlusion (coronoplasty) and fine proprioceptive refinement is required with TENS to establish a simultaneous terminal contact free of any interferences at the myocentric position.

Design Notes:

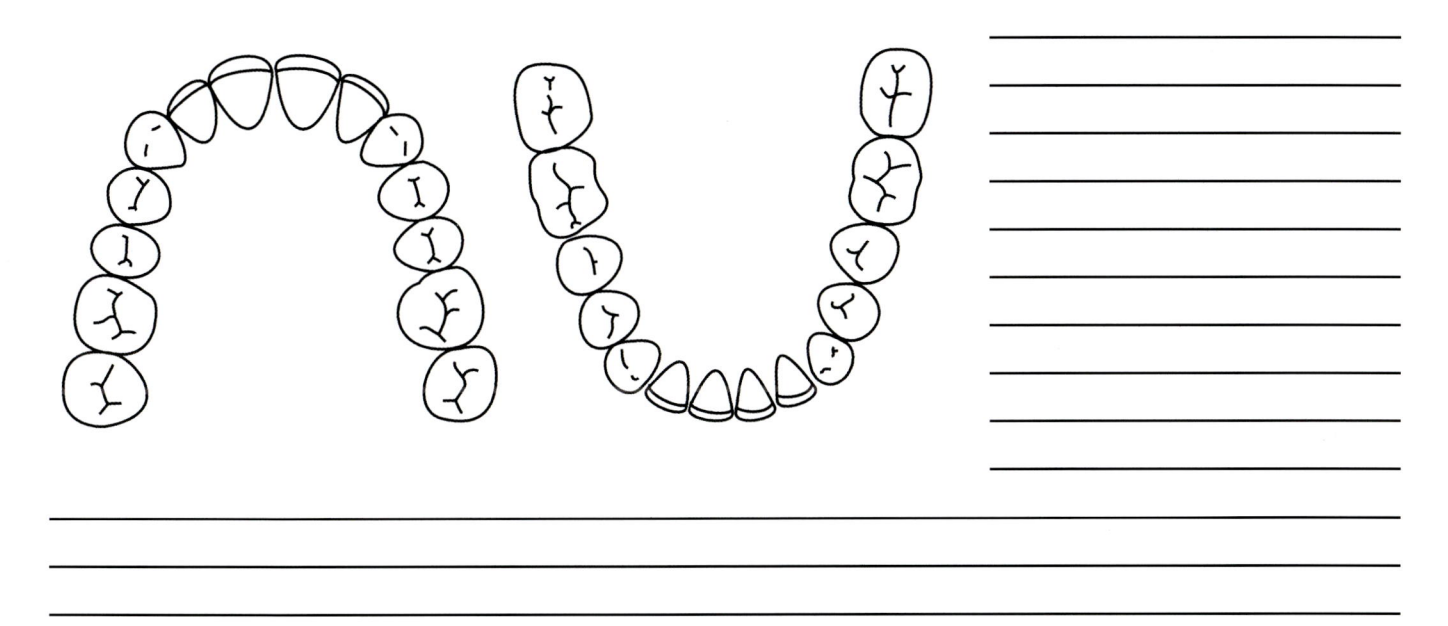

Design Notes

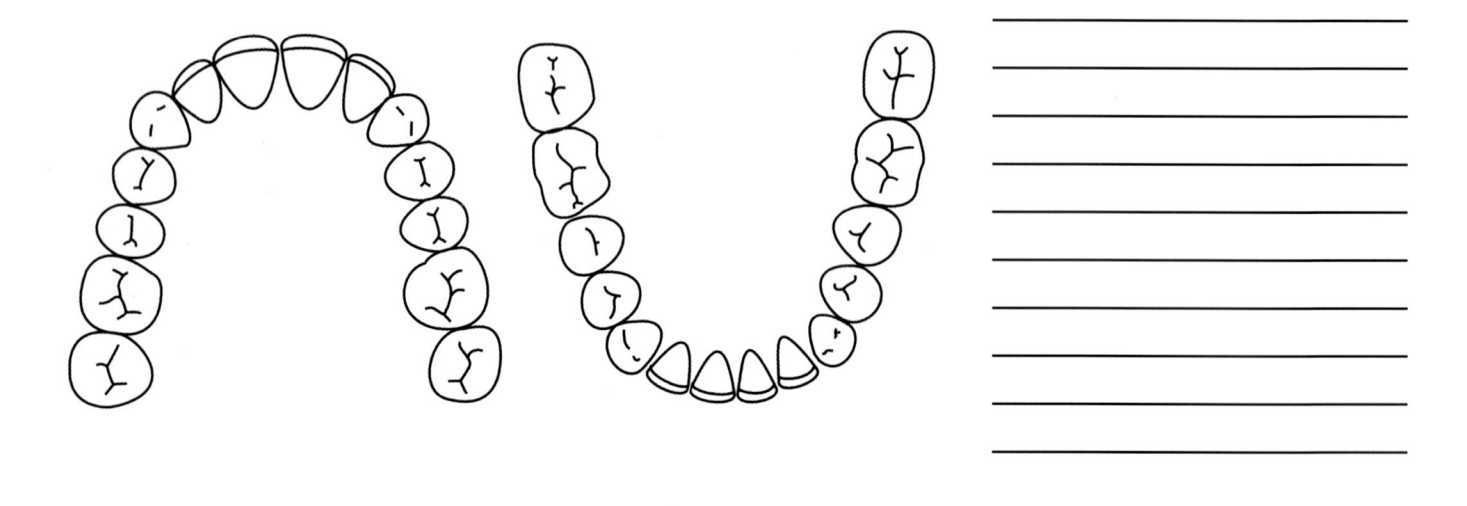

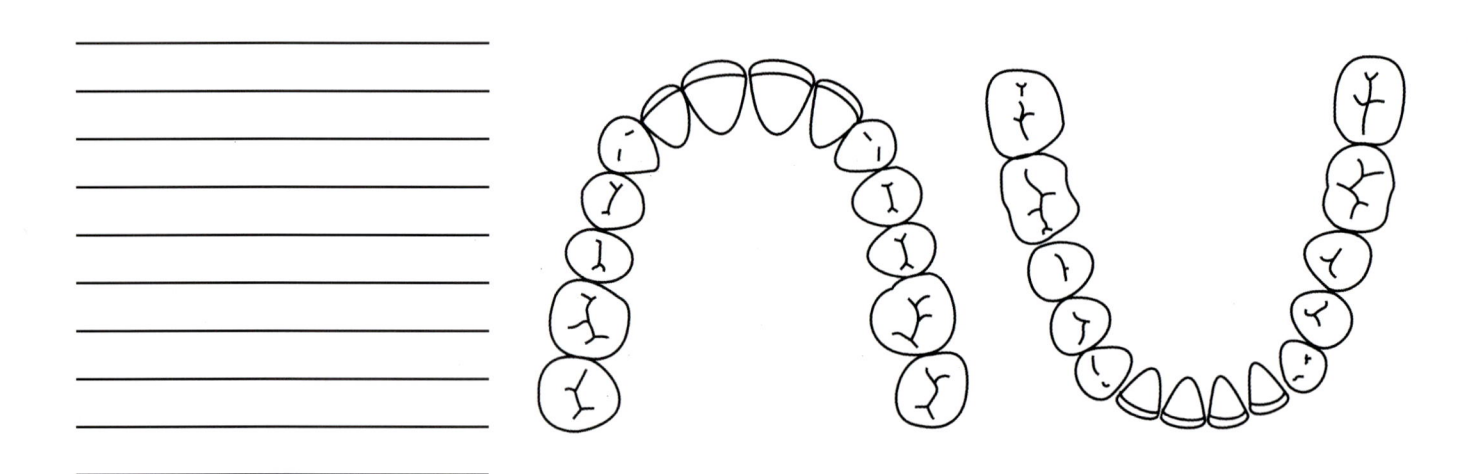

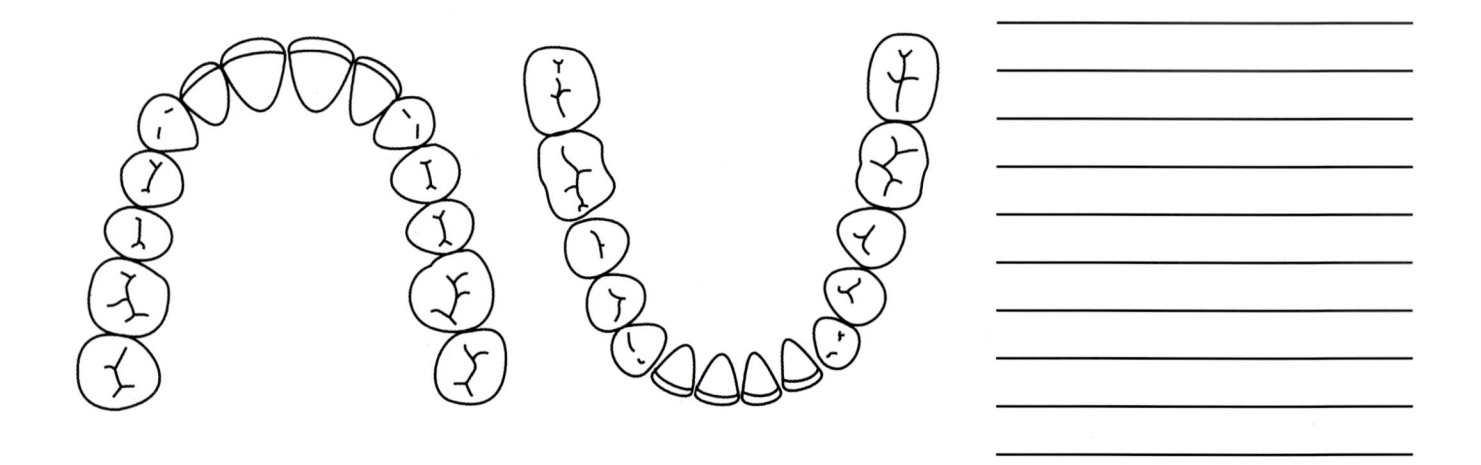

RESTORATIVE ENHANCEMENTS

an overview: RESTORATIVE ENHANCEMENTS

Chapter 14

One of the primary goals of restorative dentistry is to maintain excellent form, function, and esthetics. To offer our patients the best care possible, we must be capable of performing a variety of therapeutic approaches when trying to treat a difficult prosthetic situation. If we are not, the care we deliver will simply be compromised.

For example, an extraction followed by the placement of a bridge may appear to be your only choice for a tooth broken down below the bony crest. However, if you are able to incorporate a forced eruption technique in conjunction with periodontal surgery, this otherwise un-restorable tooth can be restored without sacrificing bone on the adjacent teeth or having to prepare them for a bridge.

It is hard to perform quality cosmetic dentistry without having the ability to move teeth. Today, our patients demand a cosmetic result, and in an effort to give them what they want, over preparation of teeth or "instant ortho" is too often performed. "Instant ortho" usually results in extremely thick veneers, and oversized crowns. You might mask their improper position and achieve a cosmetic result, but at what cost? Why compromise, when performing a small amount of tooth movement would allow you to achieve a superior outcome?

Simply put, a simple minor tooth movement procedure is often the difference between a successful prosthetic result and a failure. Teeth that are improperly positioned in the arch or have an abnormal axial inclination lead to:

- an inappropriate distribution of occlusal forces.
- an inadequate parallelism.
- a poor occlusal plane.
- a lack of interproximal space.
- adverse root proximity.
- faulty occlusal landmarks.
- excessive tooth preparation with potential pulpal involvement.
- inadequate pontic space.
- hard and soft tissue deformities of the periodontal structures.
- teeth that are more difficult to clean.
- bruxism and clenching habits.

The appliances in this chapter have been designed to help you re-establish the best restorative conditions possible, prior to starting your reconstruction procedures.

RESTORATIVE ENHANCEMENTS

1042 Removable Space Regainer   U/L

When a second bicuspid is congenitally missing or lost early, the first molar will often drift mesially. Placing a bridge without returning the molar to its ideal position will create abnormal forces on the molar that will eventually cause the bridge to fail.

By using a removable appliance with an expansion screw, you can easily return this tooth to its normal position in the arch and create the appropriate space needed for a properly sized pontic or implant.

This appliance is designed to utilize the rest of the arch as anchorage to support the forces created by the expansion screw as it moves the molar back into its normal position.

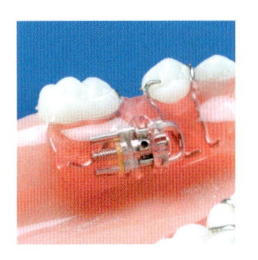

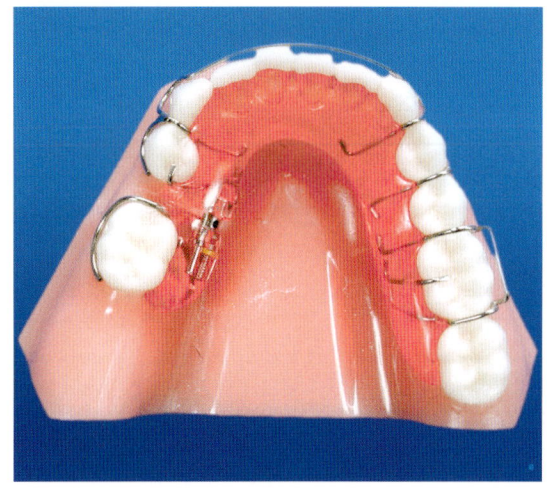

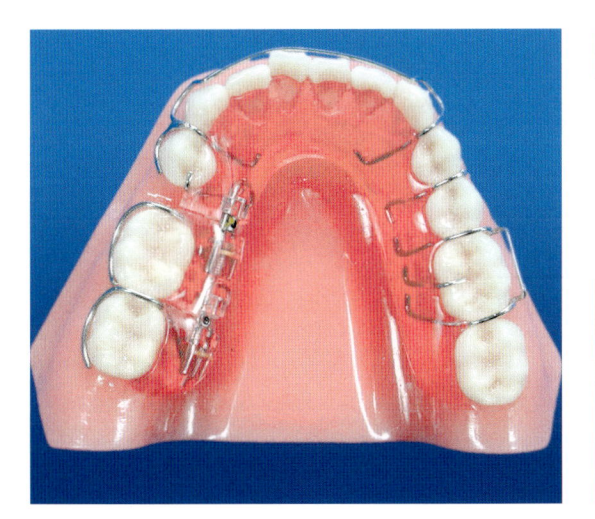

1042D Removable Molar Distalizer   U/L

To move two adjacent molars distally with a removable appliance, maximum anchorage must be utilized while each molar is moved individually. This can be accomplished with one appliance that has two screws aligned next to each other by sequentially turning the screws.

First, move the second molar by adjusting the distal most screw. Once you have achieved the desired distalization of the second molar, you may begin adjusting the mesial screw to distalize the first molar.

It is important to remember that as the mesial screw is opened one turn, the distal screw needs to be closed one turn. This will keep the second molar in its new position as the first molar is distalized to meet it.

Note - When distalizing both first and second molars, it is important to properly instruct the patient about the precise adjustment technique and sequence.

14.1

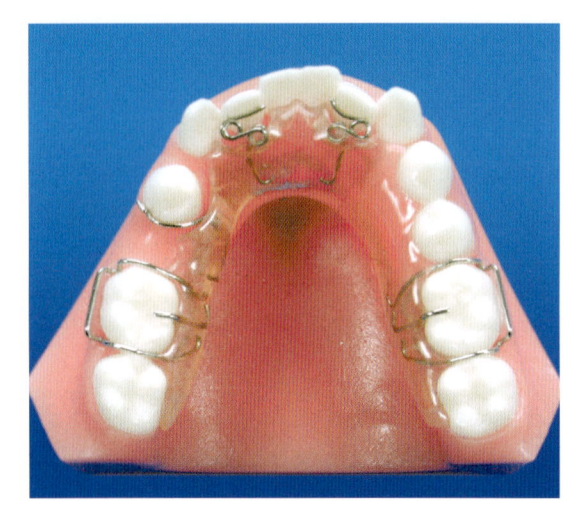

RESTORATIVE ENHANCEMENTS

4182 Lower Active Partial (any design)   L

Keeping the patient comfortable and functional while performing minor tooth movement procedures is the key to successfully treating adult patients.

In this example, a lower active partial with a mesial kicker spring is being used to move the left 1st bicuspid forward to create space for a fixed bridge or an implant. Finger springs are guiding the laterals labially after some light mesial-distal stripping has been done to gain the needed space for these anteriors, and two denture teeth are being used to maintain the space for the patient's 1st and 2nd right bicuspids. Clasps and rests are placed to stabilize the appliance and keep the patient comfortable. All of this can be accomplished with one well-designed appliance.

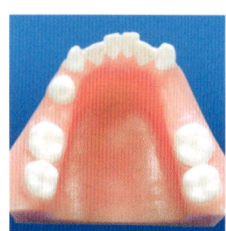

Note - For proper appliance construction, always send an opposing model and a bite registration.

4183B Upper Active Partial (any design)

This upper active partial sample was designed to treat a patient that has a peg lateral on the left side and a congenitally missing lateral on the right side. First and second bicuspids are also missing on the right side.

By using this simple appliance, space can be created for the replacement of the lateral on the right with either a bridge or an implant, and for the placement of a veneer on the left lateral.

This tooth movement is accomplished with the use of simple mesial and distal kicker springs. With an appliance like this, we are able to accomplish this essential minor orthodontic movement while still maintaining a functional occlusion.

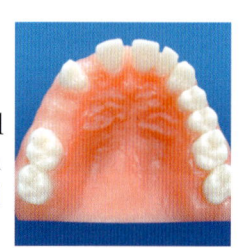

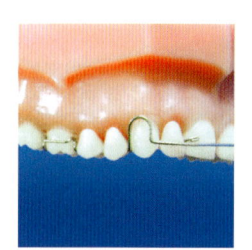

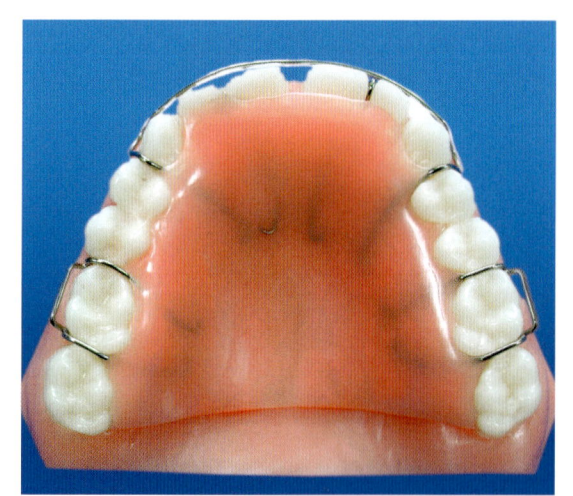

RESTORATIVE ENHANCEMENTS

1076 Multi-Spring Appliance - Mesial/Distal Anterior Positioning

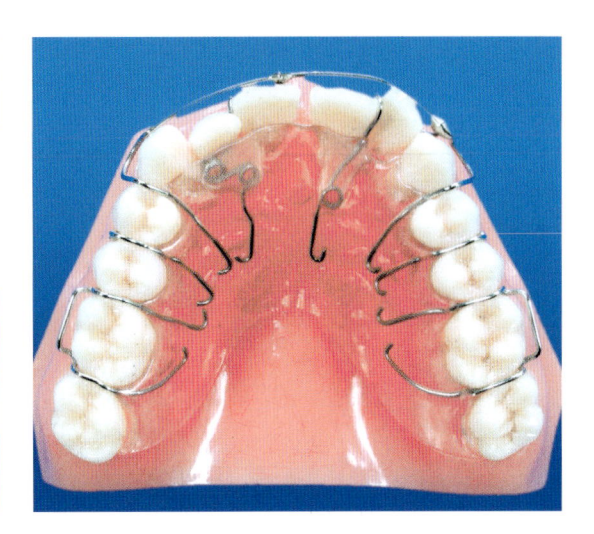

It is hard to perform cosmetic dentistry without having the ability to move teeth. Picture attempting to do veneers or crowns on this patient without first moving these teeth. The result would be extremely thick veneers, and oversized crowns. Maybe you could mask their improper position and achieve a cosmetic result but at what cost? Why compromise, when performing a small amount of tooth movement would allow you to achieve a superior outcome?

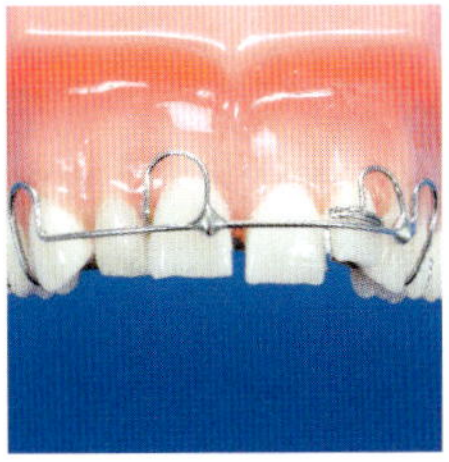

This simple appliance demonstrates the use of kicker springs for the mesial and distal movement, recurved springs for labial movement and T-springs for lingual movement. Each spring is activated by finger pressure or with a 139 bird-beak plier and can be easily adjusted to better position the teeth prior to the placement of veneers, crowns or jackets.

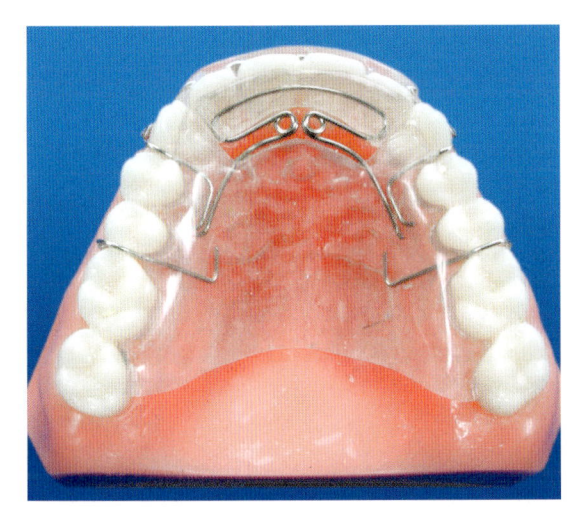

1333 Modified Spring Retainer   U/L

This design is useful for correcting minor rotations of the upper anterior teeth. The teeth are set up in the corrected position on the model and then the appliance is fabricated to this position.

On the day of appliance delivery, the dentist should complete the necessary interproximal recontouring needed to allow tooth movement. When in place, the resulting labial-lingual force will align the teeth. The helical coil in the labial wire portion, and the "mushroom" helical coil spring design of the active lingual component, make this appliance very effective for quickly aligning the incisors. Since the appliance is made to an ideal arch set-up, it may not seat well at the initial seating.

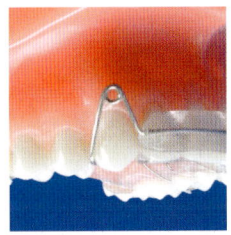

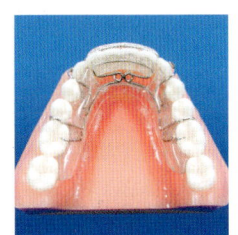

Once the teeth have adapted to their new position, the appliance will seat well. (The appliance may also be used as a final positioning retainer but is not recommended for closing spaces.)

14.3

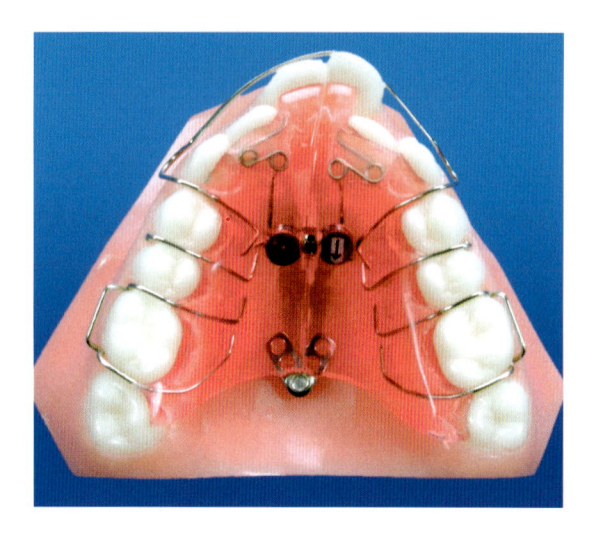

RESTORATIVE ENHANCEMENTS

1103 Swing Lock Expander   U

Many adult patients who want an anterior esthetic improvement will present with a V-shaped or Gothic arch form and anterior crowding. When this is the case, often all that is needed to improve the patient's smile is to increase the upper intercanine width enough to allow you to "round out" the incisors.

In our example, this would be accomplished by labial movement of the laterals and a small amount of lingual movement of the centrals. To create the space needed to accomplish this scenario, an appliance using an expansion screw in conjunction with a posterior hinge, as designed here, has proven very effective. It gains anterior space without disturbing the posterior bite relationship. Since the expansion screw and the hinge are separate pieces, it is possible to keep the palatal acrylic thickness at a minimum for patient comfort.

This design is only effective for a limited amount of expansion (up to 4mm). If additional expansion is required, use a larger fan screw like the one seen in appliance #1104 found in Chapter 8.

Note - As in all removable expansion appliances, activation of any of the springs should take place after space has been created through the expansion process.

2053 Diastema Closing   U/L

Peg laterals, missing teeth, and small centrals are just a few of the conditions that can create the need to realign the anteriors prior to performing the prosthetics needed to provide an ideal esthetic result.

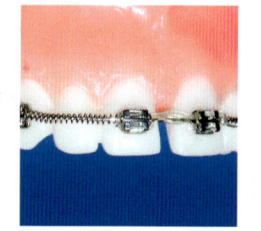

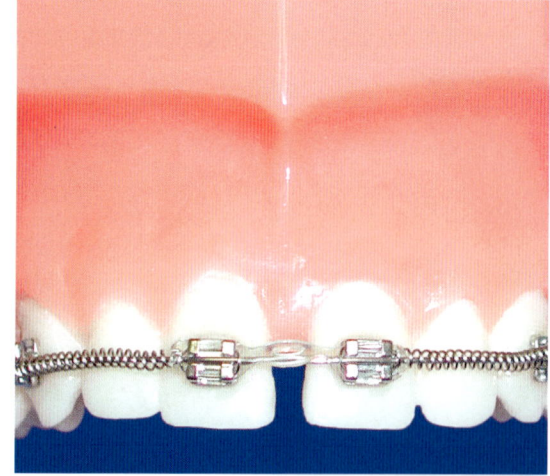

In the example shown here, excess space existing between the centrals must be closed differentially to maintain the centrals on the mid-line and equalize the lateral spaces. Once this is accomplished, veneers will be placed to restore a harmonious smile line. Here, force is applied from both chain elastics and coil springs. An arch wire has been placed from cuspid to cuspid to act as a guide and to keep the centrals from tipping. The initial length of coil spring placed distal to the central is equal to the distance between the brackets plus the width of the central bracket. This amount will typically move the tooth 1.5mm. Increasing the amount of coil spring distal to one central can move it faster than the other. However, the teeth should not be moved faster than approximately 1mm per month to prevent root resorption. Because this is such an active appliance, the patient should be seen every two weeks.

Note - To prevent unwanted movement of the cuspids, a lingual bonded 3-to-3 retainer can be placed to create an anchorage unit, holding the cuspids in place.

14.4

RESTORATIVE ENHANCEMENTS

1091 Mini-Screw Appliance   U

In an effort to meet the esthetic demands of our patients, excessively thick veneers are frequently placed on upper incisors. Although this quick fix may temporarily make the patient happy, in the long run it is a recipe for failure. When lingually placed upper anteriors are left untreated, abnormal occlusal forces can lead to periodontal problems, cause abnormal wear of the lower anteriors and even lead to an early failure of the veneer. In cases like this, where you need to move a maxillary anterior labially, the use of the mini-screw is an excellent choice.

Because the mini-screws are easy for the patient to adjust, some doctors use them in situations where the patient cannot readily return to their office on the recommended bi-weekly basis. However, these screws add a modest amount of bulk to the anterior portion of the appliance creating an anterior bite plane. Therefore, the use of this design in a patient who already has an open bite and is a vertical grower is contraindicated.

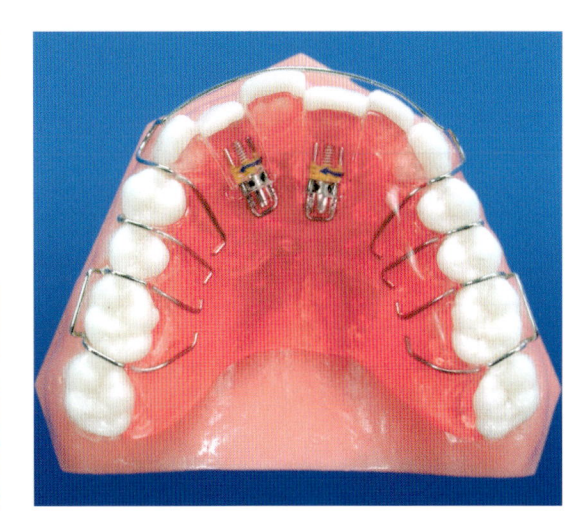

1072B   Recurved Extrusion Spring   U/L

Because teeth that are not fully erupted are harder to keep clean they tend to be more caries prone. Once this occurs, restoring them is also more difficult. In fact, it often becomes necessary to forcefully erupt the tooth prior to placing a final restoration.

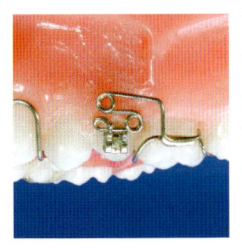

The extrusion appliance, shown here, uses a recurved finger spring to aid in the eruption of a single bicuspid. A direct bond straight wire bracket is placed on the bicuspid to create an undercut for the helical recurved spring. The patient then simply inserts the activated appliance and "snaps" the activated spring under the gingival tie wings of the bracket. This not only expedites the eruption of the tooth, but also aids in appliance retention.

RESTORATIVE ENHANCEMENTS

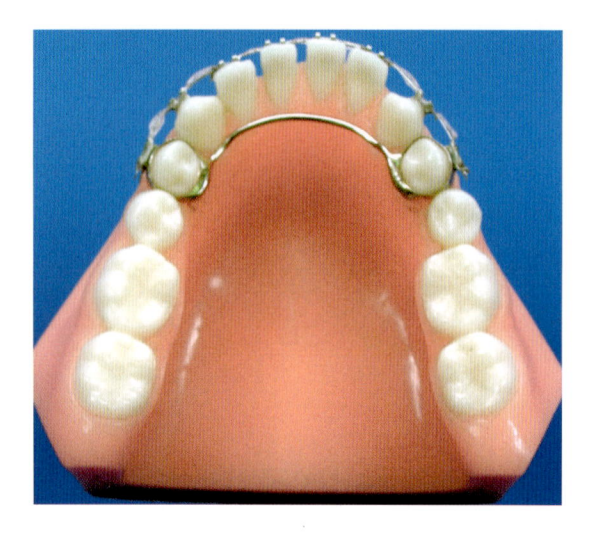

2211B Fixed Lower Retraction Appliance   L

In many adult cases with lower anterior flaring, positive individual bodily tooth movement combined with root torquing is desirable. The design offered here is very popular and effective in treating this situation. It employs limited bracketing, provides optimum anchorage, and allows for individual mesial/distal, as well as lingual, tooth movement.

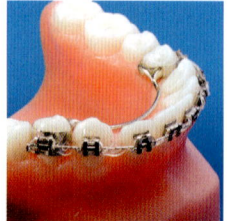

Anchorage is provided by a banded, fixed lingual arch wire from first bicuspid to first bicuspid. A sectional arch wire can then be used along with chain elastics to retract the incisors as well as control their mesial and distal positions.

Once the anteriors are retracted, they usually need to be splinted together. They can be temporarily splinted using steel ligature underties.

1122B Lower Apron Spring Retractor   L

Correcting lower anterior flaring can be achieved with this appliance in a relatively short period of time when simple lingual uprighting is required. As the Apron spring is activated to retract the incisors, the lingual acrylic must be periodically relieved to allow room for the movement to occur.

It is recommended that only 1mm of acrylic be relieved at each appointment so that a controlled retraction is achieved. This will also allow the appliance to be used as a retainer once the incisors are retracted as desired. Full time wear of this appliance is recommended.

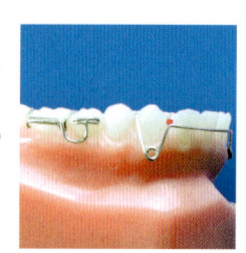

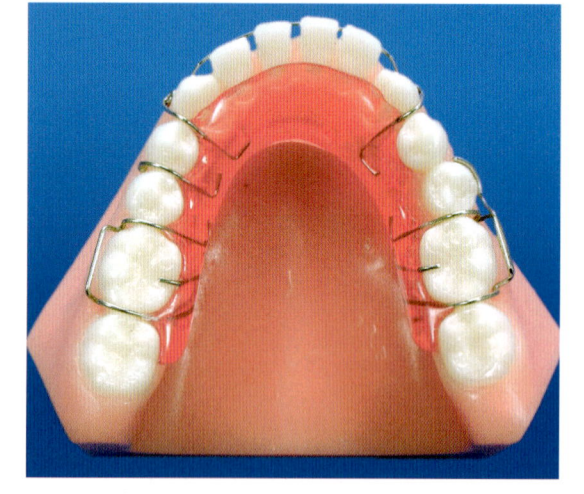

Design Notes:

RESTORATIVE ENHANCEMENTS

2081 Simple Molar Crossbite Correction w/Bands

In an adult, a single tooth crossbite can have a serious effect on your final restorative result. Too often bridges are built and partials are placed which cause abnormal forces to occur to the supporting teeth of these restorations. By simply correcting a crossbite, you can direct the occlusal forces down the long axis of the teeth and eliminate the abnormal forces.

Here maxillary and mandibular bands are made for the molars in crossbite. Hooks are placed on the buccal of the maxillary band and on the lingual of the mandibular band, so elastics can be used to correct the crossbite. Slight occlusal adjustment or the use of a bite plane is often needed as the crossbite is treated. Once the condition is corrected, normal intercuspation is usually sufficient to maintain the results.

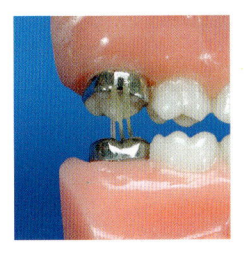

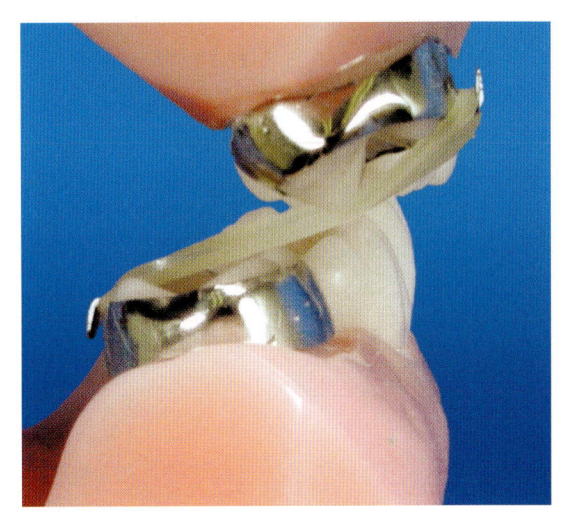

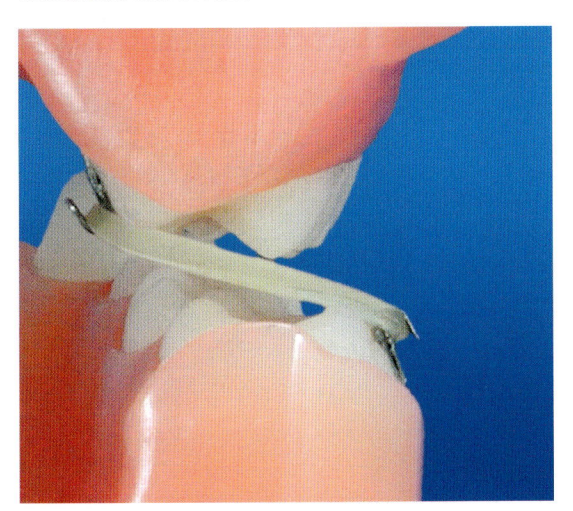

2082 Simple Molar Crossbite Correction w/Bonded Hooks

Many practitioners have found it easier to use bonded hooks instead of bands when they need to jump a molar crossbite. As mentioned above, careful attention must be paid to the occlusion until the crossbite is corrected.

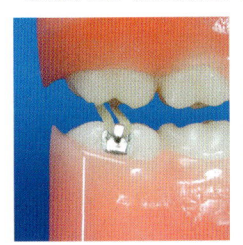

Note - It may be necessary for the patient to wear a Hawley with an anterior bite plane or a bruxism splint while this crossbite is being corrected. For further assistance in selecting an appliance call us at your Appliance Therapy laboratory.

1334 Buccal Molar Uprighting for Mandibular Molar

It is not unusual to have one molar erupt in lingual version. This special expansion screw is designed to upright the lingually inclined molar towards the buccal. It affords a precisely controlled tipping of the crown without bodily movement. A key is provided with the appliance for the weekly adjustments.

Note - This appliance also shows a micro-screw. This screw is very effective in moving a single tooth labially.

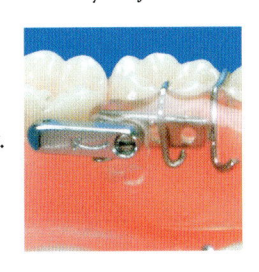

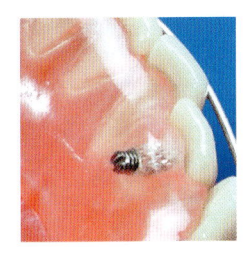

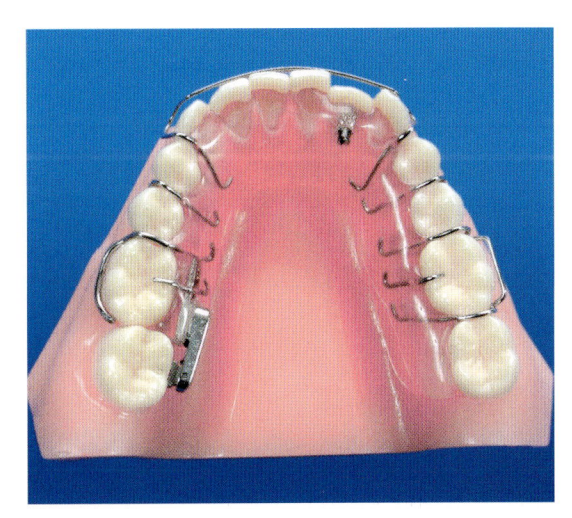

14.7

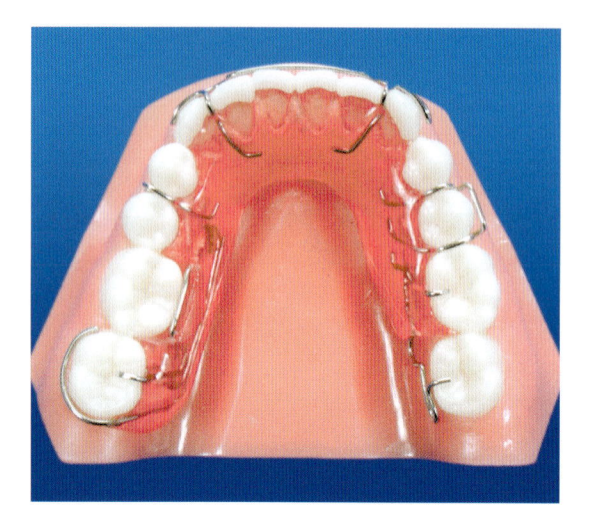

RESTORATIVE ENHANCEMENTS

1076E Multi-Spring Molar Uprighter   U/L

This appliance illustrates the use of two very effective uprighting springs: the mushroom spring and the distal recurve. These springs are easy to adjust and can very effectively tip molars upright, usually with only two or three adjustments. Placing a rest, as shown, on the molar being uprighted by the distal recurve spring, aids in controlling super-eruption when an opposing tooth is missing.

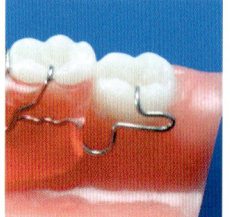

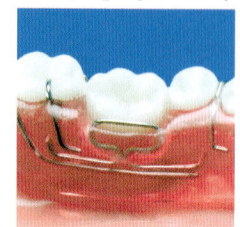

Note - When using "C" clasps, consider the use of a composite ledge for superior retention.

1084 Buccal Molar Uprighting w/Expansion Screw

Here is another design to correct a molar that is lingually positioned. With this expansion screw, you should expect to get both tipping and some bodily movement of this molar. Remember, if there is any occlusal interference during this procedure, you will need to properly adjust the bite, or use an occlusal bite plane.

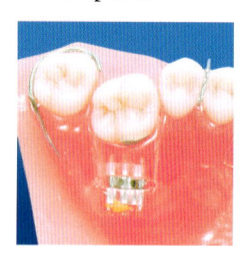

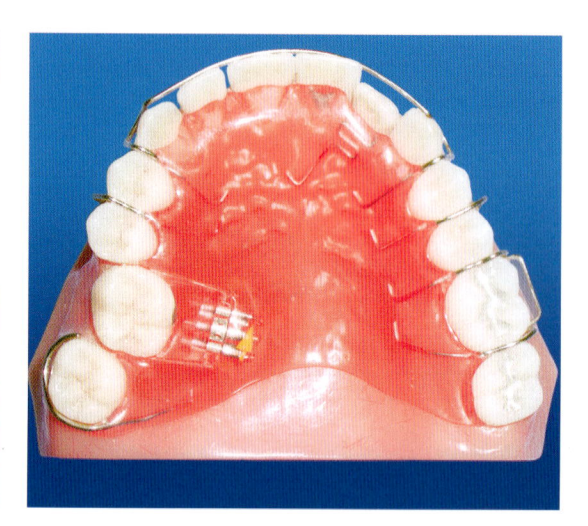

Note - As in many minor tooth movement appliances, you can often accomplish a variety of movements with one appliance. Notice the recurved spring to move the lateral labially.

Design Notes:

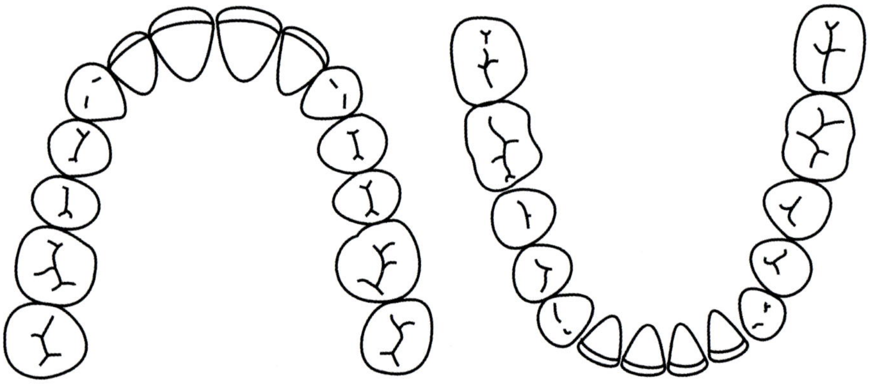

RESTORATIVE ENHANCEMENTS

Molar Uprighting

Perhaps the most common use of orthodontics to aid in restorative work is the uprighting of a second molar. A tipped molar can have a profound effect on prosthetic dentistry. After a first molar is lost, typical clinical problems include extrusion and migration of teeth, accelerated mesial drift, uneven marginal ridges, angular bony crests, altered coronal to gingival form, food impaction, caries, periodontal disease, and ultimately posterior bite collapse with loss of the occlusal vertical dimension.

Molar uprighting can be accomplished using either a fixed or a removable appliance. Both have their advantages and disadvantages. While most general practitioners find removable appliances easier to use, the removable affords less control over tooth movement.

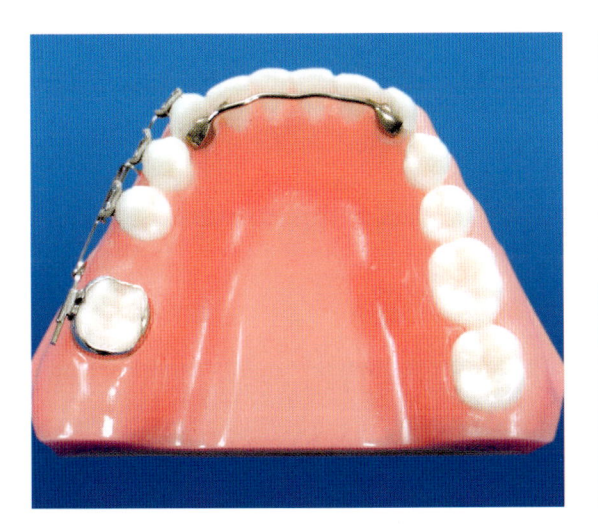

2034 Fixed Molar Uprighting Appliances   U/L

A variety of fixed appliances have been proposed to upright tipped molars. In this design, all teeth as far forward as the canine in the treatment quadrant are included to provide anchorage. The canine on the contralateral side is also linked to the anchor teeth by use of a heavy stabilizing lingual arch. This canine-to-canine stabilizing arch not only increases the anterior anchorage, but also resists buccal displacement of the anchor teeth.

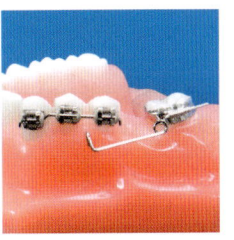

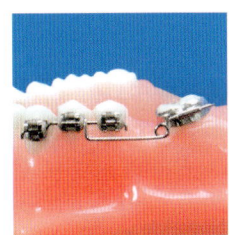

Although direct bonded brackets are suitable for all the teeth, it may sometimes be advisable to band the molar. In the simplest of cases, where the premolars and cuspids are only being used for anchorage, edgewise brackets can be placed in the position of maximum convenience where minimum wire bending will be required to engage a passive arch wire. A rigid stabilizing wire, .019 x .025 stainless steel, is placed in the area of the premolars and canine.

The molar uprighting is done with a helical uprighting auxiliary spring of .017 x .025 stainless steel wire placed in the auxiliary tube of the molar. The mesial arm of the helical spring should be adjusted to lie passively in the vestibule, and upon activation should hook over the arch wire in the stabilizing segment. It is important that the hook be positioned so that it is able to slide distally as the molar uprights. A slight lingual bend placed in the uprighting spring is needed to counteract the forces that tend to tip the anchor teeth buccally and the molar lingually.

Note - All of the component parts seen here are sent to you as a customized complete kit. Simply send upper and lower casts and a construction bite along with your lab slip.

RESTORATIVE ENHANCEMENTS

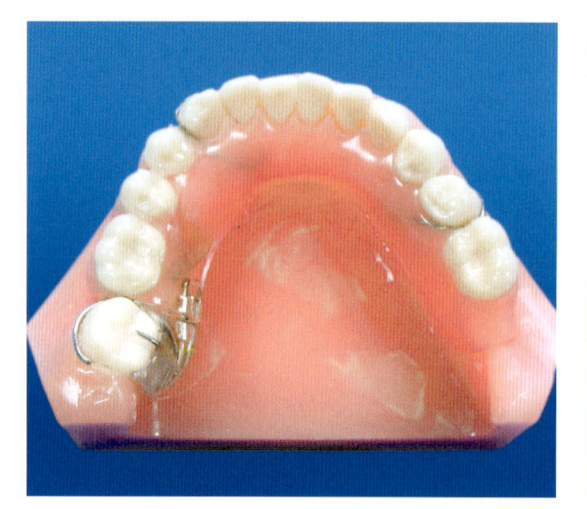

4184 Molar Uprighting Partial   U/L

There are times when the fixed appliance approach to molar uprighting is either inappropriate or not possible. Sometimes patients do not have enough teeth to use as an anchor or the stabilizing teeth are periodontally involved. A removable design allows you to use the soft tissue, teeth, and the appliance to form an anchor unit.

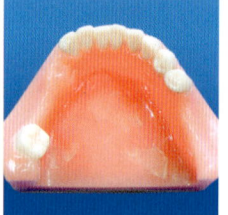

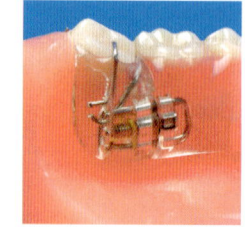

A temporary partial can be designed which incorporates a spring or an expansion screw to accomplish the desired tooth movement.

Retention and anchorage are accomplished by using two to three clasps and by having excellent tissue adaptation. This design is especially useful on adult patients with 12-year molars tipped mesially. Although not shown in this example, a labial bow is often used to prevent flaring of the anterior teeth.

Note - When using removable appliances that have an expansion screw, have your patient activate the appliance one turn per week. This is equivalent to 1mm of movement per month.

1037 Fixed/Removable Molar Uprighter   U/L

When the molar is severely inclined and bodily movement is needed to upright it, only a fixed approach will suffice. But sometimes the teeth that would normally be used for anchorage are not available. When this is the case, a removable appliance can be used for anchorage in conjunction with a fixed component on the molar.

Here, an uprighting spring inserts into a fixed molar bracket that has a tube or slot. The spring then hooks onto the removable appliance which provides the necessary anchorage and prevents lingual tipping. When using this approach, it is essential to place an occlusal rest on the distal aspect of the occlusal surface to prevent extrusion.

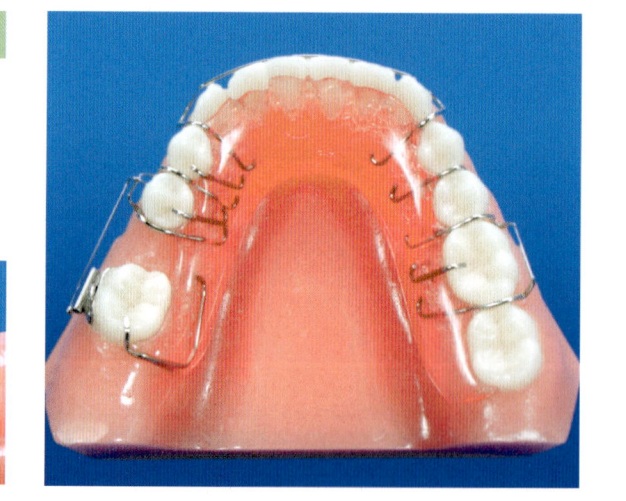

RESTORATIVE ENHANCEMENTS

2027 Elastic Halterman Appliance   U/L

We often see second molars that cannot erupt fully because they are locked under the distal aspect of the first molar. When this happens, the area becomes very difficult to maintain. Opposing molars can super erupt causing occlusal problems, and caries and periodontal disease can eventually lead to the loss of both molars. Simply moving the second molar distally and allowing it to erupt into its normal position can easily avoid this sequence of events.

One appliance to accomplish this is the Elastic Halterman. Here a button is bonded to the occlusal surface of the second molar and a band with a hook distal to this molar is cemented to the first molar. Chain elastic extending from the hook to the button is used to provide the distal force needed to unlock this tooth.

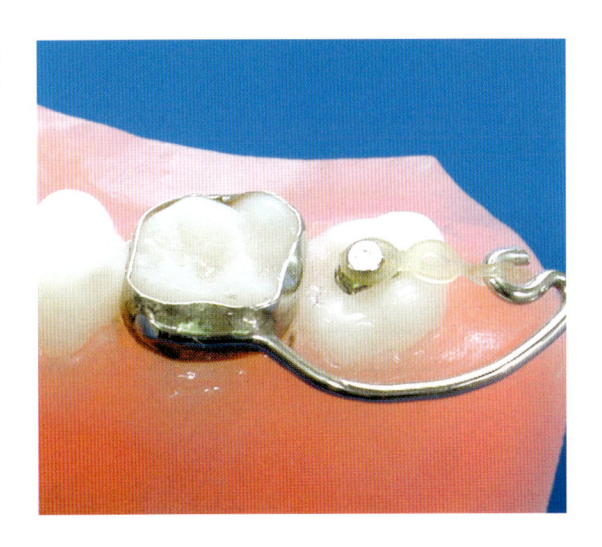

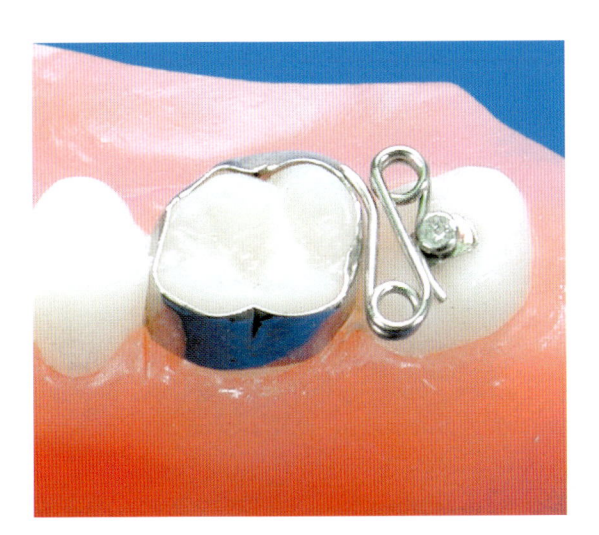

2028 Ectopic Spring Distalizer   U/L

Designed in principle to function the same as the Elastic Halterman, this appliance features a recurved wire spring to achieve the distal movement of the second molar that is caught under the first molar. Placement of the occlusal button is usually on the distal aspect of the erupting molar.

Note - This design is especially useful for uprighting lower second molars, due to restricted space in the area of the ascending Ramus.

Note - Always send an opposing cast to evaluate if there is sufficient occlusal clearance for this appliance.

Design Notes:

14.11

RESTORATIVE ENHANCEMENTS

Forced Eruption

One of the primary goals of restorative dentistry is to replace form, function, and esthetics lost due to trauma or disease. Often, clinical conditions can make a tooth appear to be unrestorable. Fractures, caries, large old restorations, osseous defects, a poor root to crown ratio, and perforations at or below the level of the crestal bone are just a few of the factors that can contribute to tooth loss. When situations like these arise, we must be equipped with alternative therapy to maintain a healthy, intact masticatory system. Forced eruption is such a therapy.

Forced eruption is appropriate when loss of tooth structure is in the region of the alveolar crest. It can be defined as an orthodontic movement in a coronal direction through the application of gentle, continuous forces.

Specifically, when a root segment is forcefully erupted, the forces stretch the gingival and periodontal fibers producing a coronal shift of gingiva and bone. If done slowly, the gingiva and supporting structures will follow to a position that is further coronal than the adjacent teeth. These gingival and osseous changes can be used to manage many restorative problems.

For example, after forced eruption, periodontal surgery can be performed exposing sound tooth structure without sacrificing bone on the adjacent teeth. The soft tissue can then be sutured to blend with the gingival margins of the adjacent teeth. Once the tissue has healed, a final restoration can be made giving you an excellent esthetic result, which could not be achieved without doing this procedure.

There are several methods for erupting teeth. As always, proper appliance selection and application requires a well thought out and thorough diagnosis and treatment plan. To select the appropriate appliance technique, use your mounted study casts to evaluate the bite relationship, the number of teeth available for anchorage, and their position in relation to the tooth needing eruption. This will allow you to select the appropriate appliance. For example, in a deep bite, clearance does not exist for bracket placement on lower anteriors. Here a removable appliance with a bite plane to open the vertical would be the appliance of choice.

Note - Inflammation must be controlled prior to initiating tooth movement. If it is not, forced eruption may contribute to the deepening of an osseous defect.

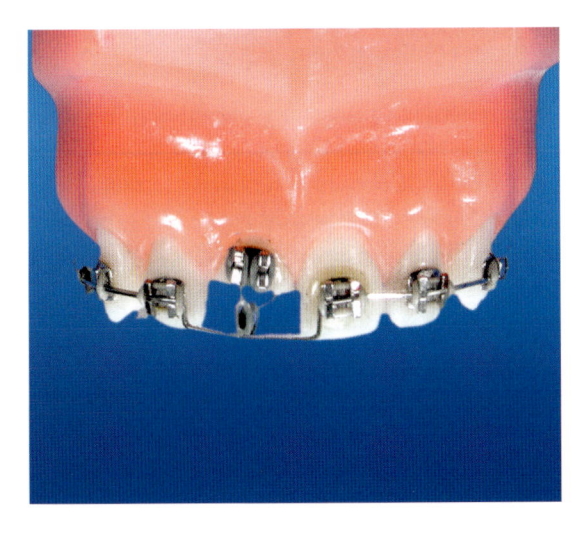

RESTORATIVE ENHANCEMENTS

2211 Fixed Forced Eruption Appliance   U/L

When using a fixed approach, the equivalent of two teeth on either side of the tooth to be erupted must be available for anchorage. The appliance is set up as follows:

The Anchorage Unit:

Edgewise brackets are bonded into place in the same horizontal plane on all of the anchor teeth. The teeth on each side of the tooth to be erupted are then tied together with metal ligature ties. This will eliminate any unwanted movement of these anchor units.

A stainless steel orthodontic wire, 0.018 inch by 0.025 inch, is then ligated into the brackets of the anchorage units with elastic ligatures. This wire has been bent by the lab to the general labial contours of the anchorage teeth and the crown of the tooth to be extruded. An occlusal offset has been placed in the wire over the tooth to be extruded. This wire, when properly positioned inciso-gingivally, will provide the needed extrusion distance between the wire and the attachment on the tooth needing eruption.

The Attachment Unit:

The attachment unit is the part of the appliance that attaches to the tooth needing eruption. The preferred method is bonding a bracket to natural tooth enamel. However, if there is no labial enamel to bond to, then the next best options are a temporary, or a final post and core, and a temporary crown. A temporary crown has the advantage of being more esthetically pleasing while retaining the tooth's original position. After the temporary crown has been constructed, an orthodontic bracket is bonded to its surface as far to the gingival as possible.

The Active Force Module:

After placing the arch wire, you can activate the appliance. An elastic is placed from the attachment, looped over the wire and back on to the attachment, to initiate the eruption. In this example, chain elastic is being used.

1079 Removable Forced Eruption Appliance - Spring Activated   U/L

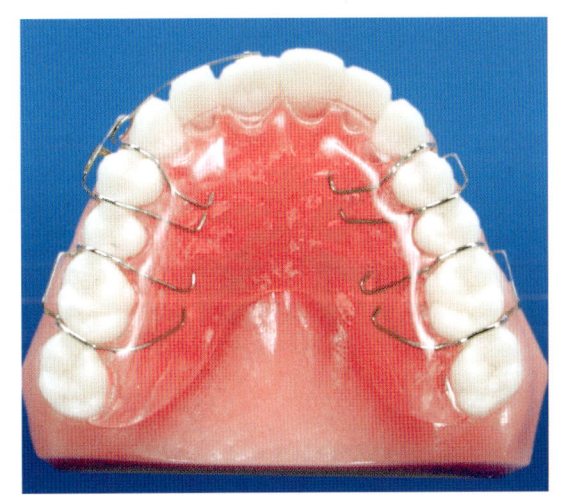

There are times when bracketing teeth for anchorage is either inappropriate or not possible. For example, placing brackets on porcelain veneers or crowns is not recommended, as the bonding process can damage the finish. Some patients simply do not have enough teeth to be the sole method of anchorage. When this is the case, a removable appliance allows you to use the soft tissue, along with remaining teeth for anchorage.

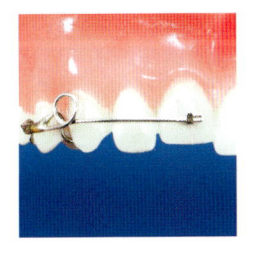

Appliance designs can be very flexible and creative. In some cases, you may be able to use a patient's existing partial by simply adding a hook over the tooth needing eruption. In the example shown here, a simple acrylic orthodontic appliance with an activating spring arm can be used. This type of appliance works by simply engaging the spring over the direct bonded attachment bracket.

RESTORATIVE ENHANCEMENTS

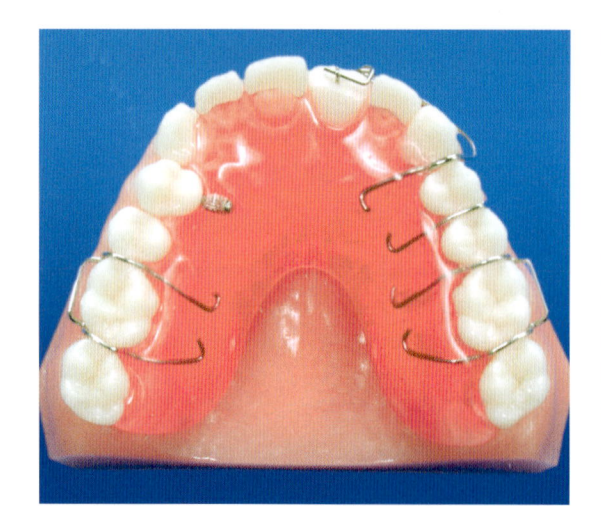

1078 Removable Forced Eruption Appliance

This appliance is appropriate when a temporary crown is not needed and a fixed approach is not possible. Forced eruption in this case is accomplished by using a very effective helical coil spring that is connected directly to a temporary post. Though not the solution for all cases, innovative removable appliance designs such as this can greatly expand the clinician's options to initiate forced eruption.

Note - Inflammation must be controlled prior to initiating tooth movement. If it is not, forced eruption may contribute to the deepening of an osseous defect.

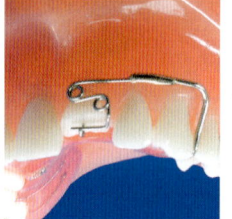

6111 Custom Fluoride Tray

All patients who are undergoing extensive restorative work need extra fluoride protection. The simplest and most effective way to deliver this protection is by using a custom tray and 1.1% neutral sodium fluoride.

Simply have the patient fill the tray with 1.1% neutral sodium fluoride and wear it for five minutes after they brush and floss. Then take the tray out and have the patient spit out the excess without rinsing. That's all it takes to give them the extra protection they need. Neutral sodium fluoride is recommended as safest for composites and porcelain restorations. Do not use acidulated fluorides.

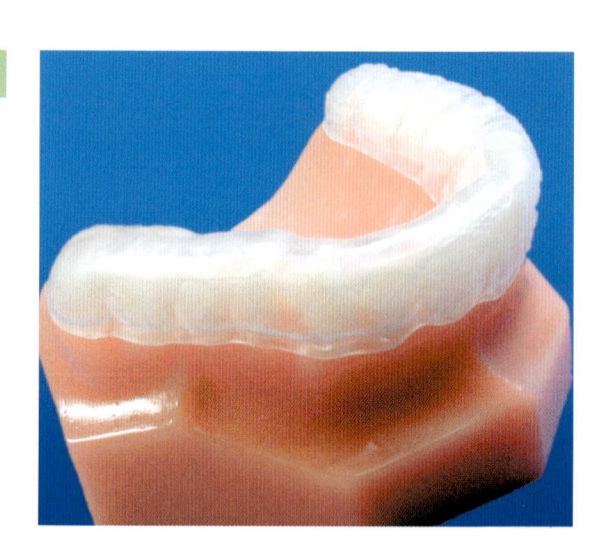

Design Notes:

RESTORATIVE ENHANCEMENTS

6111B Bleaching Trays

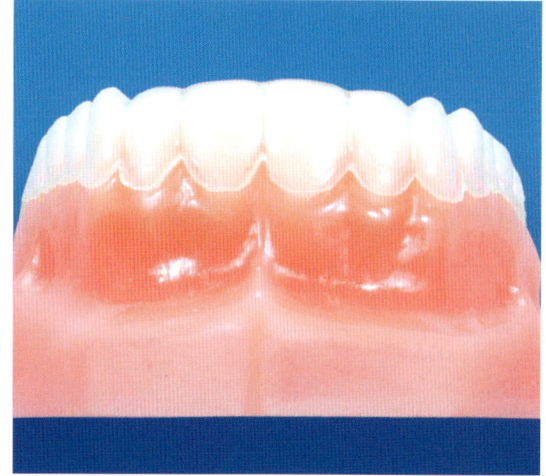

"Doctor, can you make my teeth whiter?" This is without a doubt the most asked question in the dental office today. The answer to the question is, of course, yes. But how successful your home bleaching technique will be is dependent on using a well-designed custom tray. A properly designed bleaching tray like the one shown here, conforms perfectly to the teeth and seals tightly at the gingival margin to prevent the bleach from leaking out onto the tissue. Although the thickness of the tray can be adjusted to your particular desire, the normal thickness is .040 mm.

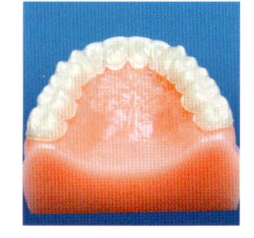

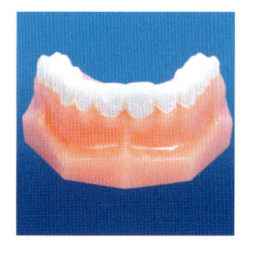

Note - Some practitioners like the lab to place a spacer on the model to create a well for the bleach. Our experience shows that this is not necessary, however you may request this design addition when you write your prescription.

Design Notes:

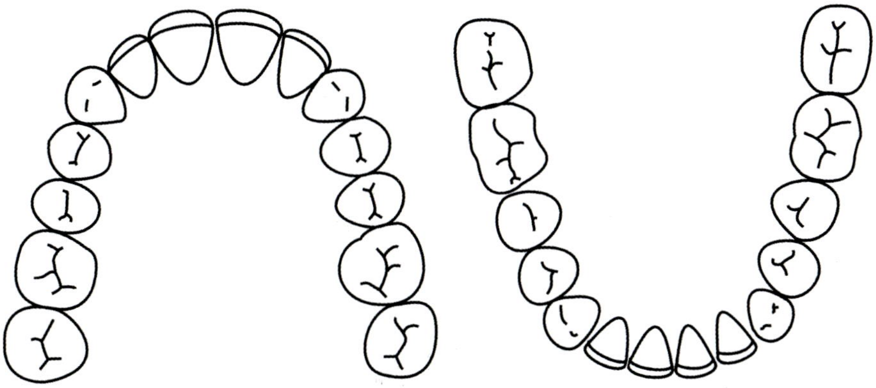

Design Notes

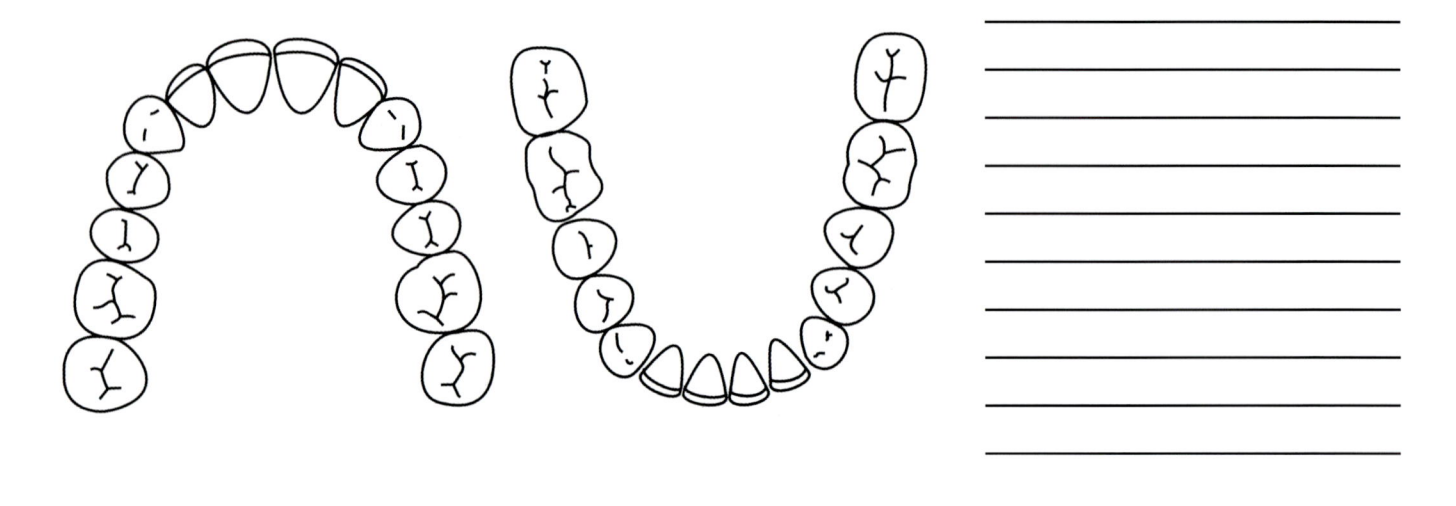

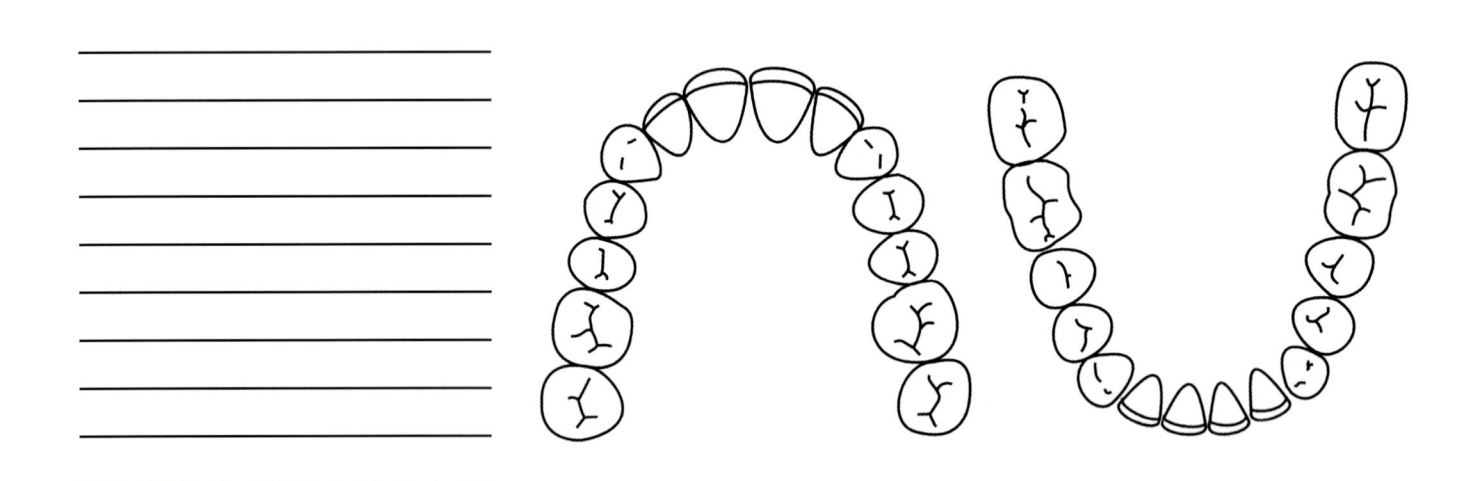

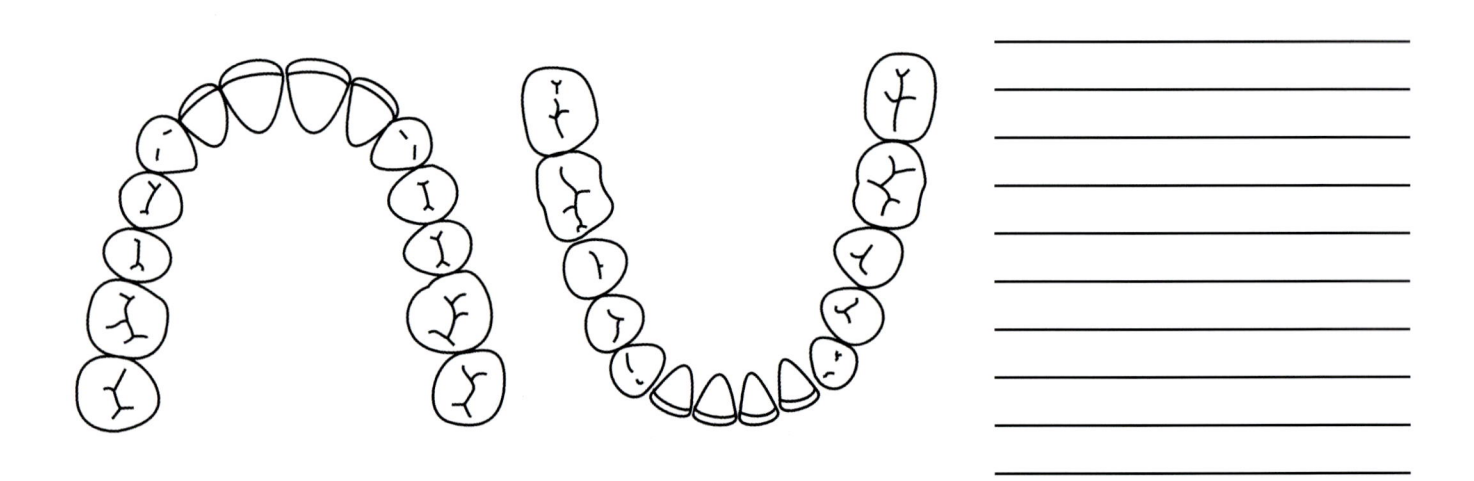

INTERIM PARTIALS / BRIDGES

an overview: INTERIM PARTIALS/BRIDGES

Chapter 15

Temporary or interim appliances serve many useful purposes and are often an integral part of a prosthetic treatment plan. They are indicated when age, health, poor finances, or lack of time precludes a more definitive treatment.

For example, an interim appliance is often used in young patients who, because of an accident, rampant caries, or hereditary partial anodontia, are missing either anterior or posterior teeth. Permanent restorations are usually contraindicated for some time in a growing child. So interim partials and bridges are an excellent method to maintain the patient's esthetics and function.

Elderly patients whose health contraindicates the lengthy and physically trying appointments needed to construct permanent fixed replacements for missing teeth, are excellent candidates for interim restorations. These patients can usually tolerate the simple clinical procedures needed to construct and insert a temporary appliance.

Another indication for the interim appliance may occur in patients who have suffered a financial set back. The cost of this service is considerably less than for the definitive treatment that will eventually be required. For example, many patients have a mouth full of teeth with large restorations that need to be replaced with crowns. When a patient like this loses a first molar, a bridge is usually the treatment of choice. However, when the patient can't immediately afford a bridge, an interim bridge can inexpensively be used to maintain the space and stabilize the area. This technique is particularly useful where the patient's large restorations make these teeth subject to fracture. Not having to prepare the teeth and being able to place bands around them will act to hold them together until the patient can afford to move on with his or her treatment.

Other indications for interim appliances, seen in the general practice on a daily basis, are:

- to maintain space.
- to re-establish occlusion.
- to replace visible missing teeth while definitive restorative procedures are being accomplished.
- to serve while the patient is undergoing periodontal or other prolonged treatment.
- to condition the patient to wearing a removable prosthesis.
- when healing is progressing after an extraction or a traumatic injury.
- to maintain function while accomplishing minor tooth movement.

These appliances can be designed to be either fixed or removable. Which approach is used is dependent on numerous factors ranging from the patients' periodontal condition, to their ability to maintain their hygiene. Regardless, having the choice gives clinicians the flexibility they need to direct and control their patients' treatment.

INTERIM PARTIALS/BRIDGES

Unilateral Interim Bridges

Interim appliances can be fixed or removable. Simple space maintainers, which are more commonly used after premature loss of primary teeth, are used quite effectively as fixed interim bridges. This is an inexpensive way to stabilize an area until a decision on the best restorative technique can be made. Temporary bridges can also maintain implant sites and are much more comfortable than a temporary partial or flipper.

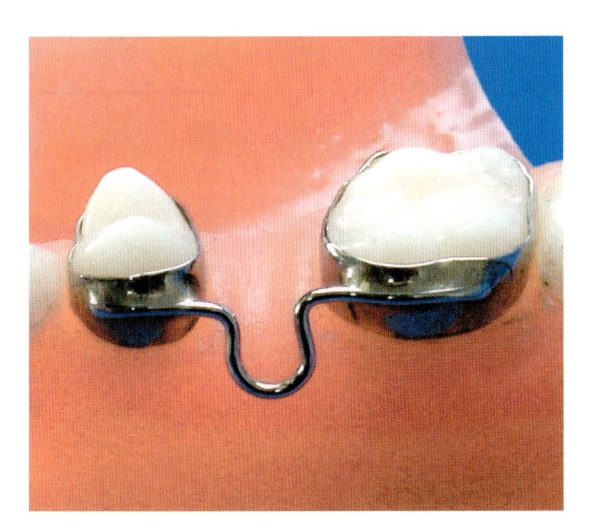

2013 Adjustable Two Band Interim Bridge   U/L

When a tooth is missing in the posterior aspect of the arch, an interim bridge can be used to maintain space and stabilize the area without having to prepare the teeth. This technique is particularly useful if buccal/lingual walls of the teeth to be banded are subject to fracture. An example of this would be teeth with very large MOD alloys. In this case, the bands would act to hold them together.

This particular appliance is designed with an adjustable buccal wire. A simple adjustment with a 139 bird-beak plier will allow you to gain a small amount of lost space or upright a tooth that has tipped slightly into the edentulous space.

2014 Two Band Interim Bridge with Occlusal Bar   U/L

This appliance is the same as appliance #2013 but features a rigid non-adjustable metal bar. Both of these appliances are used in situations where hygiene is a consideration as they are easy to clean. The occlusal metal bar makes this temporary splint ideal to maintain an implant site or protect an area that has undergone a ridge augmentation.

Note - It is important to check for a parallel path of insertion between the two abutment teeth.

Note - Adding occlusal rests to this design will prevent gingival displacement of this appliance. Bonding these rests in place will allow the patient to maintain this appliance for a longer period of time.

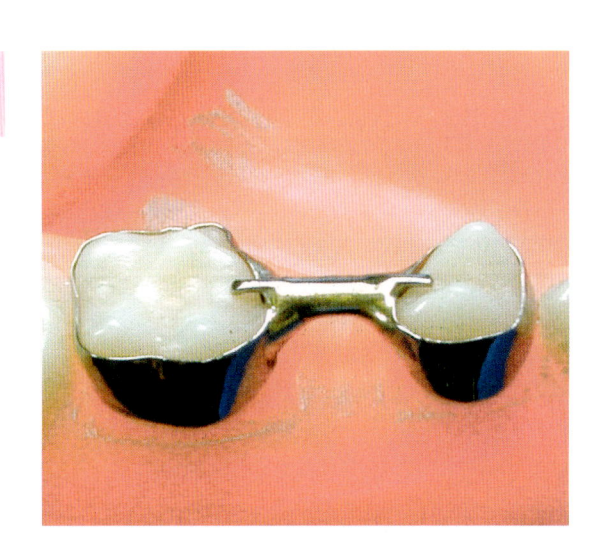

INTERIM PARTIALS/BRIDGES

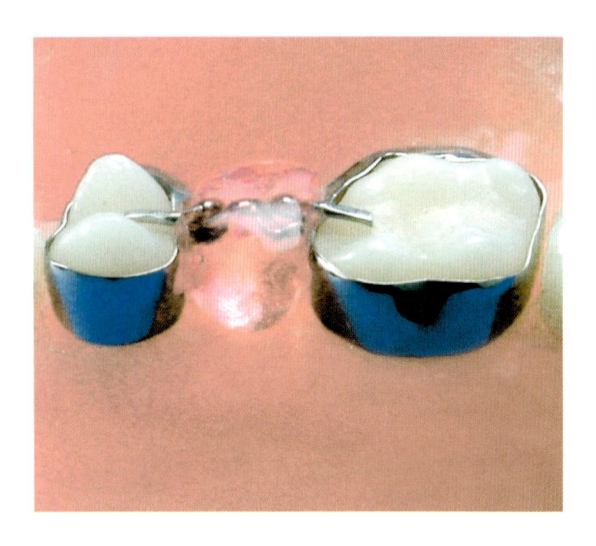

2023 Two Band Interim Bridge with Occlusal Acrylic Pad U/L

When the possibility of super-eruption is a concern, an acrylic pad can be used to make occlusal contact with the opposing dentition. This pad is designed so that it is clear of the tissue and the patient can easily floss underneath it using a floss threader. Upon delivery, it will be necessary to adjust the occlusal surface of the pad. Again, it is always important to check for a parallel path of insertion between the two abutment teeth.

Note - Adding occlusal rests to this design will prevent gingival displacement of this appliance. Bonding these rests in place will allow the patient to maintain this appliance for a longer period of time.

4023 Two Band Interim Bridge w/Pontic U/L

Bioform shade teeth can be placed instead of an acrylic pad for those patients who prefer a more natural look. This pontic is designed so that it is clear of the tissue and the patient can easily floss underneath it using a floss threader. Upon delivery, it will be necessary to adjust the occlusal surface of the pontic. Again, it is always important to check for a parallel path of insertion between the two abutment teeth.

Note - Adding occlusal rests to this design will prevent gingival displacement of this appliance. Bonding these rests in place will allow the patient to maintain this appliance for a longer period of time.

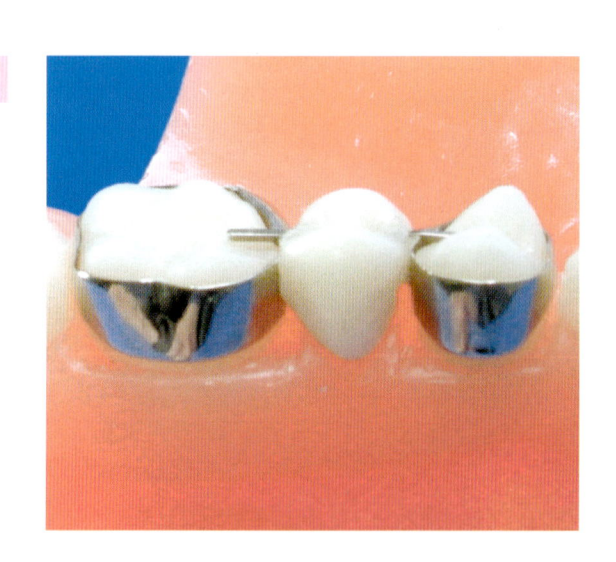

4022 Banded/Bonded Interim Bridge U/L

When esthetic considerations are important, an occlusal rest and a lingual "C" clasp may be used in place of a band on the visible abutment. Bonding material can then be placed over the lingual "C" clasp and occlusal rest to add stability and retention.

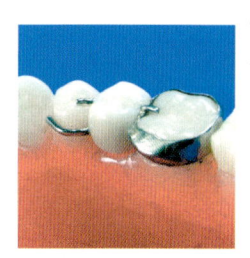

This is also useful if the path of insertion prevents the use of two bands.

INTERIM PARTIALS/BRIDGES

4021 Temporary Maryland Bridge   U/L

When a removable temporary partial cannot be tolerated, using a temporary Maryland bridge can be an effective way to maintain space and provide the patient with an esthetic result. This appliance consists of two bondable mesh pads attached to a pontic. Tooth preparation is not needed, making it ideal for the young trauma patient, but it is essential to have occlusal clearance with the opposing arch.

Note - When ordering this appliance always send an opposing model, an accurate bite registration, and a tooth shade selection.

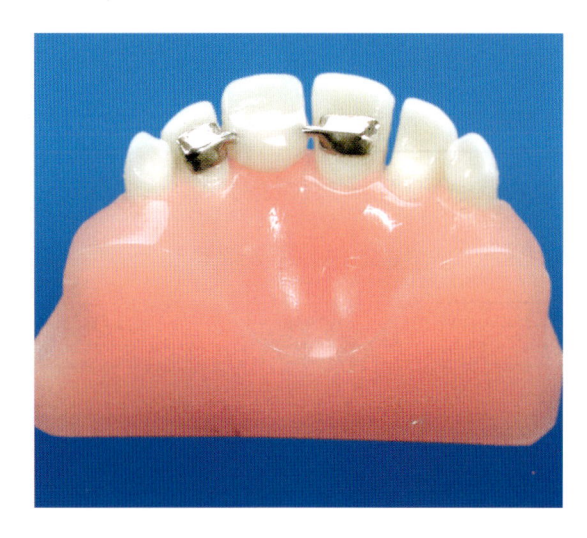

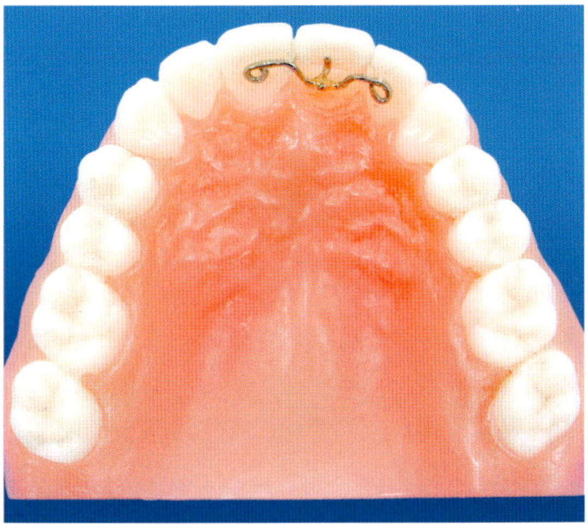

4602 Intra-coronal Interim Bridge   U/L

An intra-coronal bridge may be indicated for patients that cannot tolerate a temporary removable partial denture and whose inter-incisal space is too tight to accommodate a temporary Maryland bridge.

To prepare for this appliance, simply cut a groove deep enough in the lingual aspect of the abutment teeth to allow the supporting wire wings to be kept out of occlusion when they are bonded into place. Then take an accurate impression of the preparation. Don't forget to send the lab both upper and lower casts, a bite registration and the tooth shade you desire.

Note - This approach is not appropriate for the young trauma patient as the pulp chambers in the abutment teeth are usually still quite large.

4172 Fixed Banded Temporary Anterior Bridge   U/L

When bonding to anterior teeth is not an option, the appliance shown here is an excellent alternative. It utilizes a lingual wire soldered to bands on the first permanent molar, and occlusal rests on the premolars. Each anterior tooth (up to four) is fitted to a wire that has been soldered to the arch wire. Acrylic is then applied to bond them into a single unit. Replacement teeth are available in the appropriate Bioform shade. This appliance can give the patient very pleasing esthetics, but requires extra care as it is vulnerable to breakage.

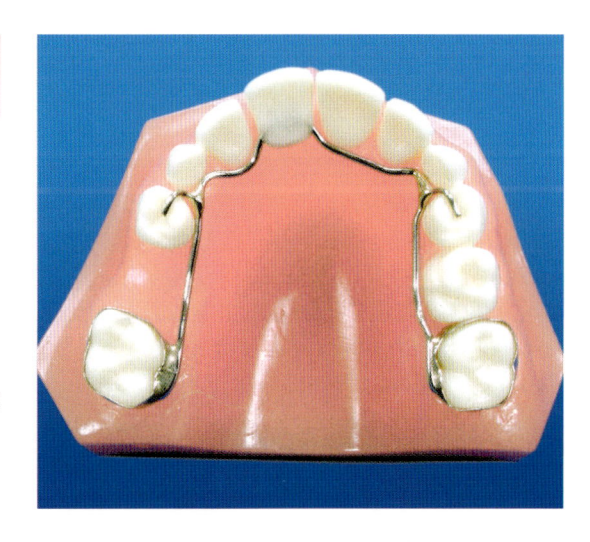

15.3

INTERIM PARTIALS/BRIDGES

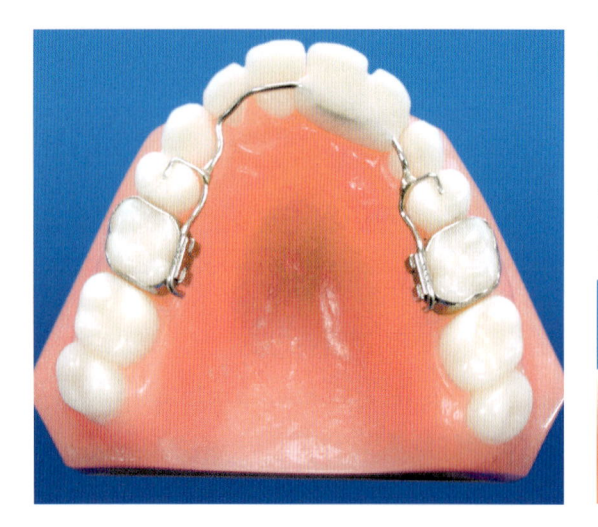

4024 Fixed/Removable Banded Temp Anterior Bridge

Designed to keep the implant patient functional throughout the integration and restorative period of treatment, the Fixed/Removable Banded Anterior Bridge has become an appliance used for any patient that has found it difficult to tolerate a traditional interim partial denture. This appliance utilizes Wilson vertical tubes soldered to bands to allow the patient to have the benefit of a palate-free fixed appliance while still allowing the dentist to easily remove it to gain access to the tissue.

Excess pressure can be kept off the ridge by allowing the wire to positively rest against the surrounding anteriors, as seen here, or by adding rest seats and rests on the bicuspids or cuspids. This appliance can give the patient very pleasing esthetics, but requires extra care as it is vulnerable to distortion and breakage.

Note - Don't forget to adjust the internal aspect of the pontics to make sure they do not put any unwanted pressure on the ridge.

4191 Essix Temporary Partial

This simple appliance is excellent for temporary replacement of anterior teeth while the patient is waiting for a permanent bridge, a partial, or implants. Traditionally, these missing anteriors would be replaced by incorporating denture teeth into a Hawley type retainer more commonly referred to by patients as a "flipper". Unfortunately, these appliances are often initially uncomfortable and affect speech because they have acrylic in the palatal region.

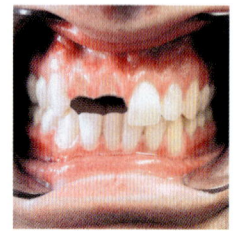

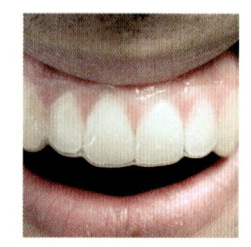

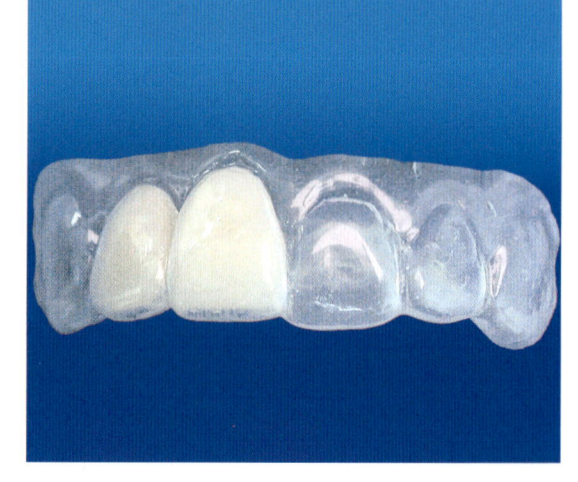

By using the new Essix technology, a simpler, more efficient method is used to retain and replace the missing teeth on a temporary basis. This removable interim bridge is made using the Essix "C-type" clear vacuum-formed material. When properly designed and fabricated, this appliance will snap into place and stay retained by using the natural undercuts gingival to the anterior contact points. They are clear, thin, run from cuspid-to-cuspid, and are clasp free and palate free. Patient acceptance and esthetics are excellent.

INTERIM PARTIALS/BRIDGES

Temporary Removable Partial Dentures

There are three types of temporary removable partial dentures. They are classified according to their purpose, either as an interim, a treatment, or as a transitional partial.

Interim Partials

Interim Partials are used in the following situations:

1. Young patients who have lost anterior or posterior teeth. Treatment usually consists of an interim partial denture or a series of dentures, if necessary, until the teeth adjacent to the space have matured sufficiently to permit abutment preparations for a fixed bridge without the risk of mechanically exposing the pulpal tissue or until implants can be placed.

2. Elderly patients whose health contraindicates the lengthy and physically trying appointments needed to construct fixed replacements for missing teeth.

3. Patients who have suffered a temporary financial set back. The cost of this service is considerably less than for the definitive treatment that will eventually be required.

4. To maintain space.

5. To re-establish occlusion.

6. To replace visible missing teeth while definitive restorative procedures are being accomplished.

7. To serve while the patient is undergoing periodontal or other prolonged treatment.

8. To condition the patient to wearing a removable prosthesis.

9. When healing is progressing after an extraction or a traumatic injury.

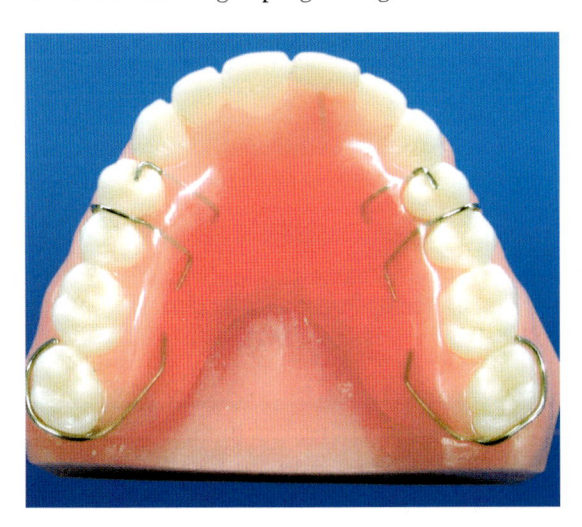

4181 Upper Interim Removable Partial

A simple, inexpensive partial is shown here to replace a single, lost permanent central. This appliance is great for the rapidly growing youngster, from pre-teen through the teenage years, as it is easily and inexpensively remade as the patient develops.

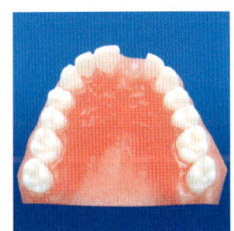

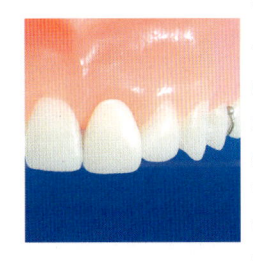

The example is shown with "C" clasps and Ball clasps. Placing occlusal rest seats and rests in the appropriate spots gives you the ability to protect tissue areas by making the appliance tooth borne. This is particularly important when the appliance is being used to protect an implant site or an area that has undergone surgery. This needs to be done prior to taking your impression for this appliance.

Note - An opposing model, wax bite, and Bioform shade are necessary for appliance construction. Please specify if the anterior teeth are to be butted up against the tissue or if an acrylic saddle is desired.

INTERIM PARTIALS/BRIDGES

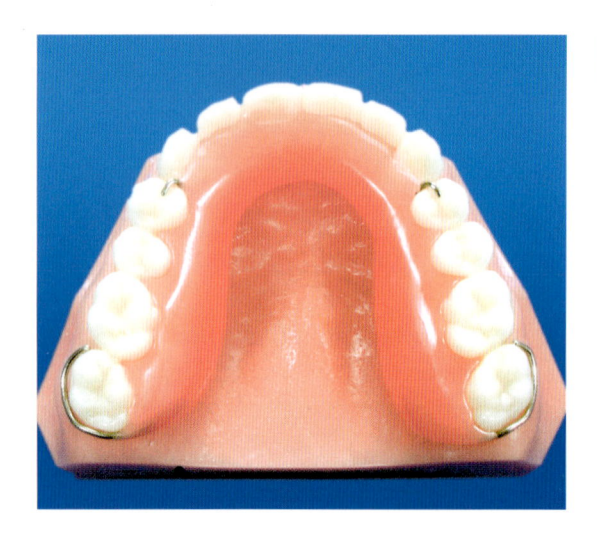

4185H Horseshoe Temporary Partial

Often an adult requiring an interim partial will find it difficult to wear a full palatal coverage appliance. Speech is adversely affected and they have a great deal of difficulty adapting. Although time is often all that is needed to adapt fully, many patients' employment requirements do not afford them the luxury of time.

In this situation, the horseshoe design indicated here will usually solve the problem. Kevlar fiber is added to the acrylic to improve its strength and make up for the minimal amount of acrylic. The use of "C" clasps on the distal-most molars and rests on the first bicuspids offers good stability and retention.

4180 Lower Interim Partial

This is a sample of a typical lower interim partial. Here it is being used to maintain space during periodontal therapy. To be effective at providing function while protecting the tissue, clasping and rests must be well placed.

Note - Taking the time to place rest seats on the appropriate teeth prior to taking a final impression will mean the difference between success and failure.

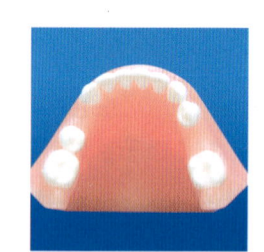

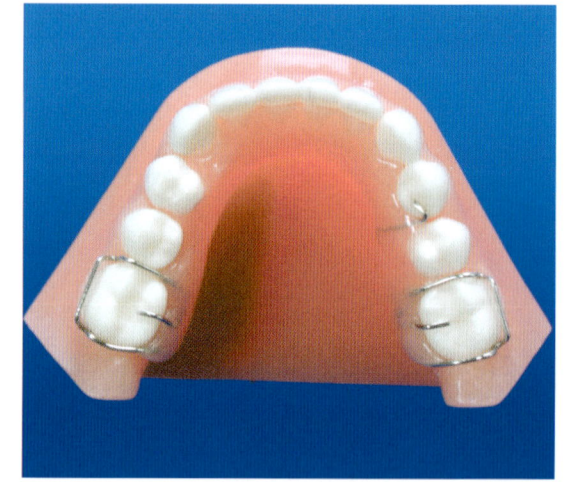

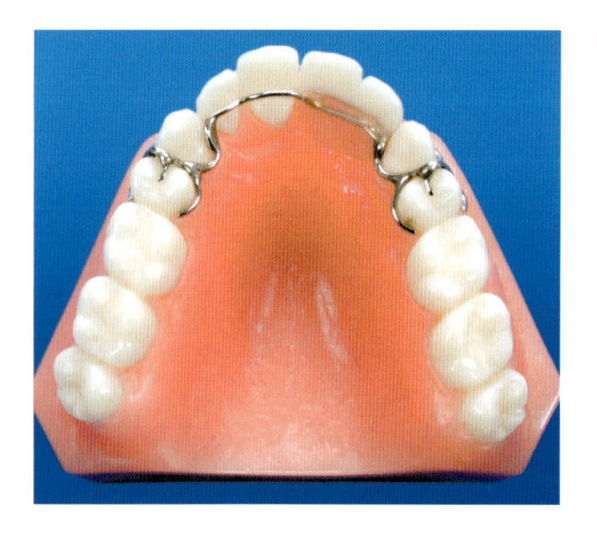

4025 Palate-Free Temp Removable Partial Denture

This appliance was originally designed as a removable interim implant site protector for patients who could not tolerate a removable partial denture. Its double clasps and rest seats are designed to give extra retention and tissue protection. But because one of the clasps is often on the cuspid, esthetics can be an issue. Therefore selecting patients with a low lip line when they smile is preferable when choosing this appliance. Fabrication requires both upper and lower casts, an interocclusal record, and a tooth shade.

Note - Don't forget to adjust the internal aspect of the pontics to make sure they do not put any unwanted pressure on the ridge.

INTERIM PARTIALS/BRIDGES

Treatment Partials

Treatment Partials are used:

- To hold space while accomplishing some minor tooth movement.
- To increase or restore the vertical dimension of occlusion on a temporary basis while the results of the increase can be observed.
- As a splint following surgical corrections in the oral cavity.
- As a vehicle to carry tissue treatment material to abused oral tissue.

Note - When a hyperplastic tissue response occurs such as papillary hyperplasia or the formation of an epulis fissuratum, a tissue conditioning treatment material supported by a treatment partial denture is usually needed to reverse these processes. The healing process of many surgical procedures can also be improved in this manner.

The clinical procedures for making a tissue treatment partial or a surgical splint are basically the same as for the interim partial. In fact, any interim partial can be used, as long as you make sure you indicate on the prescription how the appliance is being used. Indicate the design desired followed by the words "Tissue Treatment." We will then create the space necessary to hold the tissue conditioning material.

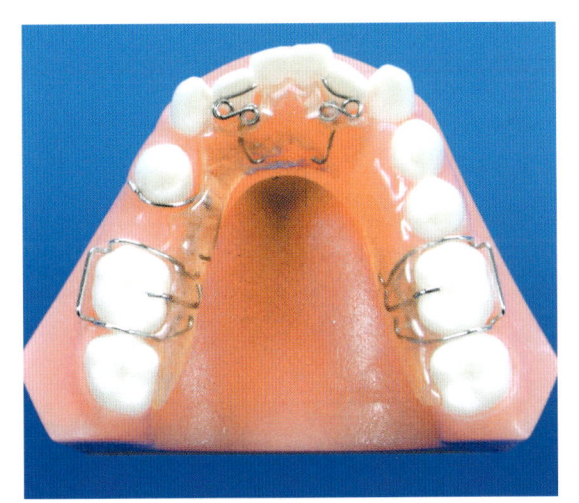

4182 Lower Treatment Partial w/Tooth Movement

This lower adult treatment partial is used to provide a functional occlusion by replacing the 1st and 2nd bicuspids on the right side. The left first bicuspid is being moved mesially prior to construction of a fixed bridge. For cosmetic improvement, the laterals are being moved labially with finger springs after some light mesial-distal stripping to gain the needed space.

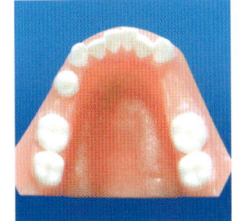

Note - Please send an opposing model and an occlusal record to ensure a proper functional relationship is established.

4183B Upper Treatment Partial with Tooth Movement

Treatment partials can facilitate some minor tooth movement prior to placing final restorations. In this example, denture teeth are replacing the right lateral and the two bicuspids. Springs are being used to close the anterior diastema and make room for the lateral. Once this has been accomplished, veneers and traditional crown and bridge will be completed to enhance the patient's function and appearance.

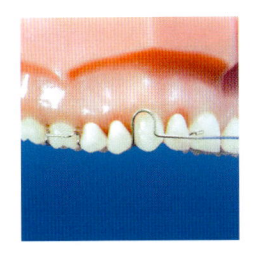

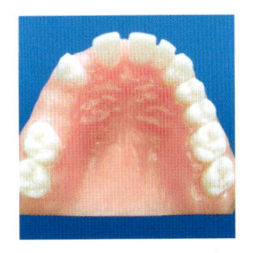

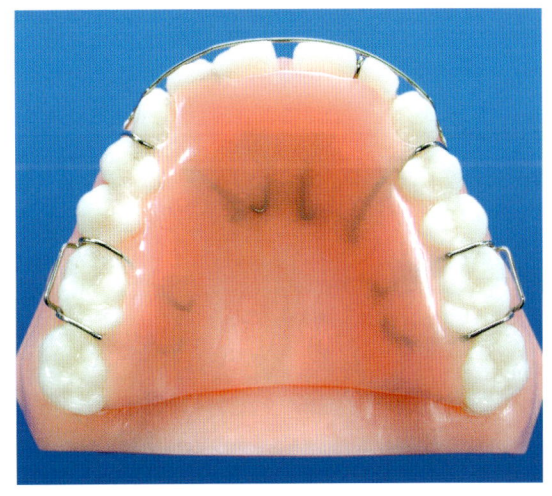

INTERIM PARTIALS/BRIDGES

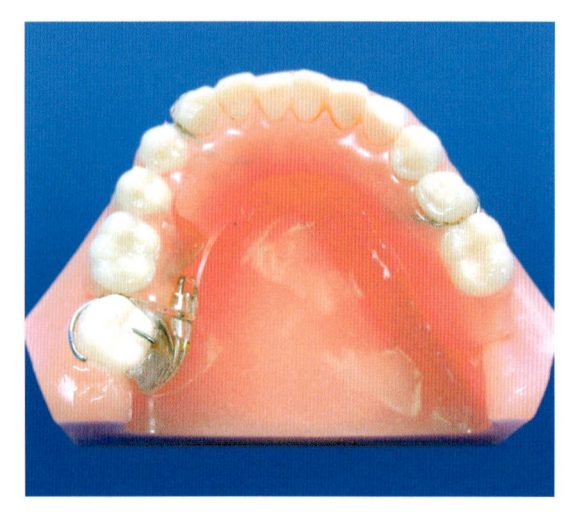

4184 Molar Uprighting Treatment Partial

A treatment partial can be designed to incorporate a spring or an expansion screw to upright or distalize a tooth. This design is especially useful on adult patients with 12-year molars that are tipped mesially. Retention and anchorage are accomplished by using two or more clasps and by having excellent tissue adaptation.

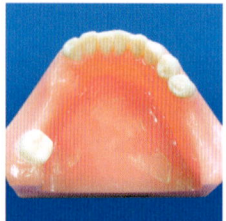

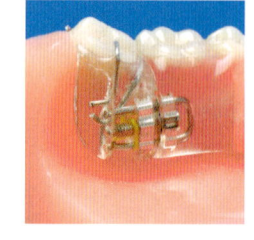

Removable expansion appliances can often be adjusted between visits by the patient. Simply instruct your patient to activate the screw mechanism in the direction of the arrow, one turn per week. This provides 1mm of movement per month.

4187 Treatment Partial To Control Vertical Dimension

Many partially edentulous patients have a decreased vertical dimension. At best, this often makes it difficult to properly restore them. At worst, it can lead to a serious TMJ problem.

A treatment partial is one of the best tools available to help you re-establish an acceptable vertical. This overlay partial may be readily altered to increase or decrease the height of occlusion until clinical signs and subjective symptoms are eliminated and you feel comfortable restoring the patient at the newly established vertical.

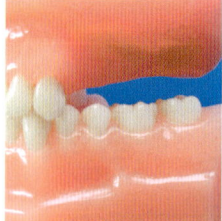

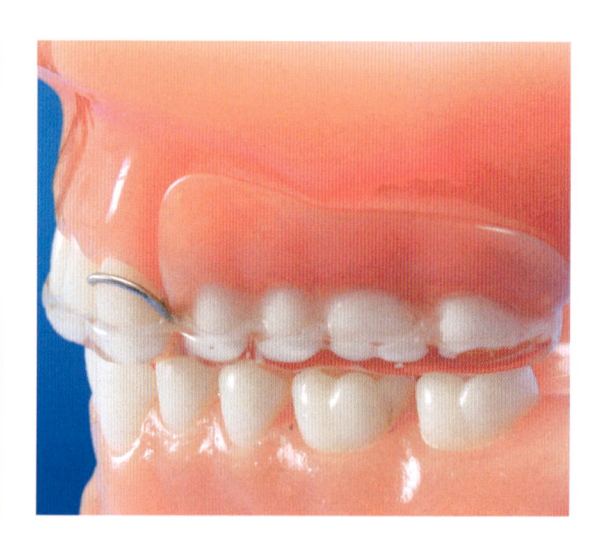

Design Notes:

INTERIM PARTIALS/BRIDGES

4183C Upper Treatment Partial To Gather Flared Anteriors

This appliance demonstrates the versatility of treatment partials. In this scenario, all of the anteriors are flared due to a loss of posterior support and periodontal disease. Specifically, both cuspids and the left lateral need to be moved lingually prior to gathering the rest of the anteriors and placing an intra-coronal splint. To accomplish this tooth movement, T-springs are used to move the cuspids and lateral lingually.

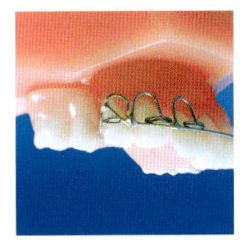

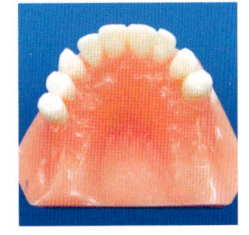

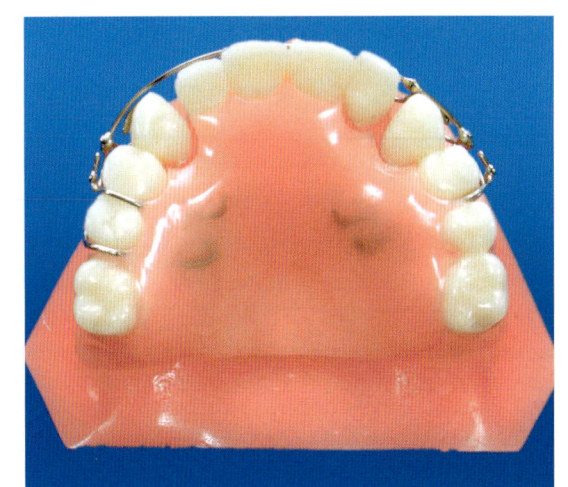

Then, to finish gathering the anteriors, an elastic is placed across the labial surface of the anteriors stretching from hooks on the labial bow at the first bicuspids. All of this tooth movement takes place using a temporary treatment partial.

Once all of the desired tooth movement is complete, an intra-coronal splint will be placed so that the splinting will not interfere with the design of the permanent partial.

Design Notes:

INTERIM PARTIALS/BRIDGES

Transitional Partial Dentures

Transitional partial dentures are used when some or all of the remaining teeth are beyond the point of restoration, but immediate extractions are not indicated for physiologic or psychologic reasons. For example, this treatment plan can be used effectively on an elderly patient suffering from a chronic debilitating disease where multiple extractions could exacerbate the basic illness.

A transitional partial may be appropriate for patients who are psychologically unable to accept the loss of their teeth. In the minds of many people, the presence of natural teeth is related to sex appeal, youth, and happiness. Patients overly concerned with this loss of their teeth can have the indicated treatment spread out over a longer period of time making the change more gradual and easier to accept.

Accurate alginate impressions are essential when making transitional dentures. The impressions should be extended sufficiently to capture all supporting tissues. In the mandibular impression, the anatomy of the ridge lingual to the natural and missing teeth must be captured. In the maxillary impression, the impression tray must be altered to eliminate any excessive space between the tray and the hard palate. If this is not done, the impression material may sag resulting in a poor fitting appliance.

4185 Upper Transitional Partial

The key to the design of a transitional partial is to allow for teeth to be added to the original framework without the necessity of remaking the partial denture.

Also in this example, note the full palate coverage to give maximum tissue support and the presence of rests which are inset into prepared rest seats to keep them out of occlusion.

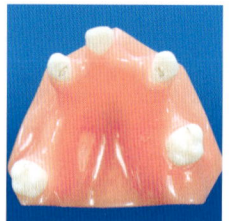

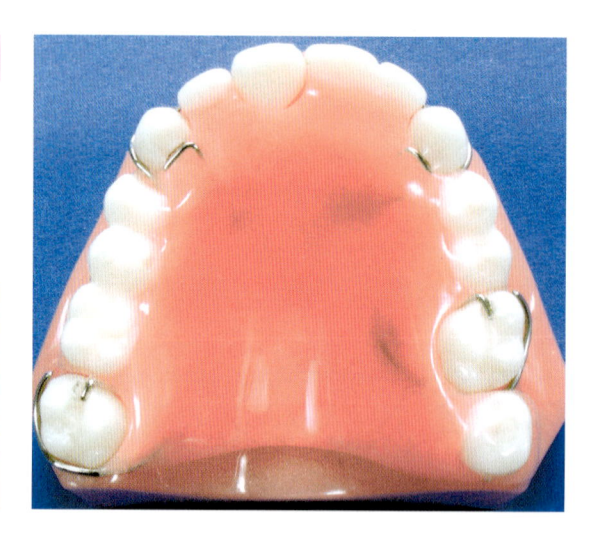

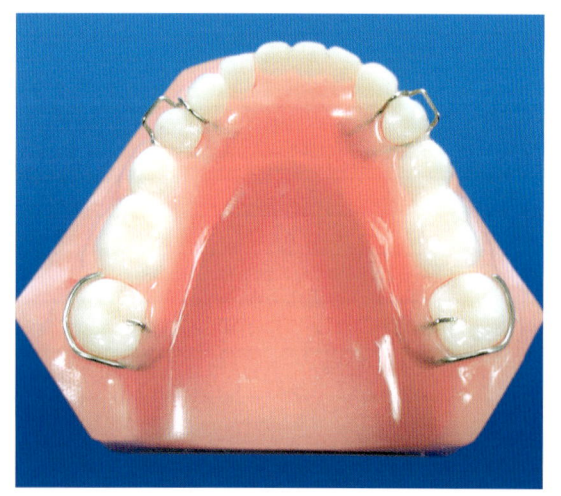

4186 Lower Transitional Partial

Supplying the lab with accurate impressions of the soft tissue, as mentioned above, permits use of the full extensions on this transitional partial.

In this sample, Adams clasps and "C" clasps are used to provide extra retention, and rest seats prevent tissue trauma during function. Patients receiving transitional partial denture service should be seen on a regular recall system so that the remaining teeth can be closely monitored.

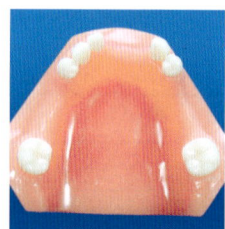

IMPLANT SERVICES

an overview: IMPLANT SERVICES

Chapter 16

When creating a treatment plan for a patient who is missing teeth, it is essential to offer the patient all of the options that are available to help restore them to ideal function. This may include a denture, a partial denture, a fixed bridge, implants, and numerous interim fixed and removable appliances.

Today, it is considered the standard of care to offer the option of having an implant to patients when they have lost a tooth. In fact, implantology remains one of the fastest growing fields in dentistry.

Placing and restoring an implant requires planning. Because there are both surgical and prosthetic considerations that have to be taken into account before placing an implant, it is critical that the restorative dentist and the surgeon work together as a team to properly plan its placement. Not doing so will lead to failure.

Simply put, for an implant to succeed it must have excellent bony support and be placed in a position where the occlusal forces placed upon it will be ideal. The most common mistake made is placing an implant in a position that causes it to constantly bear abnormal occlusal forces. To prevent this, pre-prosthetic surgical planning is a must. Many appliances are now available to help you plan for the ideal implant placement.

Implant stents can be used with CT scans to aid in the proper placement of implants. It is generally accepted that a CT scan, used in conjunction with special imaging, can produce invaluable information for pre-surgical planning of osseointegrated implants.

When properly designed a CT appliance can:

- immobilize a patient's jaws helping the patient to remain motionless during the scan.
- allow the technologist to properly align the patient.
- be used to create practical reference points from which accurate measurements can be taken.
- show the angulation of the proposed restorations and how they relate to the available bone.

Because the ideal placement of the implant is so critical to its success, a surgical stent, that is an exact replication of the position of the final restorations, is used as a guide for implant placement at the time of the surgery. This will allow the surgeon the best opportunity to place the implants down the long axis of the teeth being restored.

Interim implant appliances ranging from temporary partials to fixed temporary bridges have been designed to give you flexibility in your treatment. Appliance selection will depend on the stage of treatment and the desires of the patient. For example, when a removable temporary partial cannot be tolerated, using a temporary Maryland Bridge can be an effective way to protect an implant site during the period of integration.

IMPLANT SERVICES

6520A CT Scan Appliance for the Fully Edentulous Patient

Relating scan slices to clinical locations becomes very difficult in the completely edentulous mandible and maxilla. The mandible measurements can be made from the mental foramen, but in the maxilla, there are no practical reference points from which to make measurements.

This scanning appliance is designed to give a clear indication of the occlusal plane, the long axis of the teeth, and the location of the center of the proposed restoration.

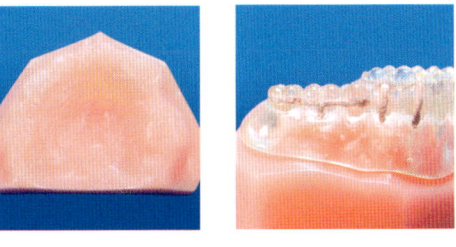

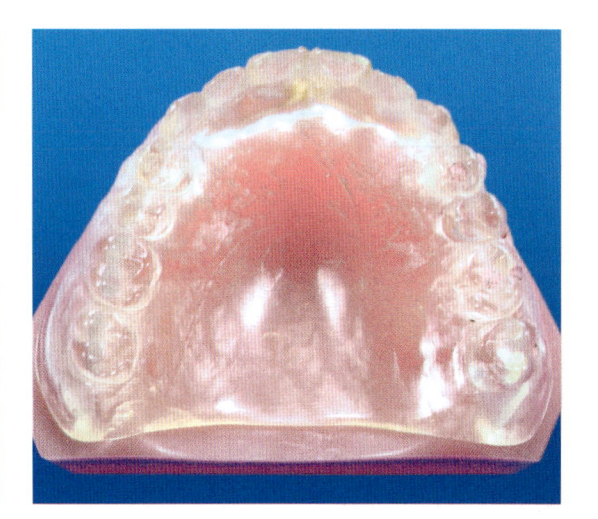

To fabricate this appliance, we will need to replicate the patient's trial denture or existing denture in clear acrylic. Gutta Percha is used to place the radiopaque markers.

Remember this appliance is a representation of your desired prosthetic result. It is important to take the time to make sure the denture set-up is correct.

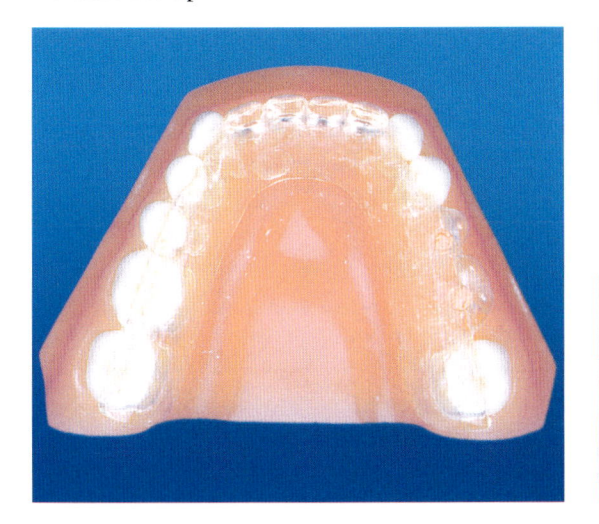

6520B CT Scan Appliance for the Partially Edentulous Patient

When a partially edentulous patient is scanned, many measurements can be made relative to the position of the existing teeth. However, it is still necessary to make an appliance that will replicate the diagnostic set-up of your planned restorative work.

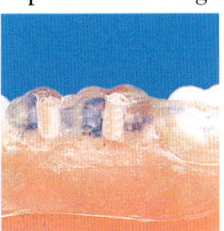

Not doing so may lead to an implant placement that compromises the final prosthetic result.

Again, radiopaque markers are used to evaluate the position of the proposed restoration to the existing bone.

Design Notes:

_____
_____
_____
_____
_____

IMPLANT SERVICES

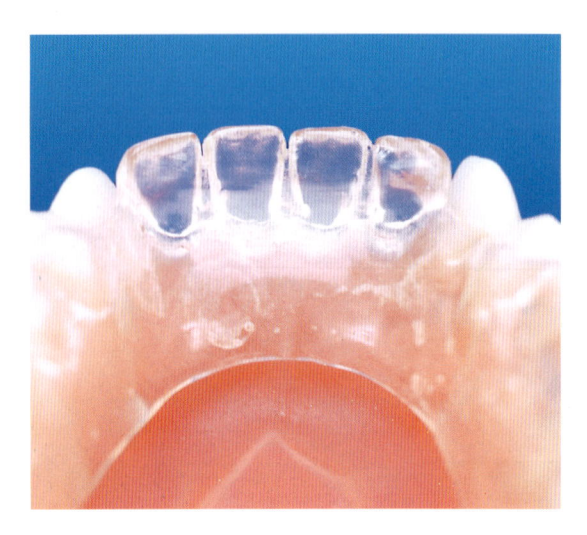

6520C Surgical Stent for Implant Placement

Surgical stents are designed in the same manner as a scanning appliance with the exception that radiopaque markers are not needed. In fact, most surgeons simply modify their CT stent and use it during surgery.

Surgical stents can be modified in many ways. For example, some surgeons prefer occlusal coverage over the existing teeth, while others want the appliance to have full palatal coverage. Your laboratory will construct your stent to your exact specifications.

2013 Adjustable Two-Band Interim Bridge

Simple space maintainers, which are more commonly used after premature loss of primary teeth, are used quite effectively as fixed interim bridges in the adult dentition. Specifically, these appliances can provide an inexpensive way to maintain implant sites and are much more comfortable than a temporary partial or flipper.

When a tooth is missing in the posterior aspect of the arch and a slight amount of uprighting or lost space needs to be regained, the Adjustable Two-Band Interim Bridge is ideal. This appliance can be used to maintain space and stabilize the area without having to prepare the teeth. This technique is particularly useful when buccal/lingual walls of the banded teeth are subject to fracture.

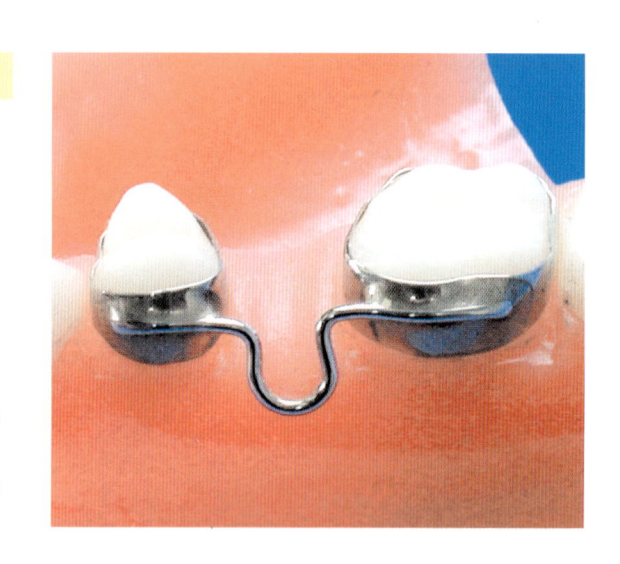

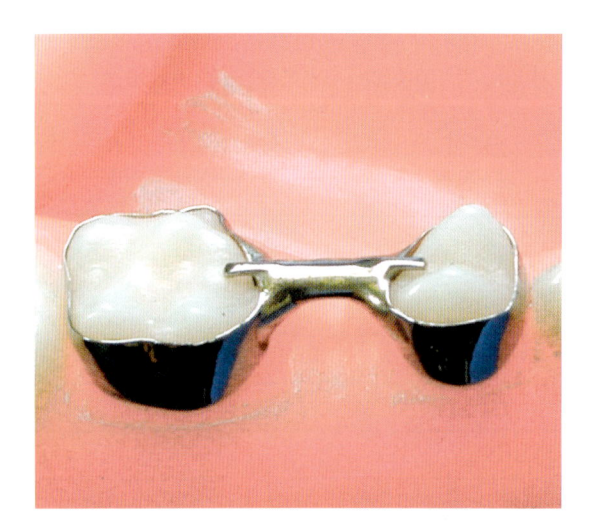

2014 Two-Band Interim Bridge w/Occlusal Bar

This appliance is the same as appliance #2013 but features a rigid non-adjustable metal bar. Both of these appliances are used in situations where hygiene is a consideration as they are easy to clean. The Occlusal metal bar makes this temporary splint ideal to maintain an implant site. However, before choosing this appliance, it is important to make sure there is a parallel path of insertion between the two abutment teeth.

Note - Adding occlusal rests to this design will prevent gingival displacement of this appliance. Bonding these rests in place will allow the patient to maintain this appliance for a longer period of time.

16.2

IMPLANT SERVICES

2023 Two-Band Interim Bridge w/Occlusal Acrylic Pad

When the possibility of super-eruption into the edentulous space is a concern, an acrylic pad can be used to make occlusal contact with the opposing dentition. This pad is designed so that it is kept clear of the tissue, eliminating any chance of abnormal pressure being placed on the implant site. Upon delivery, it will be necessary to adjust the occlusal surface of the pad. Again, it is always important to check for a parallel path of insertion between the two abutment teeth.

Note - Adding occlusal rests to this design will prevent gingival displacement of this appliance. Bonding these rests in place will allow the patient to maintain this appliance for a longer period of time.

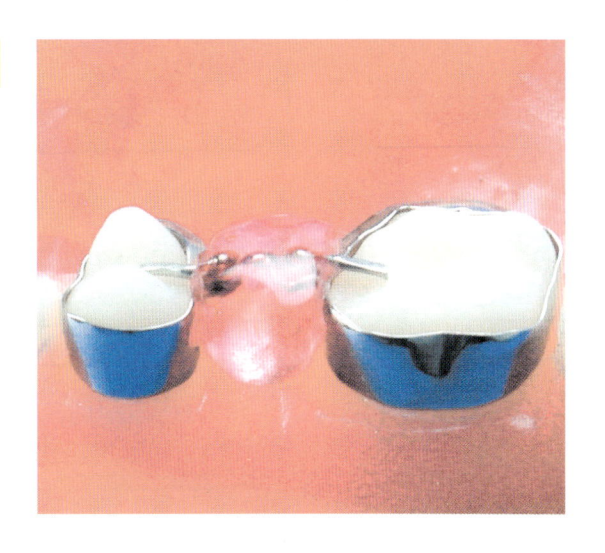

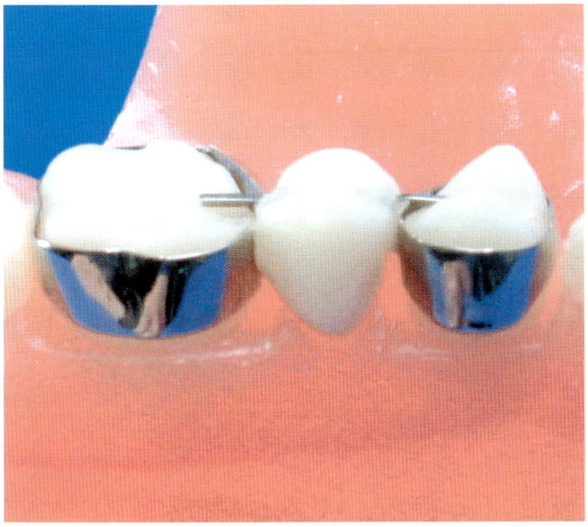

4023 Two-Band Interim Bridge w/Pontic

Bioform shade teeth can be placed instead of an acrylic pad for those patients who prefer a more natural look. This pontic is designed so that it is kept clear of the tissue, eliminating any chance of abnormal pressure being placed on the implant site. The patient should also be able to easily floss underneath it using a floss threader.

Upon delivery, it will be necessary to adjust the occlusal surface of the pontic. Again, it is always important to check for a parallel path of insertion between the two abutment teeth.

Note - Adding occlusal rests to this design will prevent gingival displacement of this appliance. Bonding these rests in place will allow the patient to maintain this appliance for a longer period of time.

4022 Banded/Bonded Interim Splint

When esthetic considerations are important, an occlusal rest and a lingual "C" clasp may be used in place of a band on the visible abutment. Occlusal rests are essential when using this design to help control forces which could cause bond failure between the "C" clasp and the tooth.

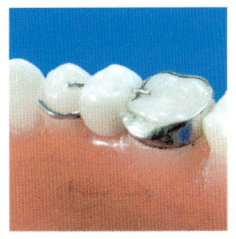

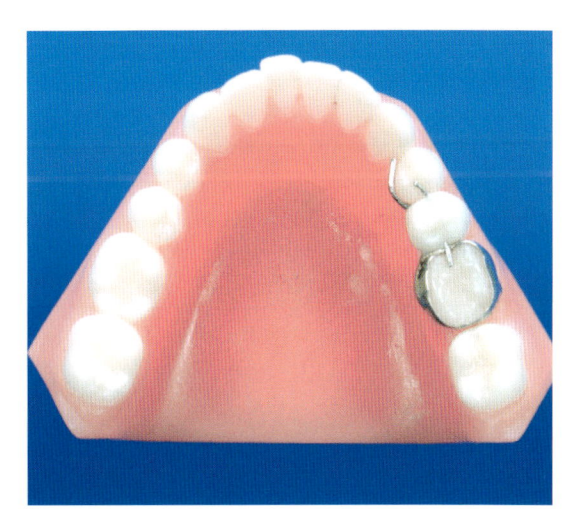

16.3

IMPLANT SERVICES

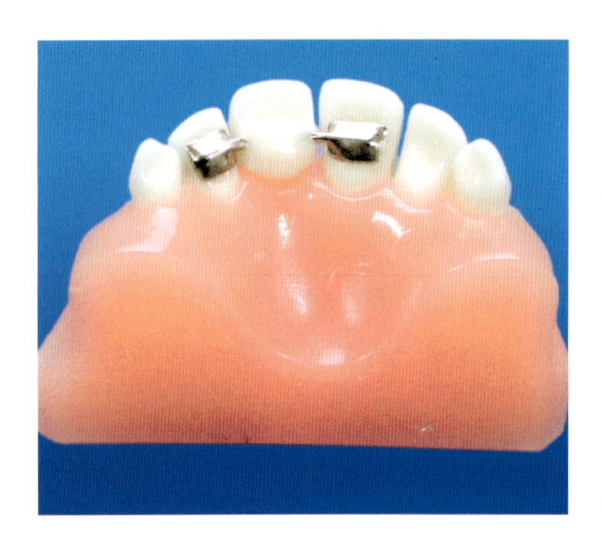

4021 Temporary Maryland Bridge

When a removable temporary partial cannot be tolerated, using a temporary Maryland bridge can be an effective way to protect an implant site during the period of integration.

This appliance consists of two bondable mesh pads attached to a pontic. Tooth preparation is not needed, but it is essential to have occlusal clearance with the opposing arch.

Note - When ordering this appliance always send an opposing model, an accurate bite registration, and a tooth shade selection.

4602 Intra-Coronal Interim Bridge

An intra-coronal bridge may be indicated for patients that cannot tolerate a temporary removable partial denture and whose inter-incisal space is too tight to accommodate a temporary Maryland bridge. Because this is a fixed restoration, it is only appropriate to use during the period of osseointegration.

When it is time to restore the implant, another method of temporization will need to be accomplished. To prepare for this appliance, simply cut a groove deep enough in the lingual aspect of the abutment teeth to allow the supporting wire wings to be kept out of occlusion when they are bonded into place. Then take an accurate impression of the preparation.

Please send us both upper and lower casts, a bite registration and the tooth shade you desire.

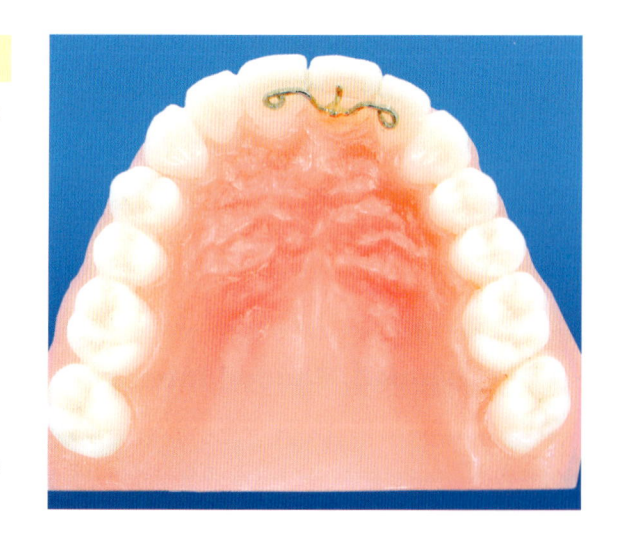

16.4

IMPLANT SERVICES

4024 Fixed/Removable Banded Temp Anterior Bridge

Many implant patients have found it difficult to tolerate interim partial dentures, so more innovative methods have had to be devised to keep an implant patient functional throughout the integration and restorative period of treatment.

The Fixed/Removable Banded Anterior Bridge is one such device. This appliance utilizes Wilson vertical tubes soldered to bands to allow the patient to have the benefit of a palate-free fixed appliance while still allowing the dentist to easily remove it to gain access to the implants.

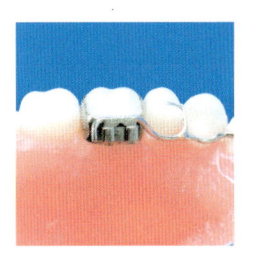

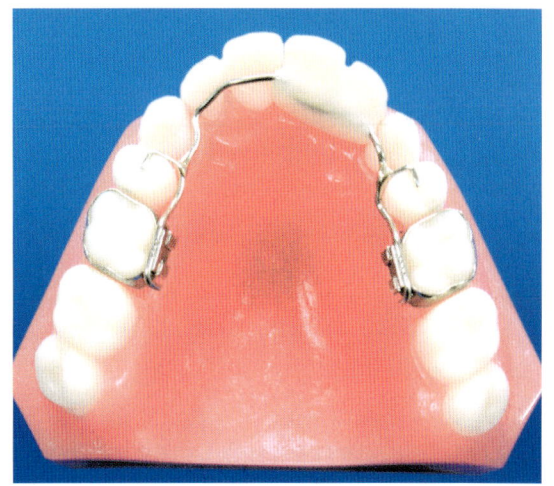

Pressure can be kept off the implant site by allowing the wire to positively rest against the surrounding anteriors as seen here or by adding rest seats and rests on the bicuspids or cuspids.

Note - Don't forget to adjust the internal aspect of the pontics to make sure they do not put any unwanted pressure on the implant site.

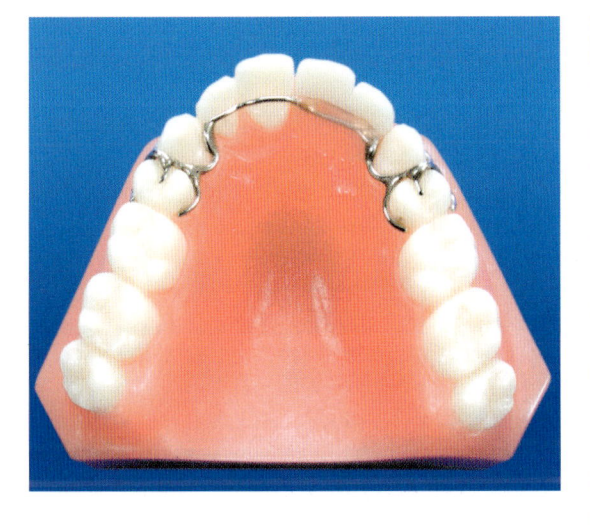

4025 Palate-Free Temp Removable Partial Denture

This appliance was originally designed as a removable interim implant site protector for patients who could not tolerate a removable partial denture. Its double clasps and rest seats are designed to give extra retention and tissue protection. But because one of the clasps is often on the cuspid, esthetics can be an issue. Therefore selecting patients with a low lip line when they smile is preferable when choosing this appliance.

Don't forget to adjust the internal aspect of the pontics to make sure they do not put any unwanted pressure on the implant site.

Note - Fabrication requires both upper and lower casts, an interocclusal record, and a tooth shade.

16.5

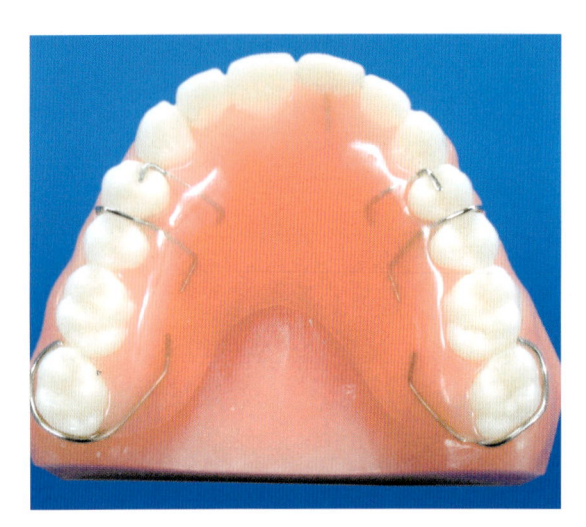

IMPLANT SERVICES

4181 Upper Interim Removable Partial

The simple, inexpensive interim partial shown here replaces a single, lost permanent central. This example is shown with "C" clasps and ball clasps to provide the patient with retention. Occlusal rests are placed to protect the implant site by making the appliance tooth borne.

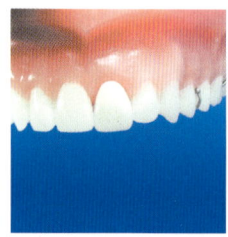

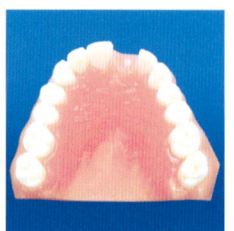

To keep these wires out of occlusion, it may be necessary to prepare small rest seats in the teeth. This preparation needs to be done prior to taking the impression for this appliance. An opposing model, wax bite and Bioform shade are necessary for appliance construction. Also, please specify if the anterior teeth are to be butted up against the tissue or if an acrylic saddle is desired.

4185H Horseshoe Temporary Partial

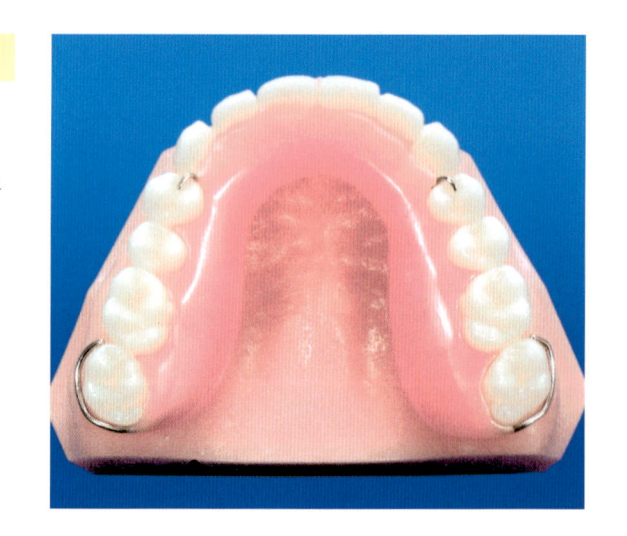

Often an adult requiring an interim partial will find it difficult to wear a full-palatal coverage appliance. Speech is adversely affected and they have difficulty adapting. Although time is often all that is needed to adapt fully, many patients' employment requirements do not afford them the luxury of time. In this situation, the Horseshoe design indicated here will usually solve the problem.

Kevlar fiber is added to the acrylic to improve its strength and make up for the minimal amount of acrylic. Occlusal rests are placed to protect the implant site by making the appliance tooth borne.

To keep these wires out of occlusion, it may be necessary to prepare small rest seats in the teeth. This preparation needs to be done prior to taking the impression for this appliance. The use of "C" clasps on the distal-most molars and rests on the first bicuspids offers good stability and retention. An opposing model, wax bite and Bioform shade are necessary for appliance construction. Please specify if the anterior teeth are to be butted up against the tissue or if an acrylic saddle is desired.

IMPLANT SERVICES

4191 Essix Temporary Partial

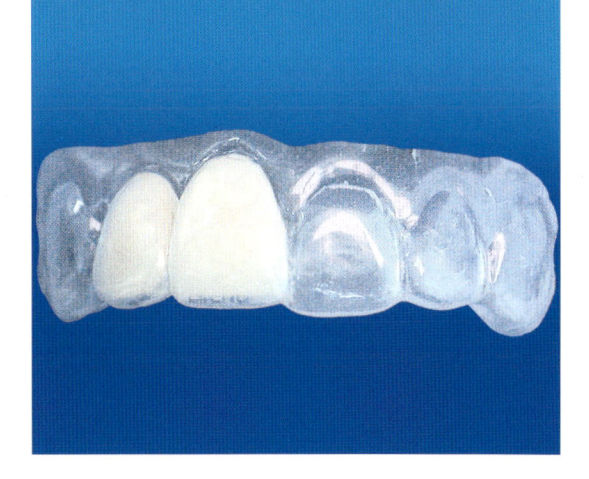

This simple appliance is excellent for temporary replacement of anterior teeth while the patient is waiting for a permanent implant. Traditionally, these missing anteriors would be replaced by incorporating denture teeth into a Hawley type retainer more commonly referred to by patients as a "flipper". Unfortunately, these appliances are often initially uncomfortable and affect speech because they have acrylic in the palatal region. Partials can also place unwanted pressure on the implant site and on the surrounding healing tissue.

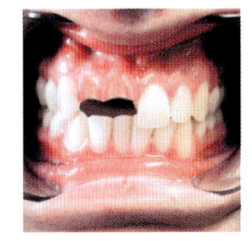

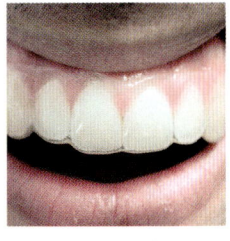

By using the new Essix technology, a simpler, more efficient method is used to retain and replace the missing teeth on a temporary basis. This removable interim bridge is made using the Essix "C-type" clear vacuum-formed material. When properly designed and fabricated, this appliance will snap into place and stay retained by using the natural undercuts gingival to the anterior contact points. They are clear, thin, run from cuspid-to-cuspid, and are clasp free and palate free. Patient acceptance and esthetics are excellent.

Design Notes:

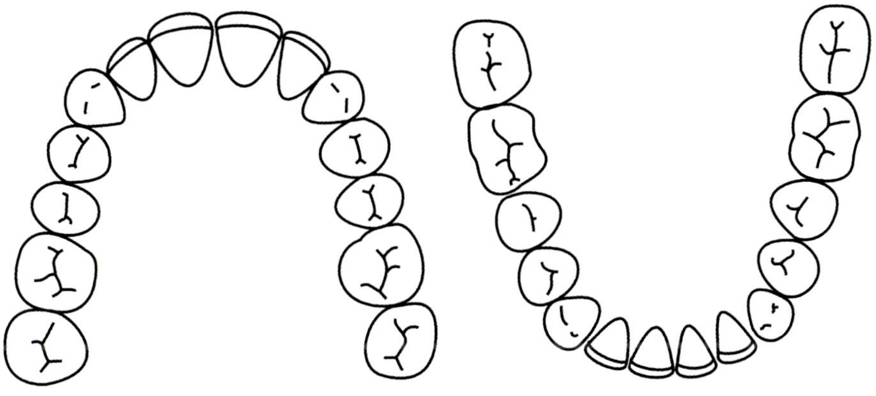

Design Notes

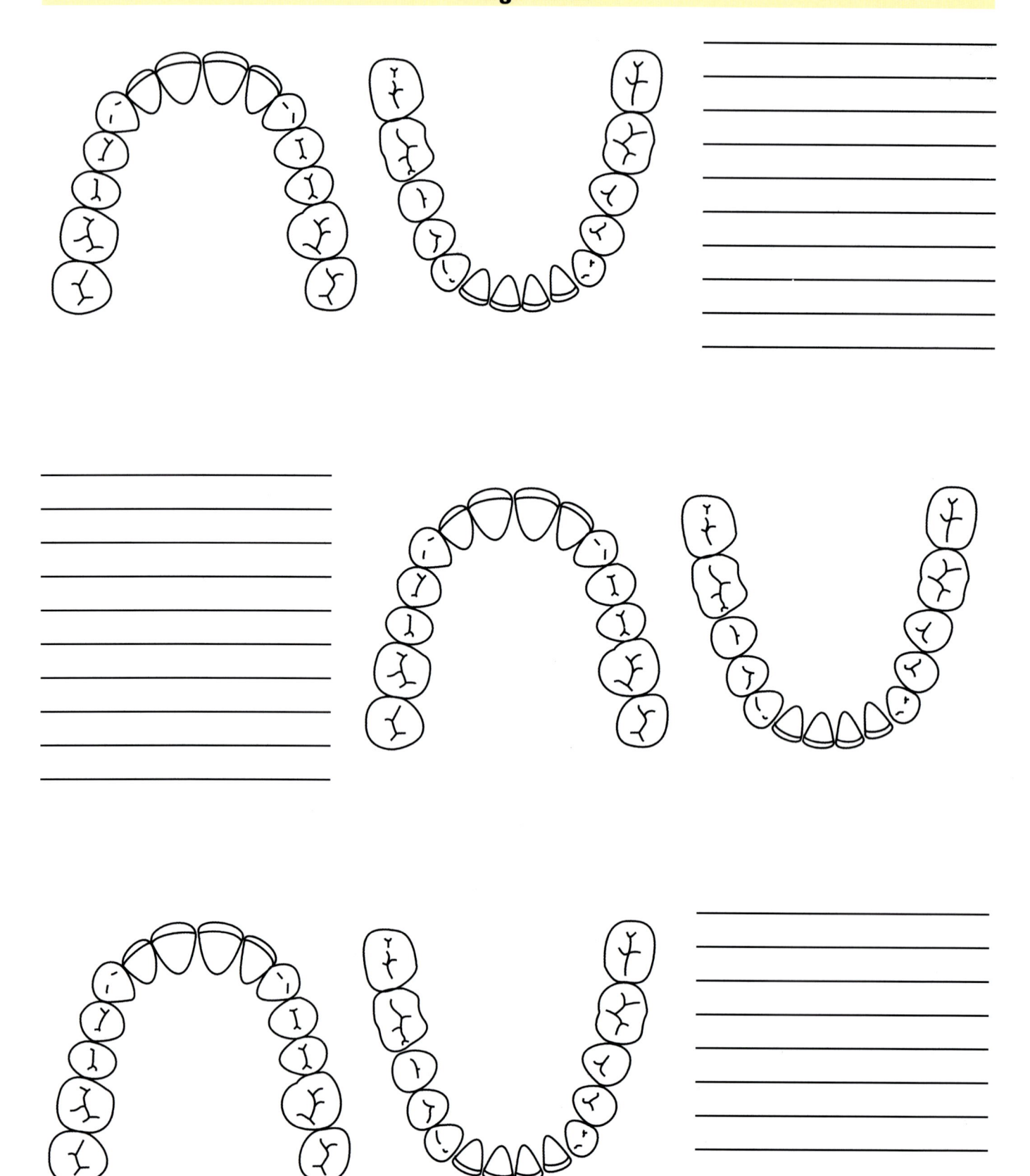

PERIODONTAL SERVICES

an overview: PERIODONTAL SERVICES

Chapter 17

In today's dentistry, periodontal, occlusal, and restorative needs must all be taken into consideration to properly manage the stomatognathic system. Tooth loss, drifting teeth, tipped molars, posterior bite collapse, anterior flaring, and occlusal trauma are some of the problems that are associated with periodontal disease.

Periodontal disease must be controlled and the results of it remedied to the best of your ability before attempting to complete the patient's restorative work. For example, when a periodontal patient has a loss in vertical dimension and flared anteriors, it is not enough to just control the disease process. The loss in vertical and flared anteriors must also be addressed.

Because your treatment approach is case dependent, it is important to have many tools at your disposal. You can gather the anteriors with either a removable appliance or fixed brackets. The vertical can be improved either by orthodontically erupting the posteriors or using crown and bridge techniques. What is important here, is that with the use of some simple appliances, you will be able have greater control of your treatment plan.

These appliances can realign teeth, level infrabony defects, create a harmonious gingival lip line relationship, maintain and stabilize a compromised dentition, and re-establish a proper occlusal plane. Just remember, before beginning any active appliance therapy, thorough root planing and curettage must be completed to eliminate the active disease process.

Maintenance of our periodontal care is also often overlooked. When patients have lost some of their bony support, mechanical retention is often needed to maintain a stable occlusion. This can easily be accomplished with intra-coronal and extra-coronal splinting techniques. Instances where mechanical retention may be necessary are:

- after periodontal surgery to distribute forces, decrease trauma, and aid in healing.
- in adult orthodontics where restoration of a broken down dentition coincides with the need for stabilization.
- in cases of secondary occlusal trauma where changes in the attachment apparatus reduce its ability to resist the functional forces.
- in a mutilated dentition, where there is both the loss of attachment and the presence of tooth mobility.

Orthodontic therapy can often be used to enhance a patient's periodontal health. It can be used to eliminate a bony defect through forced eruption or correct the axial inclination of a molar to properly distribute occlusal forces down the long axis of the tooth.

In this chapter, we will show you some of the basic approaches being used to aid in the treatment of periodontal disease. The wide variety of appliances that are available even include fluoride trays to give daily fluoride treatments to control root sensitivity after root planing or periodontal surgery. For the best results, the generalist and the specialist should work closely together. Only through this integrated method of treatment can we deliver the best possible care to the patient.

PERIODONTAL SERVICES

Removable Extra-Coronal Splints

6191 Maxillary Splint w/Full Palatal Coverage

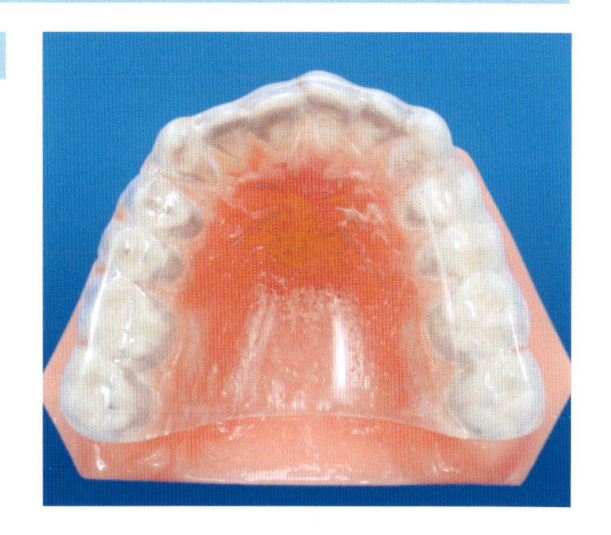

Splints are valuable in periodontal therapy because they distribute forces, decrease trauma, aid in healing, and control and protect against excess tooth mobility due to primary or secondary occlusal trauma.

This design has clear acrylic over the entire arch and is finished with full palatal coverage. The palatal coverage provides the extra stability needed in a periodontally involved case. The occlusal surface can be finished in whatever manner desired, i.e. smooth with point contact, positive facets for opposing dentition, cuspid rise, and/or anterior guidance to disarticulate the teeth in protrusive or excursive movements.

Note - Careful finishing is required so that each opposing tooth will make equal contact on the acrylic biting surface. To avoid unnecessary chair time adjusting an extra-coronal splint, always provide the lab with an accurate set of working casts and a construction bite that precisely represents the vertical and horizontal occlusal relationship of the splint.

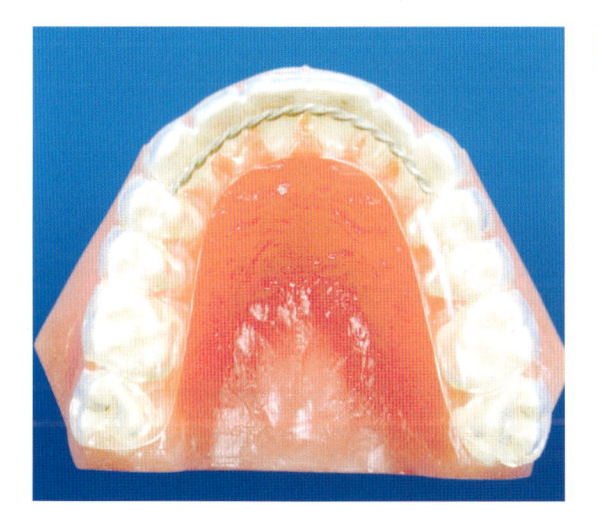

6193 Upper Removable Acrylic Splint

The maxillary horseshoe splint is the most common splint made because of its comfort and ease of adjustability. Just like the full palatal splint, this design can distribute forces, decrease trauma, aid in healing, and control and protect against excess tooth mobility due to primary or secondary occlusal trauma. It is also the most common design used to provide post-orthodontic stabilization.

The occlusal surface can be finished in whatever manner desired, i.e. smooth with point contact, positive facets for opposing dentition, cuspid rise, and/or anterior guidance to disarticulate the teeth in protrusive or excursive movements.

Note - To avoid unnecessary chair time adjusting an extra-coronal splint, always provide the lab with an accurate set of working casts and a construction bite that precisely represents the vertical and horizontal occlusal relationship of the splint.

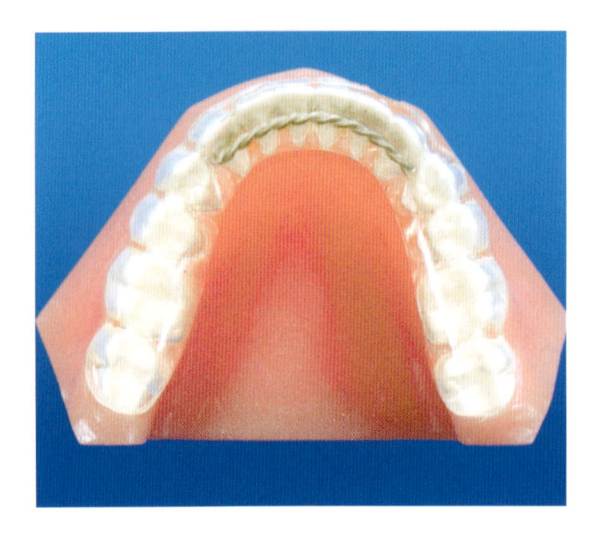

PERIODONTAL SERVICES

6192 Lower Removable Acrylic Splint

Although 80% of the splints made today are designed for the upper arch, periodontal therapy often demands the use of a full coverage lower splint to stabilize that arch. In fact, it is not uncommon for an upper and lower splint to be used at the same time, especially after orthodontic treatment has been completed in a periodontally compromised case.

Note - To avoid unnecessary chair time adjusting an extra-coronal splint, always provide the lab with an accurate set of working casts and a construction bite that precisely represents the vertical and horizontal occlusal relationship of the splint.

1165 The San Antonio Retainer w/Full Palate

Removable appliances are often used to stabilize an arch. In this design, the labial arch wire extends from molar to molar and is kept in contact with the buccal surfaces of all of the teeth. This, along with the intimate acrylic contact on the lingual surfaces, provides excellent retention and control of the entire arch.

When using removable appliances during periodontal therapy it is essential to make sure that all of the wires are kept out of occlusion. To accomplish this, "C" clasps are extended around the distal aspect of the 12-year molars and two small interproximal support wires are carried between the cuspids and the laterals to stabilize the labial bow.

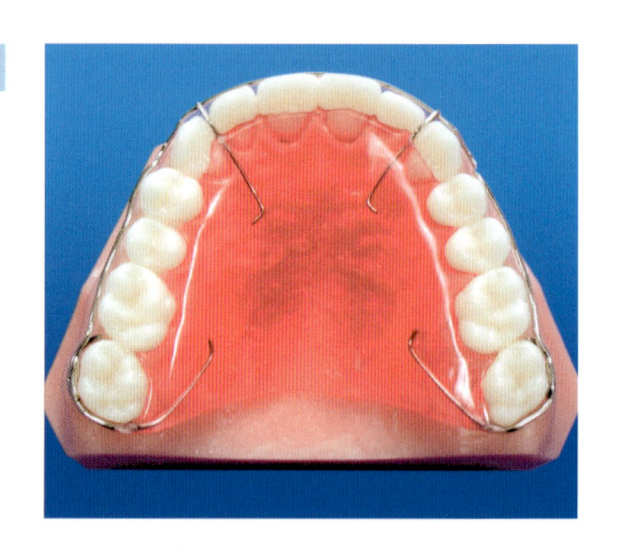

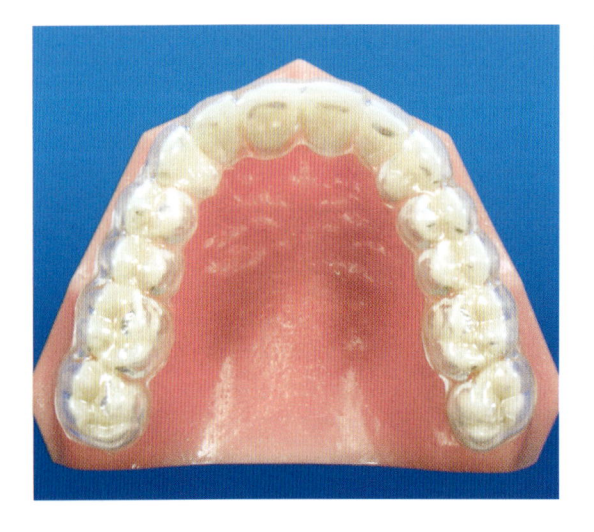

1116P The Invisible Retainer

Many patients complain that their teeth feel loose after periodontal surgery. This may occur even in those patients who do not clench or grind. When mobility does exist, a simple vacuum-formed hard splint can be used to stabilize the arch and enhance healing. This splint only covers the teeth and does not rest on the tissue at all. Because it is clear, it can be worn 24-hours a day.

Note - This splint is meant to be used only for a short period of time after surgery. It is very thin and is not appropriate for patients who grind their teeth.

PERIODONTAL SERVICES

Fixed Extra-Coronal Splints

6401 Mesh/Composite Lingual Splints

Posterior bite collapse, bone loss, and abnormal tongue habits are just some of the conditions that can cause excessive mobility of the lower anteriors. To control these forces and stabilize the anteriors, a mesh composite extra-coronal splint is commonly used because it is easy to place and is esthetically pleasing.

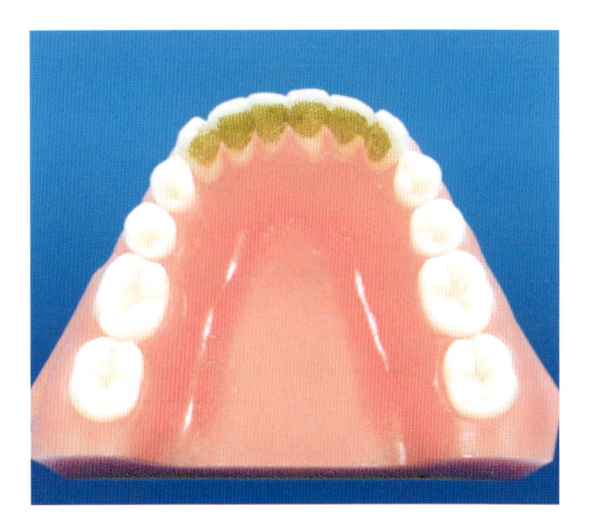

The laboratory will use your working model to cut and adapt the mesh to fit the lingual surfaces so that nothing can be seen from the facial aspect. The clinician will etch the teeth and secure the mesh in place with composite.

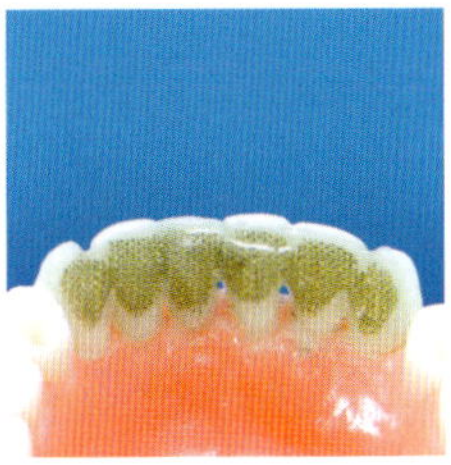

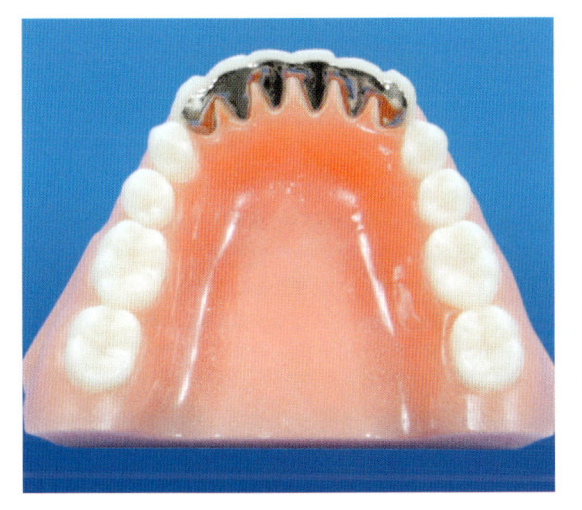

6402 Etched Metal Cast Bar Splint

A cast metal bar splint is the most rigid method of splinting and is commonly used when there is a significant amount of mobility. Although this appliance is bonded into place with a resin cement, its resistance to displacement cannot be solely dependent upon the composite bond. Therefore, each tooth must be individually prepared with vertical stops and in a manner to encompass the greatest surface area possible. This will ensure maximum retention and resistance to dislodging forces.

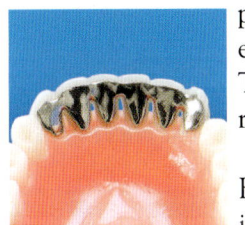

Because this is a cast metal splint, accurate impressions are essential to assure the desired fit.

Note - There are two tricks to successfully splinting these highly mobile periodontally involved teeth. The first is to get an accurate impression. To do this you must stabilize the teeth to be splinted by temporarily bonding their facial surface together with composite. Once this is accomplished, block out any interproximal undercuts that might cause your impression to become locked in place. The second trick is to keep these teeth splinted together with composite until the final splint is cemented.

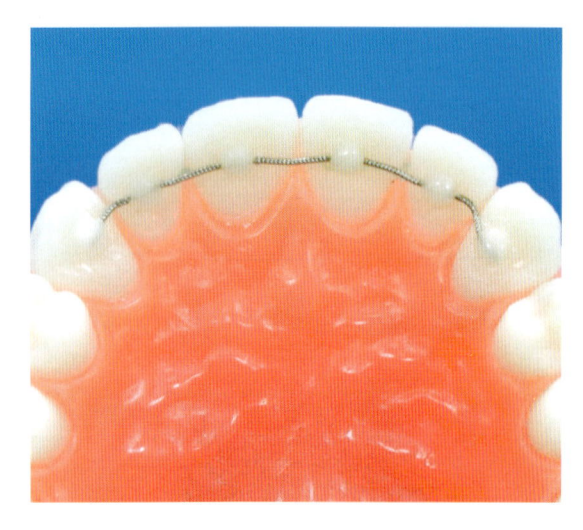

PERIODONTAL SERVICES

2212 E-Z Bond Lingual Retainer

This extra-coronal splint is constructed of a multi-stranded, lingual wire retainer that is carefully contoured to the lingual of the six anterior teeth and is light-cured with composite to each of the six anterior teeth.

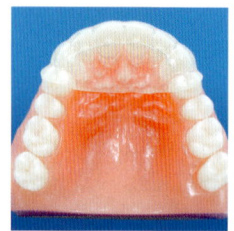

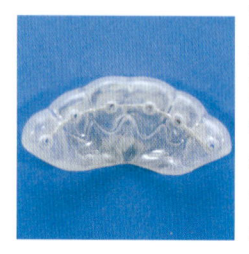

The key advantage to this appliance is use of a laboratory fabricated transfer tray that makes correct placement of the wire easy with a minimum of chair time.

The transfer tray has small reservoirs at each bonding site with an excess material escape channel directly lingual to each of the anterior teeth. This assures a complete wrap of bonding cement around the lingual wire.

To place the appliance, the reservoirs are filled with composite by use of a syringe. The tray is then gently seated by finger pressure, allowing any excess composite to flow out of the escape channels. Then it is light cured. After curing the material, any excess cement is removed from the tray with a high speed hand piece and a diamond. Then the tray is slowly and carefully lifted off of the teeth. The top of the individual composite buttons can then be polished for patient comfort with a composite diamond or disc. Complete, step-by-step, chairside instructions are provided with your first E-Z Bond Retainer.

Note - When requesting an E-Z Bond Retainer for the maxillary anteriors, it is important to send an opposing model and a wax bite. Sufficient overbite and overjet is essential to provide clearance for the maxillary E-Z Bond Retainer.

2165 Direct Bond Fixed Retainer

This appliance is bonded to the lingual of the cuspids by the use of custom contoured, direct bond pads. These pads have a metal-mesh backing for superior retention. The lingual wire is carefully contoured and routinely placed 2mm below the incisal edges unless prescribed otherwise. Additionally, many choose to add the first bicuspids into the retentive unit as illustrated in the inserted photo.

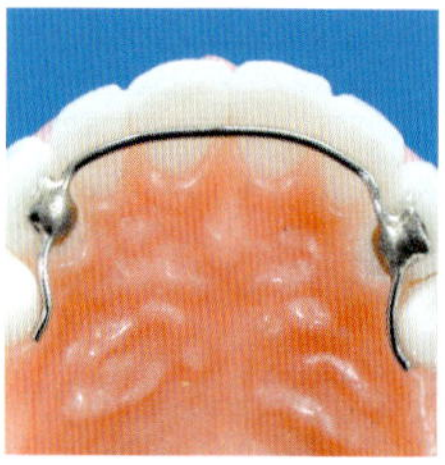

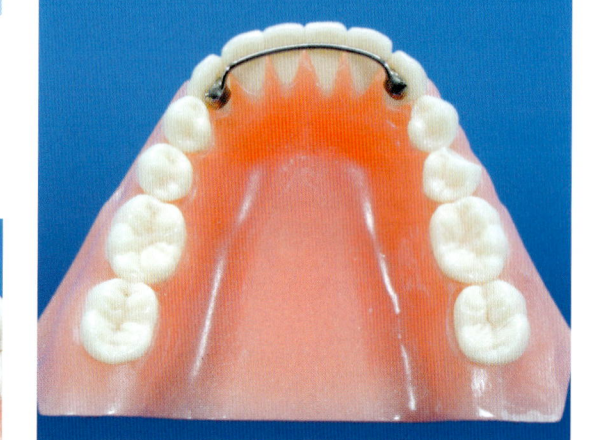

Note - Recent research shows that it is necessary to bond each tooth individually to maintain them in their corrected position. Individual anterior teeth can be secured to the lingual wire by simply adding composite over the lingual wire.

17.4

PERIODONTAL SERVICES

2166M Bonded Fixed Lingual Retainers

When splinting anteriors together, each tooth must be individually bonded to maintain them in their corrected position. This is hard to accomplish without making it more difficult for patients to maintain their hygiene. Typically patients who have lingual bonded retainers have to use floss threaders to clean interproximally.

The lingual bonded retainer shown here is designed to allow the patient to floss normally making it much easier for them to maintain a healthy oral condition. Using Australian wire, loops are placed between all the teeth except in the lower incisor region where the interproximal distances are too close. These loops avoid the interproximal areas allowing the patient to floss. A floss threader is recommended for use between the lower incisors.

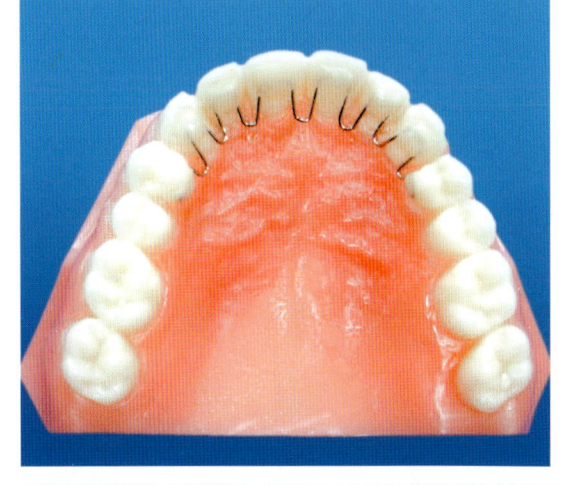

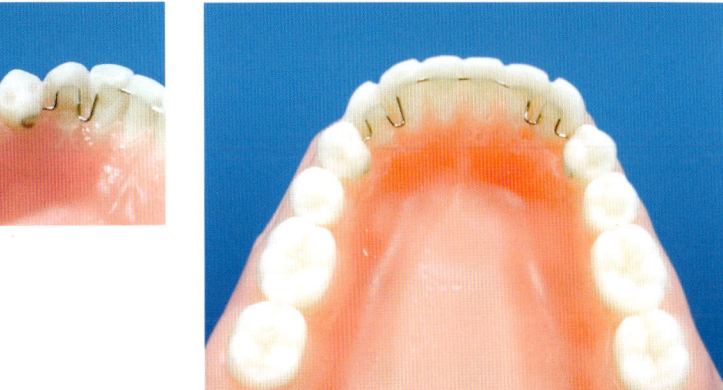

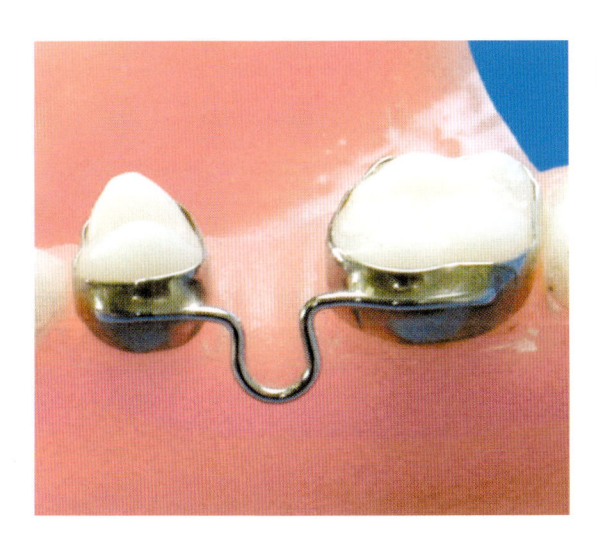

2013 Adjustable Two-Band Interim Splint

Simple space maintainers can be used quite effectively as interim splints in periodontally involved areas. They are an inexpensive way to stabilize an area and enhance healing until periodontal therapy is complete and a decision on the best restorative technique can be made. This technique is particularly useful when the teeth that are to be banded are subject to fracture, as the bands will act to hold them together.

This particular appliance is designed with an adjustable buccal wire. A simple adjustment with a 139 bird-beak plier will allow you to gain a small amount of lost space or upright a tooth that has tipped slightly into the edentulous space.

Note - When using a space maintainer as a periodontal splint, always ask the lab to use custom-made bands. This will ensure that they are made in a manner that keeps them away from the tissue and eliminates any chance for an inflammatory response.

PERIODONTAL SERVICES

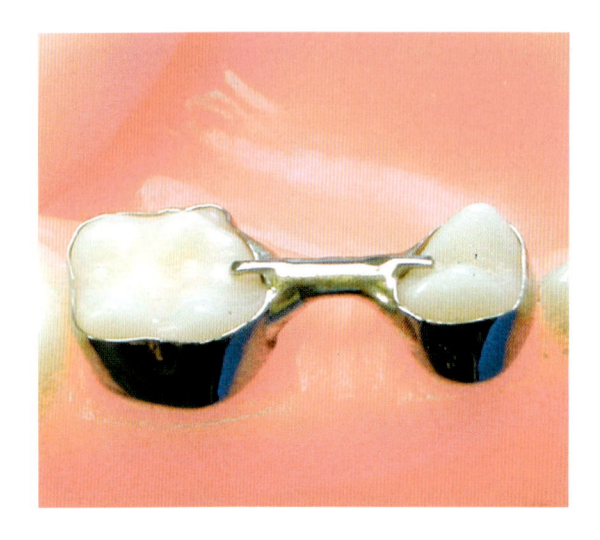

2014 Two-Band Interim Splint w/Occlusal Bar

This appliance is the same as appliance #2013 but features a rigid non-adjustable metal bar. Both these appliances are used in situations where hygiene is a consideration as they are easy to clean.

The Occlusal metal bar makes this temporary splint ideal to maintain an implant site or protect an area that has undergone a ridge augmentation. Adding occlusal rests to this design will prevent gingival displacement of this appliance. Bonding these rests in place will allow the patient to maintain this appliance for a longer period of time. It is also important to check for a parallel path of insertion between the two abutment teeth.

2023 Two Band Interim Splint w/Occlusal Acrylic Pad

When the possibility of super-eruption is a concern, an acrylic pad can be used to make occlusal contact with the opposing dentition. This pad is designed so that it is clear of the tissue and the patient can easily floss underneath it using a floss threader.

Upon delivery, it will be necessary to adjust the occlusal surface of the pad. Adding occlusal rests to this design will prevent gingival displacement of this appliance. Bonding these rests in place will allow the patient to maintain this appliance for a longer period of time. Again, it is always important to check for a parallel path of insertion between the two abutment teeth.

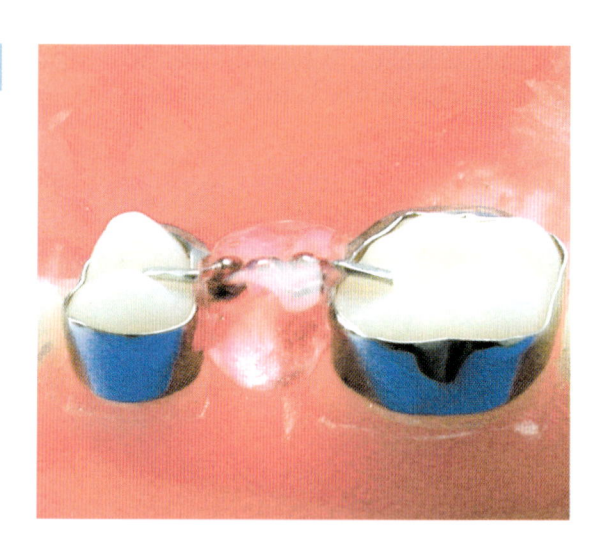

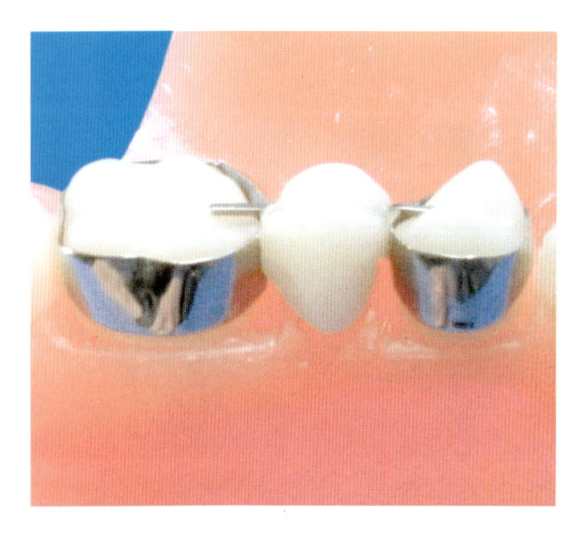

4023 Two-Band Interim Splint w/Pontic

Bioform shade teeth can be placed instead of an acrylic pad for those patients who prefer a more natural look. This pontic is designed so that it is clear of the tissue and the patient can easily floss underneath it using a floss threader.

Upon delivery, it will be necessary to adjust the occlusal surface of the pontic. Adding occlusal rests to this design will prevent gingival displacement of this appliance. Bonding these rests in place will allow the patient to maintain this appliance for a longer period of time. Again, it is always important to check for a parallel path of insertion between the two abutment teeth.

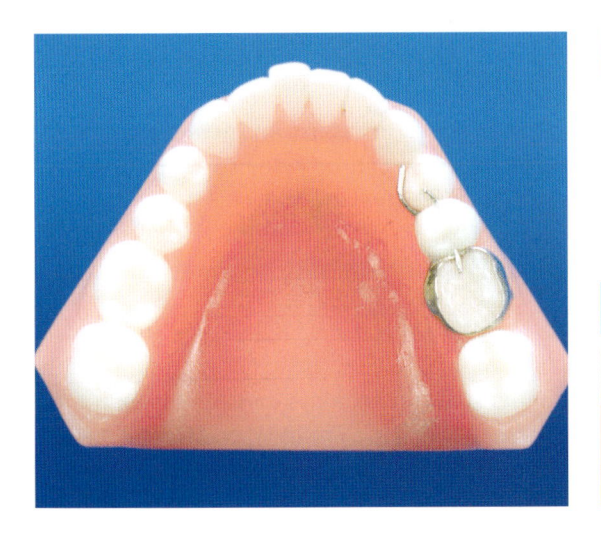

PERIODONTAL SERVICES

4022 Banded/Bonded Interim Splint

When esthetic considerations are important, an occlusal rest and a lingual "C" clasp may be used in place of a band on the visible abutment. Bonding material can then be placed over the lingual "C" clasp and occlusal rest to add stability and retention.

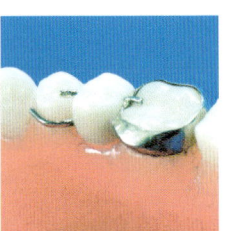

Note - When using a space maintainer as a periodontal splint, always ask the lab to use custom-made bands. This will ensure that they are made in a manner that keeps them away from the tissue and eliminates any chance for an inflammatory response.

Intra-Coronal Splints

2320 Wire/Composite Splint

An intra-coronal composite/wire splint is made by bonding a wire into a prepared channel. This channel must be deep enough to keep the wire out of occlusion once it is bonded into place. Because these splints are intra-coronal, they will not interfere with other restorative procedures such as partial design and placement.

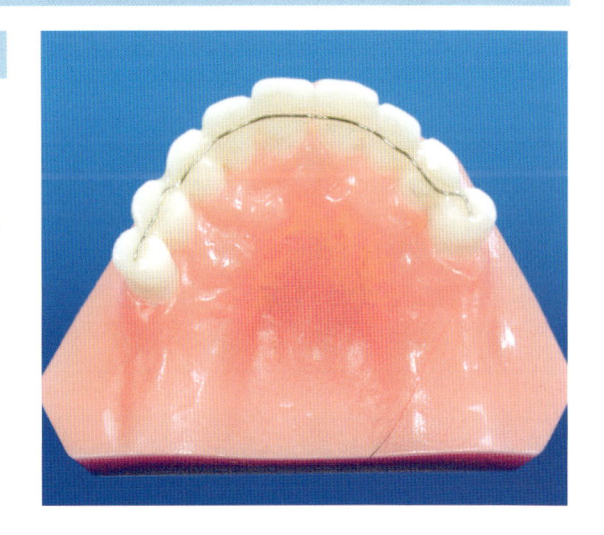

17.7

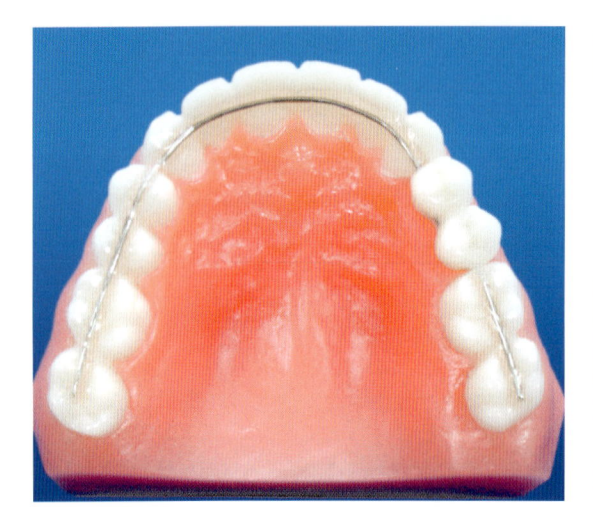

PERIODONTAL SERVICES

4603 Intra-Coronal Splint w/Pontics

An entire arch can be splinted together using an intra-coronal approach. As shown here, the splint can be made to support pontics allowing it to be used as an interim bridge.

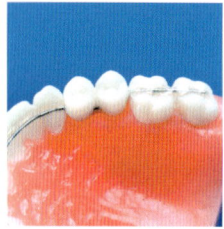

Note - To properly fabricate this appliance, the lab must have an accurate cast of your prepared teeth, an opposing cast, an occlusal registration and the Bioform shade of the teeth to be replaced.

4602 Intra-Coronal Interim Bridge

When a patient cannot tolerate a temporary removable partial denture and the inter-incisal space is too tight to accommodate a temporary Maryland splint, an Intra-coronal interim bridge can be used to maintain the space and protect the tissue site.

To prescribe this appliance, simply cut a groove deep enough in the lingual aspect of the abutment teeth to allow the supporting wire wings to be kept out of occlusion when they are bonded into place. Then take an accurate impression of your preparation. Please supply the lab with both upper and lower casts, a bite registration and the tooth shade you desire.

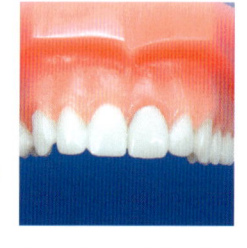

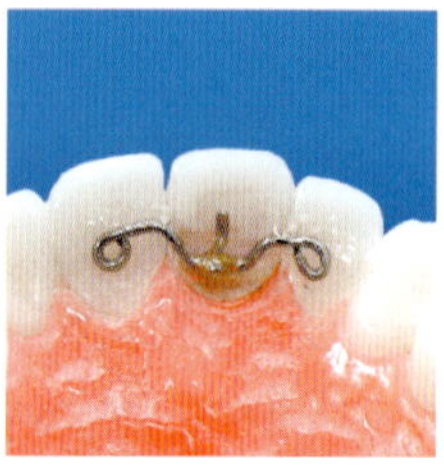

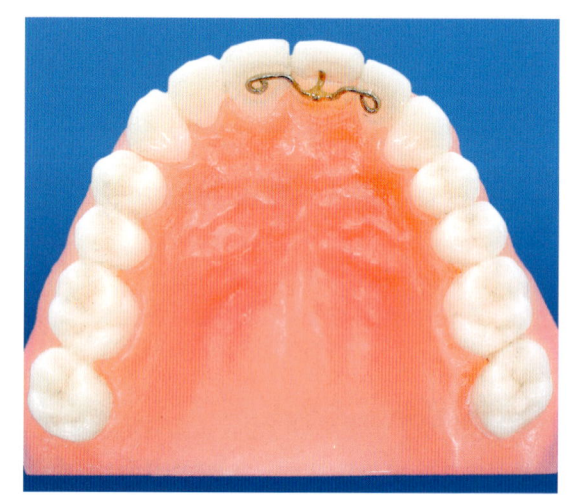

Design Notes:

_____
_____
_____
_____

PERIODONTAL SERVICES

Forced Eruption

There are several common methods available to manage a tooth that is severely broken down or periodontally involved. These include extraction of the remaining root followed by a prosthetic replacement or techniques to expose sound tooth structure such as osseous surgery and forced eruption.

Forced eruption is appropriate when the loss of tooth structure is in the region of the alveolar crest. It can be defined as an orthodontic movement in a coronal direction through the application of gentle, continuous forces. Specifically, when a root segment is forcefully erupted, the forces stretch the gingival and periodontal fibers producing a coronal shift of gingiva and bone. If done slowly, the gingiva and supporting structures will follow to a position that is further coronal than the adjacent teeth. These gingival and osseous changes can be used to manage many restorative problems. For example, after forced eruption, periodontal surgery can be performed to expose sound tooth structure without sacrificing bone on the adjacent teeth. The soft tissue can then be sutured to blend with the gingival margins of the adjacent teeth that produces an acceptable esthetic result.

Forced eruption can also be used to eliminate a bony defect. For example, if a bicuspid has a 7mm mesial defect, you can eliminate it by erupting the tooth in a manner that the bone comes with it. This is a very effective technique as long as you do not violate a 1-to-1 crown root ratio. Before initiation of forced eruption, the restorability of the tooth, after this phase of orthodontic care is completed, must be considered. Make sure the root to crown ratio will be sufficient once forced eruption is complete. A minimum of 3 to 4mm of tooth structure coronal to the alveolar crest of bone must be provided for the reformation of the biologic width and to allow the final restoration to embrace at least 1 to 2mm of solid tooth structure.

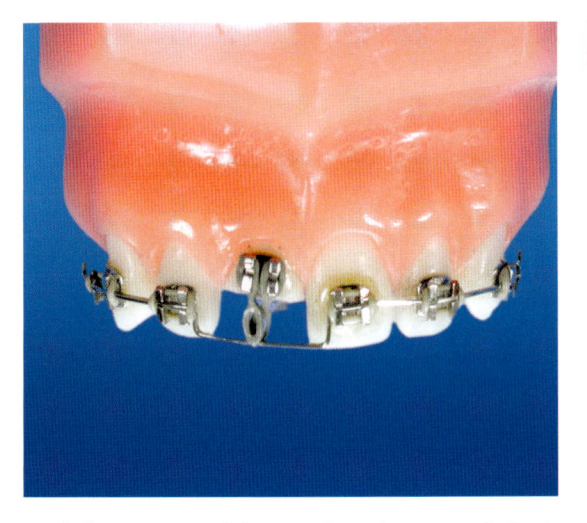

2211 Fixed Appliances

When using a fixed approach, the equivalent of two teeth on either side of the tooth to be erupted must be available for anchorage. The appliance is set up as follows:

The Anchorage Unit:
Edgewise brackets are bonded into place in the same horizontal plane on all of the anchor teeth. The teeth on each side of the tooth to be erupted are then tied together with metal ligature ties to create the two anchor units. This will eliminate any unwanted movement of these anchor units. A stainless steel orthodontic wire, 0.018 inch by 0.025 inch, is then ligated into the brackets of the anchorage units with elastic ligatures. This wire has been bent by the lab to the general labial contours of the anchorage teeth and the crown of the tooth to be extruded. An occlusal offset has been placed in the wire over the tooth to be extruded. This wire, when properly positioned inciso-gingivally, will provide the needed extrusion distance between the wire and the attachment on the tooth needing eruption.

The Attachment Unit:
The attachment unit is the part of the appliance that attaches to the tooth needing eruption. The preferred method is bonding a bracket to natural tooth enamel. However, if there is no labial enamel to bond to then the next best options are a temporary, or a final post and core, and a temporary crown. A temporary crown has the advantage of being more esthetically pleasing while retaining the tooth's original position. After the temporary crown has been constructed, an orthodontic bracket is bonded to its surface as far to the gingival as possible.

The Active Force Module:
After placing the arch wire, you can activate the appliance. An elastic is placed from the attachment, looped over the wire and back on to the attachment, to initiate the eruption. In this example, chain elastic is being used.

PERIODONTAL SERVICES

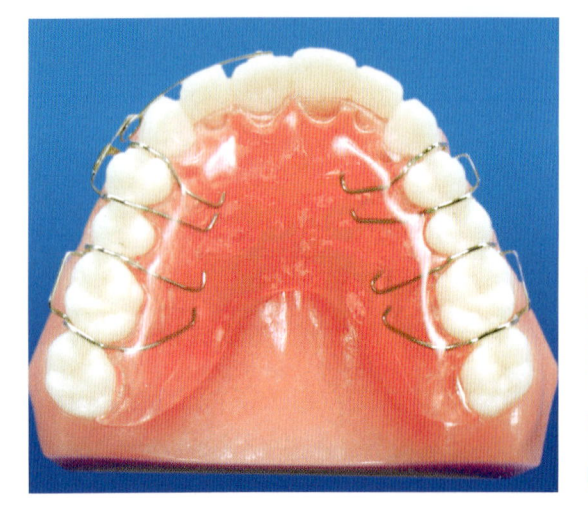

1079 Removable Forced Eruption Appliance - Spring Activated

There are times when bracketing teeth for anchorage is either inappropriate or not possible. For example, placing brackets on porcelain veneers or crowns is not recommended, as the bonding process will damage the finish.

Some patients simply do not have enough teeth to be the sole method of anchorage. When this is the case, a removable appliance allows you to use the soft tissue, along with remaining teeth, for anchorage.

Appliance designs can be very flexible and creative. In some cases, you may be able to use a patient's existing partial by simply adding a hook over the tooth needing eruption. In the example shown here, a simple acrylic orthodontic appliance with an activating spring arm can be used. This type of appliance works by simply engaging the spring over the direct bonded attachment bracket.

1078 Removable Forced Eruption Appliance

Forced eruption can be accomplished by using this very effective helical coil spring that is connected directly to a temporary post. This appliance is appropriate when a temporary crown is not needed and a fixed approach is not possible. Though not the solution for all cases, removable appliances can expand the clinicians options to initiate forced eruption.

Note - Inflammation must be controlled prior to initiating tooth movement. If it is not, forced eruption may contribute to the deepening of an osseous defect.

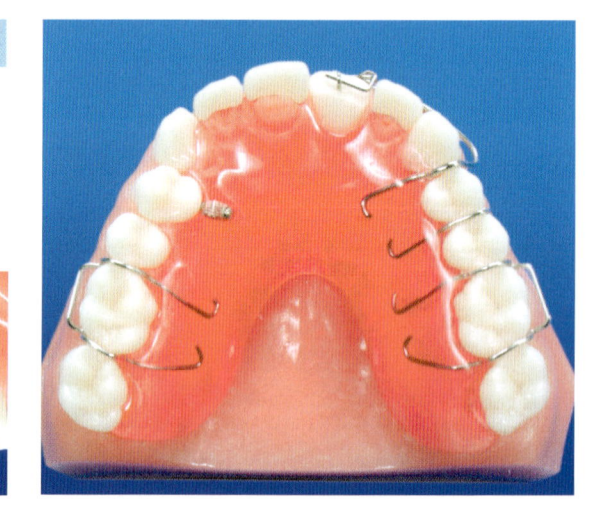

Design Notes:

17.10

PERIODONTAL SERVICES

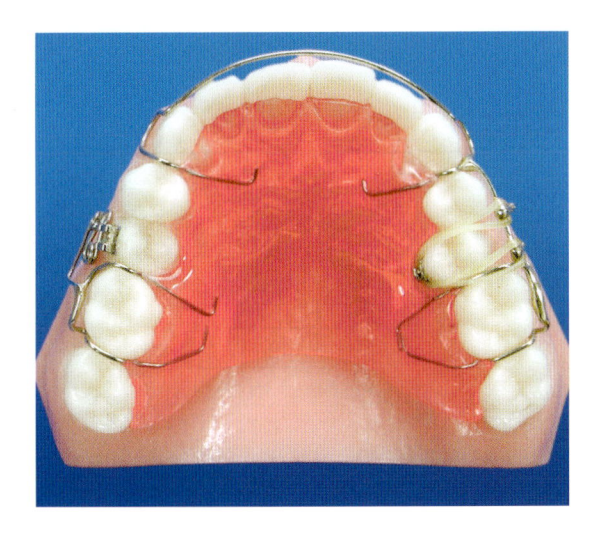

1072B Recurved Extrusion Spring

When you find it necessary to forcefully erupt a posterior tooth to correct a vertical defect or, as in this example, guide a submerged tooth back into occlusion, this technique offers a simple solution.

This unique appliance uses a recurved finger spring to aid in the eruption of a single bicuspid. A direct bond straight wire bracket is placed on the bicuspid to create an undercut for the helical recurved spring.

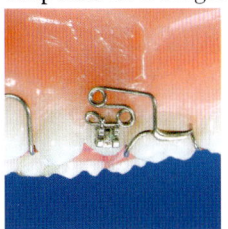

The patient then simply inserts the activated appliance and "snaps" the activated spring under the gingival tie wings of the brackets. This not only expedites the eruption of the tooth, but also aids in appliance retention.

Design Notes:

17.11

PERIODONTAL SERVICES

Molar Uprighting

It is clear that some patients are periodontally resistant and can tolerate tooth malposition. For these patients, uprighting of a mesially inclined molar may seem optional, unless it is necessary to accomplish optimal restorative treatment.

Even so, tipped teeth are more difficult to clean than teeth that are properly aligned in the dental arch. When prosthetic work is done without first uprighting a molar, oral maintenance can become very difficult.

Patients most likely to benefit from molar uprighting are those with active periodontal disease. This is the case because teeth with an abnormal axial inclination do not properly distribute occlusal forces, and in the presence of bacteria, these parafunctional forces can lead to an increase in bone loss. Furthermore, as bony support becomes reduced, normal functional forces that would not move a tooth with adequate support can cause movement of a tooth without it. For these reasons, it is appropriate to upright tipped teeth.

Before beginning tooth movement procedures, any tissue inflammation must be eliminated. A thorough root planing and curettage as well as surgery may be necessary. During tooth movement, the clinician must accept responsibility for keeping this area free of inflammation. This will require regular maintenance visits throughout treatment. In fact, the frequency of visits during tooth movement will not be determined by orthodontic adjustments alone but by the necessity to keep the soft tissue free of all inflammation and to prevent crestal bone loss during appliance therapy. Weekly appointments may be necessary.

Molar uprighting can be accomplished using either a fixed or a removable orthodontic approach. Both have their advantages and disadvantages.

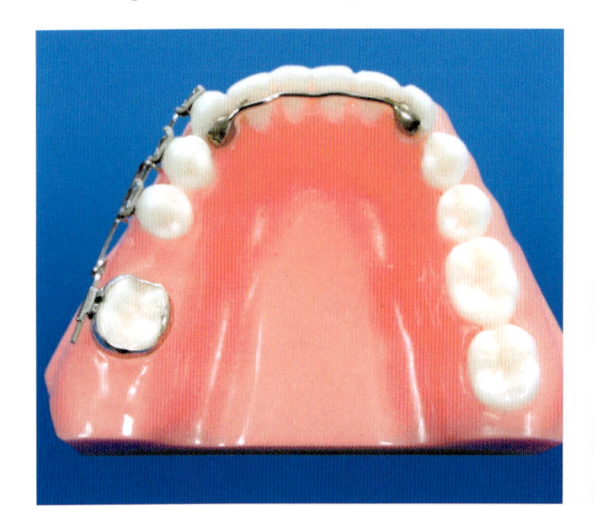

2034 Molar Uprighting Fixed Appliance   U/L

A variety of fixed appliances are available to upright tipped molars. Although the design and application may vary slightly, the principles are the same.

The key to success is to set up adequate anchorage. In this example, an anchorage unit is created by placing edgewise brackets on all teeth as far forward as the canine. These are then tied together with a segmental guide wire and metal ligature ties. The canine on the contralateral side is also included in the anchorage unit by using a lingual arch, to not only increase the anterior anchorage, but to also help resist against any buccal displacement of the anchor teeth.

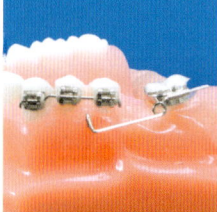

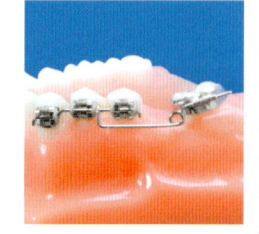

Although direct bonded brackets are available for the molar as well, it is advisable to band the molar. The actual uprighting of the molar is done with a rectangular helical uprighting spring by first placing the distal side of the spring in the special rectangular slot on the molar band so that the mesial arm will lie passively in the vestibule. Then, simply lift the mesial arm of the spring and hook it over the arch wire in the stabilizing segment.

It is important that the hook be positioned so that it is able to slide distally as the molar uprights. A slight lingual bend, placed in the uprighting spring, is needed to counteract the forces that tend to tip the anchor teeth buccally and the molar lingually.

PERIODONTAL SERVICES

4184 Removable Uprighting Partial   U/L

Uprighting of mesially inclined molars can often be accomplished with a removable appliance. This appliance should be designed to give maximum retention and anchorage. This is accomplished by using two to three clasps and by having excellent tissue adaptation.

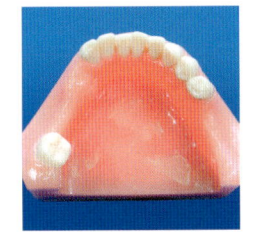

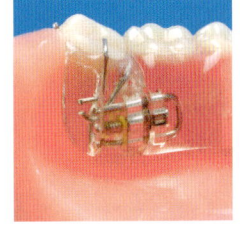

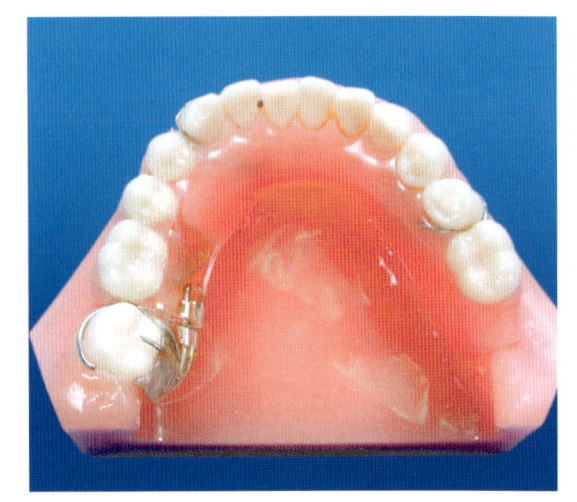

Although not shown in this example, a labial bow is often used to prevent flaring of the anterior teeth. The appliance can utilize either a spring or an expansion screw to accomplish the desired tooth movement.

When using removable appliances that have an expansion screw, the patient can activate the appliance. One turn per week is equivalent to 1mm of movement per month.

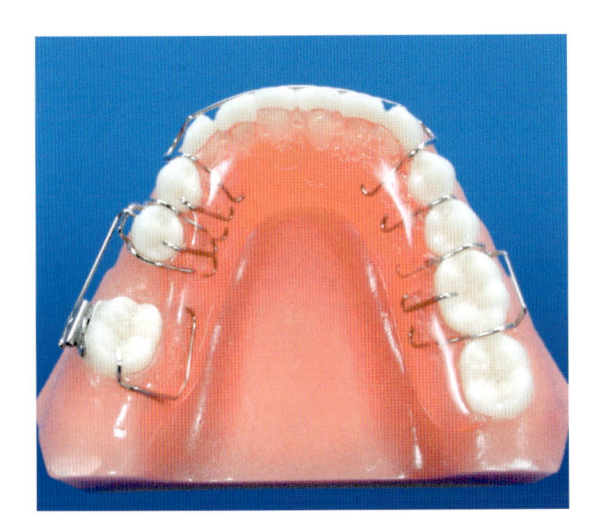

1037 Fixed/Removable Molar Uprighter   U/L

When the molar is severely inclined and bodily movement is needed to upright it, only a fixed approach will suffice. If the teeth that would normally act as an anchorage unit cannot be used because they are periodontally involved, a removable appliance can be used for anchorage in conjunction with a fixed component on the molar. Here an uprighting spring inserts into a fixed molar bracket which has a tube or slot. The spring then hooks onto the removable appliance which provides the necessary anchorage and prevents lingual tipping. When using this approach it is essential to place an occlusal rest on the distal aspect of the occlusal surface to prevent extrusion.

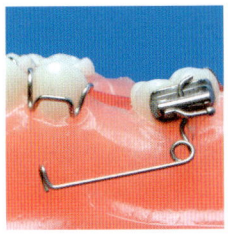

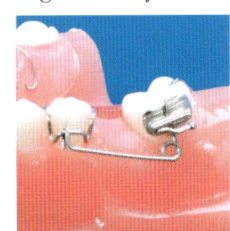

PERIODONTAL SERVICES

Space Management

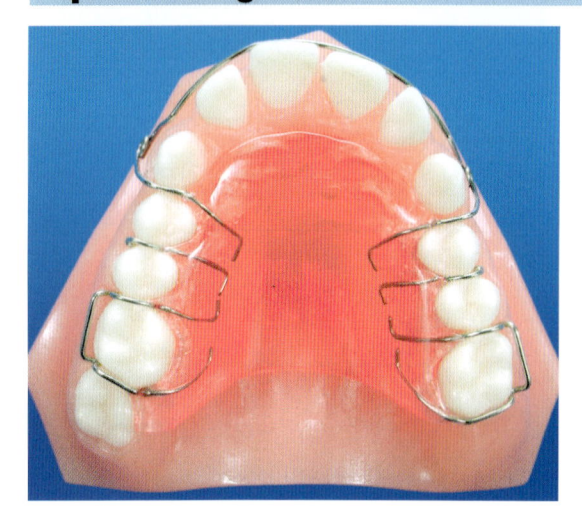

1122 Apron Spring Appliance   U

Bone loss, habits, posterior bite collapse, and a decrease in the vertical dimension are some of the factors that cause anterior flaring to occur in the periodontal patient. After scaling, root planing, and periodontal surgery are completed, anteriors often need to be brought back to their normal position.

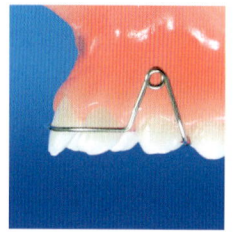

An apron spring can be used to provide light pressure to gently guide flared anteriors lingually. Minimal adjustment is required to keep this appliance active. When a tongue habit also exists, loops can easily be added to help control this problem.

Once the anteriors have been returned to their normal position, an intra-coronal or extra-coronal splint can be used to maintain the corrected position.

1122B Lower Apron Spring Retractor   L

Correcting lower anterior flaring can be achieved with this appliance in a relatively short period of time when simple lingual uprighting is required. As the Apron spring is activated, a retraction force is applied to the incisors. All that is required is that the lingual acrylic be periodically relieved to allow room for the movement to occur.

It is recommended that only 1mm of acrylic be relieved at each appointment so that a controlled retraction is achieved. This will also allow the appliance to be used as a retainer once the incisors are retracted as desired. Full time wear of this appliance is recommended.

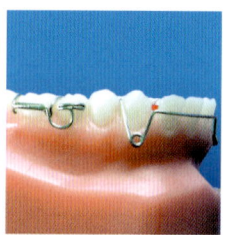

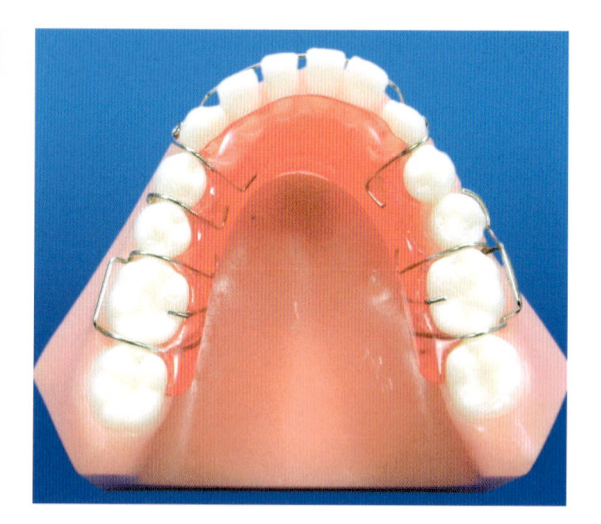

2110 Spinning Bead Tongue Retrainer   U

Anterior flaring is often associated with a tongue habit. This myofunctional device is used to retrain proper tongue position. The appliance evokes a spontaneous reaction to play with the spinner and position the dorsum of the tongue against the soft palate.

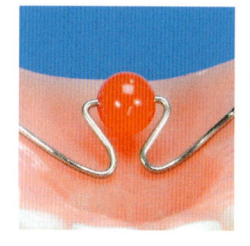

This appliance is often used in conjunction with fixed mechanics or a removable appliance to retract the anteriors.

PERIODONTAL SERVICES

2211B Fixed Lower Retraction Appliance   L

In many adult cases with lower anterior flaring, positive bodily tooth movement combined with root torquing is desirable. The design offered here is very popular and effective in treating this situation. It employs limited bracketing, provides optimum anchorage, and allows each tooth to be moved mesially, distally, as well as lingually.

The anchorage is provided by a banded, fixed lingual arch wire from first bicuspid to first bicuspid. The active tooth movement occurs by using a sectional arch wire and chain elastic. Once the anteriors are retracted the correction can be maintained by temporarily splinting them using steel ligature underties.

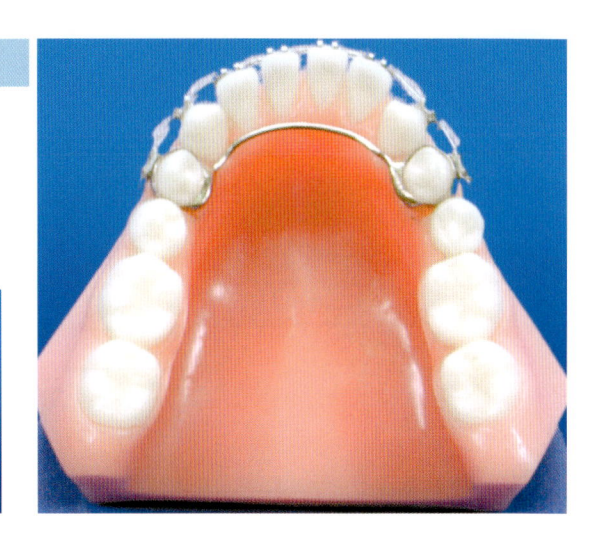

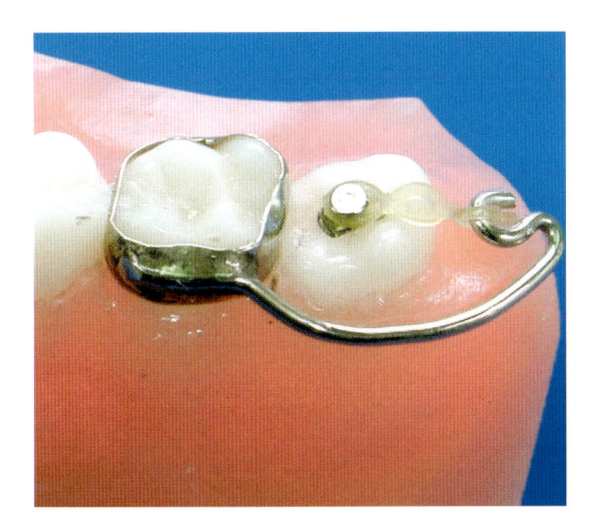

2027 Elastic Halterman Appliance   U/L

We often see second molars that cannot fully erupt because they are locked under the distal aspect of the first molar. When this happens, opposing molars can super erupt causing occlusal problems. The area also becomes very difficult to maintain. Eventually caries and periodontal disease can lead to the loss of both molars. Simply moving the second molar distally and allowing it to erupt into its normal position can easily avoid this sequence of events.

One appliance to accomplish this is the Elastic Halterman. Here a button is bonded to the occlusal surface of the second molar, and a band with a hook distal to this molar is cemented to the first molar. Chain elastic extending from the hook to the button is used to provide the distal force needed to unlock this tooth.

2028 Ectopic Spring Distalizer   U/L

When second molars cannot fully erupt, opposing molars can super-erupt causing occlusal problems. The area between the first and second molar also becomes very difficult to maintain. Eventually caries and periodontal disease can lead to the loss of both molars.

Designed in principle to function the same as the Elastic Halterman, this appliance features a recurved wire spring to achieve the distal movement of the second molar that is caught under the first molar. Placement of the occlusal button is usually on the distal aspect of the erupting molar. This design is preferred in the lower arch where space is limited in the Ascending Ramus area.

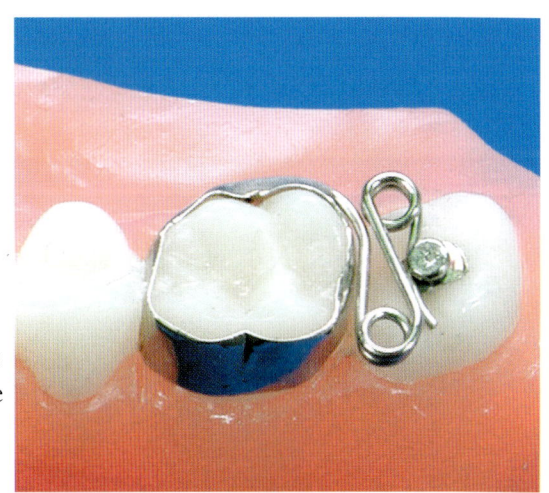

Note - Always send an opposing cast to evaluate if there is sufficient occlusal clearance for this appliance.

17.15

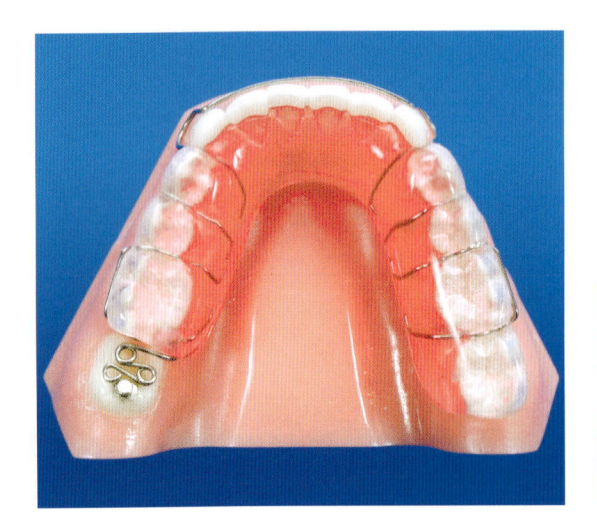

PERIODONTAL SERVICES

1044 Removable Ectopic Distalizer   U/L

This appliance is quite effective in distalizing an ectopically erupting molar when there is insufficient vertical clearance to use the fixed Ectopic Spring Distalizer #2028. In this case, vertical clearance is achieved by adding occlusal coverage to the removable appliance. Activating the finger spring soldered to the molar clasp places a positive distal driving force against the button that is bonded to the occlusal of the second molar. Typically, this appliance needs to be worn for a relatively short period of time.

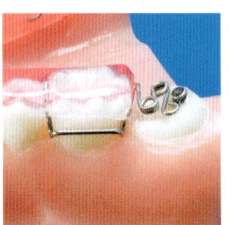

1125 Posterior Space Closure   U/L

Abnormal occlusal forces, periodontal disease and poor restorative work are just a few factors that can cause interproximal spacing to occur in the posterior segments. This often leads to food impaction that is not only annoying but can also contribute to a worsening of the periodontal condition. This excess space can be easily reversed with an appliance like the one shown here.

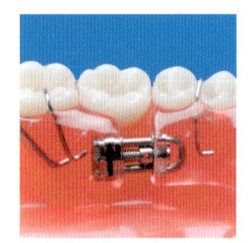

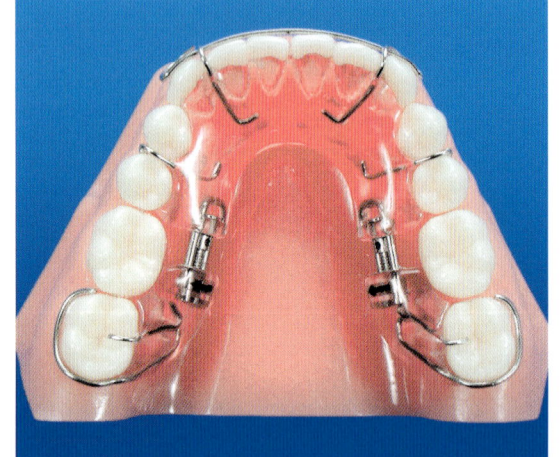

Anchorage is the key to successfully closing this space. The appliance typically requires anterior retention using a combination of bilateral clasping and a labial bow. Then, "retraction" screws are placed bilaterally and activated as needed to close the interproximal spaces through mesial movement of the molars.

Typically, heavy "C" clasps are placed around the distal of the last molars and the acrylic is removed from the interproximal areas around the teeth needing mesial movement.

Design Notes:

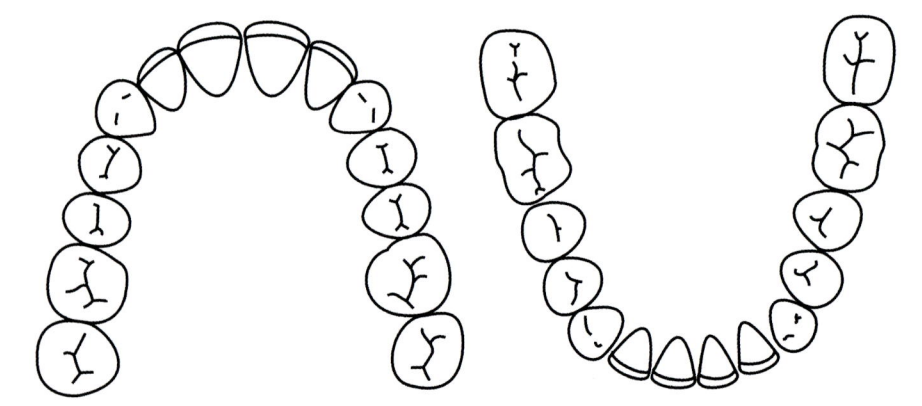

PERIODONTAL SERVICES

Periodontal Surgical Appliances

6510 Gingival Grafting Stent

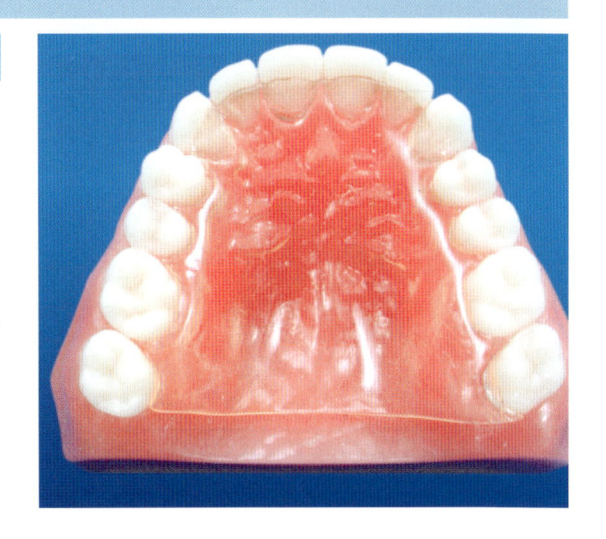

A frequent periodontal procedure is to do a gingival graft by harvesting palatal tissue and transplanting it in areas that lack attached or keratinized tissue. This procedure creates an open wound that heals by secondary intention, and can be quite uncomfortable for the patient.

A properly designed surgical stent can protect the open wound and make the procedure much more tolerable for the patient. When it is used in conjunction with a dressing it also helps control bleeding. These stents can be designed to meet your exacting specifications.

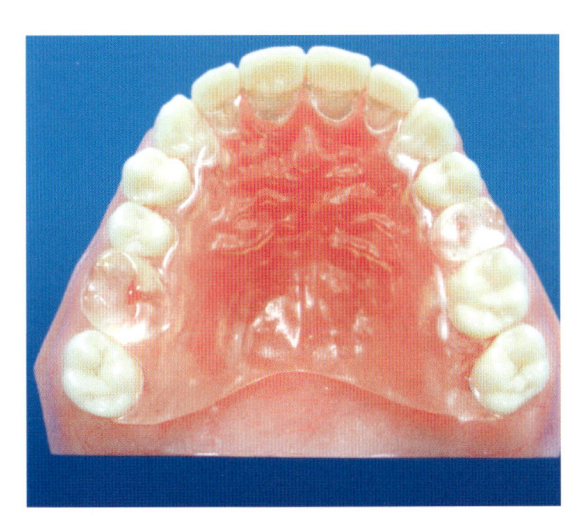

6520D Implant Stents

Implant stents are used with CAT scans and during surgical procedures to aid in the proper placement of implants. First an ideal tooth set-up is accomplished on your properly articulated models. This set-up is then duplicated and processed into a clear acrylic stent. Depending on your needs, it will be modified for use during surgery or for a CAT scan procedure. For more information, see the chapter on Implant Services.

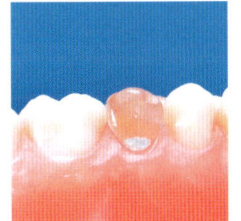

Note - It is always necessary to send upper and lower casts and a construction bite to properly fabricate this appliance.

4021 Temporary Maryland Bridge

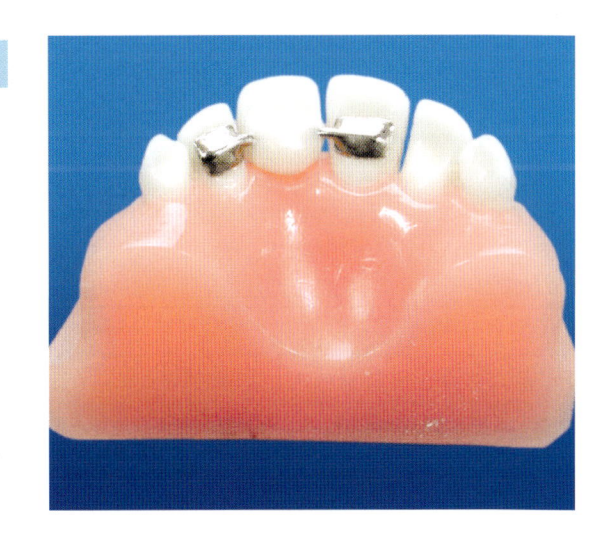

After trauma has caused the loss of a tooth, it is often necessary to do a ridge augmentation procedure to re-establish a normal bony architecture. When this is done, a method of temporization must be accomplished that will prevent any abnormal forces from being placed on the surgical site. In this situation, a bonded bridge is an excellent alternative to a removable temporary. This appliance can also be used during the period of implant integration.

Note - This appliance must have anterior occlusal clearance. If it does not, please see the section on Interim partials and Bridges for other appliance designs. Remember, it is always necessary to send upper and lower casts and a construction bite to properly fabricate this appliance.

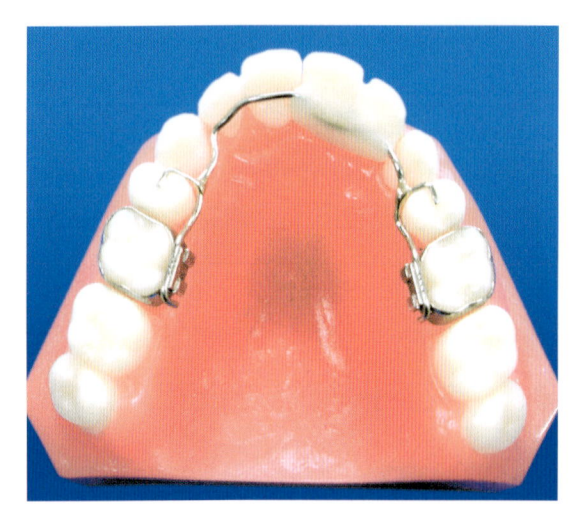

PERIODONTAL SERVICES

4024 Fixed/Removable Banded Temp Anterior Bridge

Many periodontal surgical patients have found it difficult to tolerate interim partial dentures, so more innovative methods have had to be devised to keep a patient functional throughout the the healing process. The Fixed/Removable Banded Anterior Bridge is one such device. This appliance utilizes Wilson vertical tubes soldered to bands to allow the patient to have the benefit of a palate-free fixed appliance while still allowing the dentist to easily remove it to gain access to the surgical site. Pressure can be kept off the implant site by allowing the wire to positively rest against the surrounding anteriors as seen here or by adding rest seats and rests on the bicuspids or cuspids.

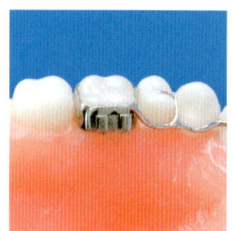

Note - Don't forget to adjust the internal aspect of the pontics to make sure they do not put any unwanted pressure on the surgical site.

4025 Palate-Free Temp Removable Partial Denture

This appliance was originally designed as a removable interim implant site protector for patients who could not tolerate a removable partial denture. Its double clasps and rest seats are designed to give extra retention and tissue protection. But because one of the clasps is often on the cuspid, esthetics can be an issue. Therefore selecting patients with a low lip line when they smile is preferable when choosing this appliance. Fabrication requires both upper and lower casts, an interocclusal record, and a tooth shade.

Note - Don't forget to adjust the internal aspect of the pontics to make sure they do not put any unwanted pressure on the surgical site.

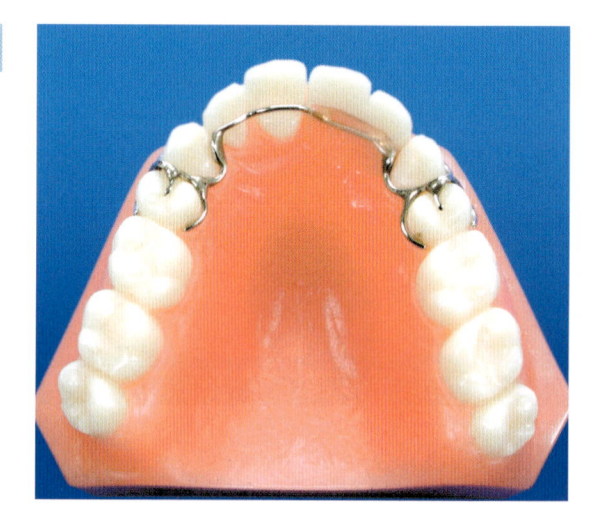

Design Notes:

_____
_____
_____
_____
_____
_____

PERIODONTAL SERVICES

4181 Upper Interim Removable Partial

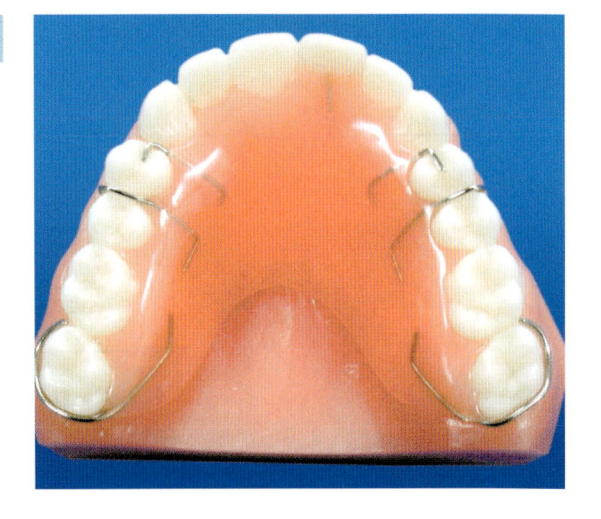

The simple, inexpensive interim partial shown here replaces a single, lost permanent central. This example is shown with "C" clasps and ball clasps to provide the patient with retention. Occlusal rests are placed to protect the surgical site by making the appliance tooth borne. To keep these wires out of occlusion, it may be necessary to prepare small rest seats in the teeth. This preparation needs to be done prior to taking of the impression for this appliance. An opposing model, wax bite and Bioform shade are necessary for appliance construction. Please specify if the anterior teeth are to be butted up against the tissue or if an acrylic saddle is desired.

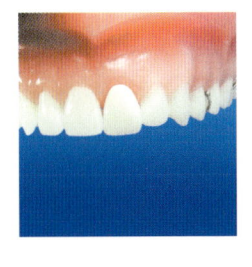

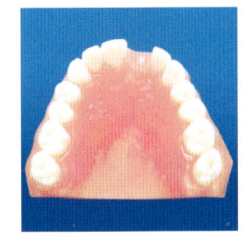

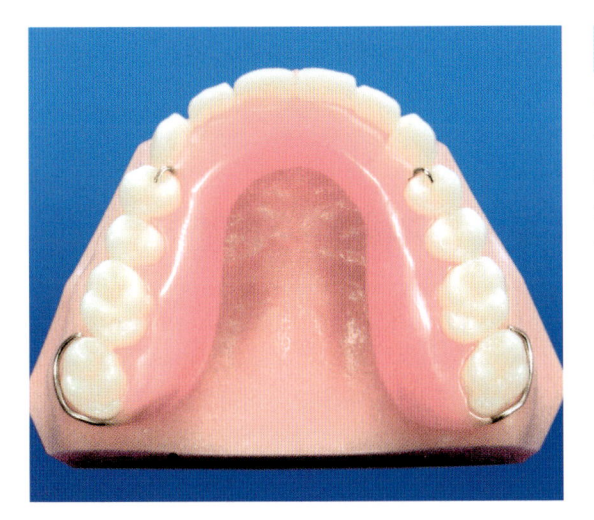

4185H Horseshoe Temporary Partial

Often an adult requiring an interim partial will find it difficult to wear a full-palatal coverage appliance. Speech is adversely affected and they have difficulty adapting. Although time is often all that is needed to adapt fully, many patients' employment requirements do not afford them the luxury of time.

In this situation, the Horseshoe design indicated here will usually solve the problem. Kevlar fiber is added to the acrylic to improve its strength and make up for the minimal amount of acrylic. Occlusal rests are placed to protect the surgical site by making the appliance tooth borne. To keep these wires out of occlusion, it may be necessary to prepare small rest seats in the teeth.

This preparation needs to be done prior to taking the impression for this appliance. The use of "C" clasps on the distal-most molars and rests on the first bicuspids offers good stability and retention. An opposing model, wax bite and Bioform shade are necessary for appliance construction. Please specify if the anterior teeth are to be butted up against the tissue or if an acrylic saddle is desired.

PERIODONTAL SERVICES

4191 Essix Temporary Partial   U/L

After trauma has caused the loss of a tooth, it is often necessary to do a ridge augmentation procedure to re-establish a normal bony architecture. When this is done, a method of temporization must be accomplished that will prevent any abnormal forces from being placed on the surgical site. This simple appliance is excellent for temporary replacement of anterior teeth while the patient is waiting for a permanent bridge, a partial, or implants.

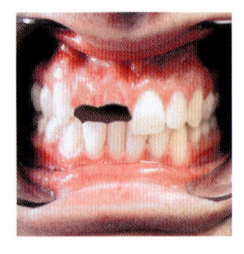

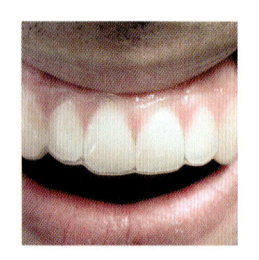

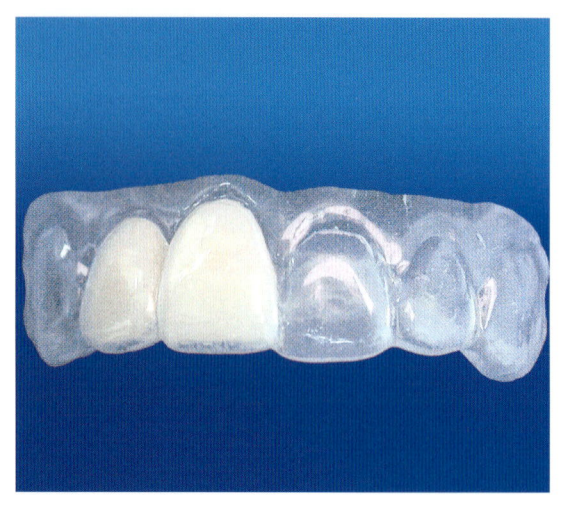

Traditionally, these missing anteriors would be replaced by incorporating denture teeth into a Hawley type retainer more commonly referred to by patients as a "flipper". Unfortunately, these appliances are often initially uncomfortable and affect speech because they have acrylic in the palatal region. Partials can also place unwanted pressure on a surgical site and on the surrounding healing tissue.

By using the new Essix technology, a simpler, more efficient method is used to retain and replace the missing teeth on a temporary basis. This removable interim bridge is made using the Essix "C-type" clear vacuum-formed material. When properly designed and fabricated, this appliance will snap into place and stay retained by using the natural undercuts gingival to the anterior contact points. They are clear, thin, run from cuspid-to-cuspid, and are clasp free and palate free. Patient acceptance and esthetics are excellent.

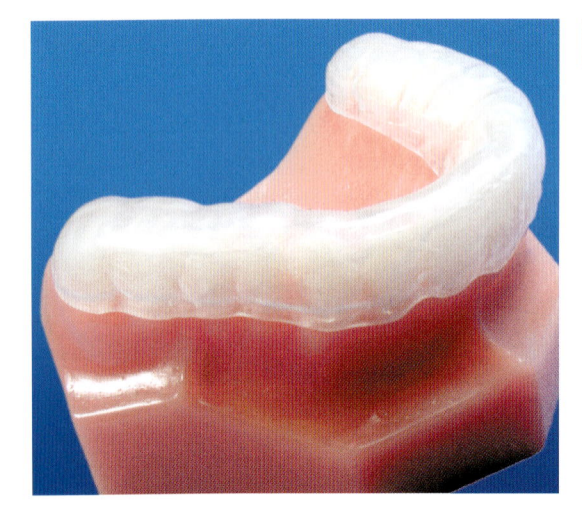

6111 Fluoride Delivery System   U/L

Many patients need extra fluoride protection on a daily basis. Unfortunately just giving them fluoride and telling them to use it after they brush usually doesn't work. Patients clearly need a tool that will help them follow your instructions. One of the best methods of motivating patients to use fluoride every day is to give them a tray delivery system. Simply have the patient fill the tray with 1.1% neutral sodium fluoride and wear it for five minutes after they brush. Then take the tray out and spit out the excess without rinsing. That's all it takes to give them the extra protection they need. Neutral sodium fluoride is recommended as safest for composites and porcelain restorations. Do not use acidulated fluorides.

This technique can effectively help:
a) patients with a high caries index.
b) patients undergoing periodontal therapy.
c) chemotherapy and radiation therapy patients.
d) patients with tissue recession, exposed roots, and root caries.
e) overdenture patients.
f) patients with extensive restorative work.
g) orthodontic patients.
h) patients with a high level of tooth sensitivity.
i) anyone who needs extra hygiene motivation.

SLEEP APNEA / SNORING

an overview: SLEEP APNEA/SNORING

Chapter 18

Dentists are now able to play a very important role in the treatment of snoring problems as well as in the recognition and treatment of the life threatening condition known as Sleep Apnea.

Patients may complain of snoring problems and be unaware of the presence of sleep apnea. Such common complaints as headaches, daytime drowsiness, lack of energy, low resistance to disease, and hypertension may actually be the result of numerous sleep apnea episodes during the night. During these episodes, breathing temporarily stops causing reduced oxygen levels in the blood. If left untreated apnea can cause serious medical conditions ranging from increased hypertension to cardiac changes that can lead to sudden death.

During an obstructive sleep apnea episode, a blockage of the airway occurs when there is a collapse of the nasopharyngeal, oropharyngeal, and hypopharyngeal tissues. Research has shown that many dental appliances are quite effective at alleviating this blockage and can now be considered an alternative when choosing a treatment modality. In fact, sleep appliances offer several advantages over other therapy choices. They are inexpensive, non-invasive, easy to fabricate, reversible, and quite well accepted by patients.

Sleep appliances seem to work in one or a combination of three ways. Appliances can reposition the tissues by lifting up the soft palate, bringing the tongue forward, or lifting the hyoid bone. As they reposition, they also act to stabilize these tissues, preventing airway collapse. Lastly, appliances seem to increase muscle tone. Specifically, there seems to be an increase in pharyngeal and genioglossus muscle activity. The key to successful appliance therapy is to properly identify the cause and location of the obstruction. If this is not done, your rate of successful appliance therapy will drop to less than 50% regardless of the appliance chosen.

Variations in design range from the method of retention, the type of material being used, the method and ease of adjustability, the ability to control the vertical dimension, differences in mandibular movement and whether it is lab fabricated or made in the office. The appliance design that you choose will be dependent upon your knowledge of these variations and the oral conditions of the patient. Several of the more frequently used designs are shown on the pages that follow.

OBSTRUCTIVE SLEEP APNEA & SNORING

6321 The Soft Palatal Lift Appliance

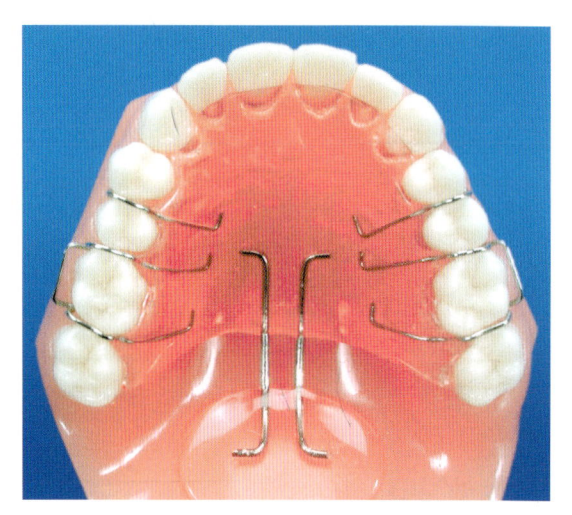

Many patients have excessive or pendulous tissue in the oral pharyngeal region that obstructs the airway and causes snoring. The Palatal Lift appliance has an adjustable acrylic button that extends distally to the midpoint of the soft palate and gently lifts this tissue, preventing it from vibrating as air passes during sleep.

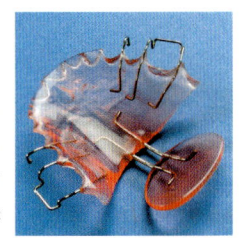

This appliance is hard for most patients to tolerate for any length of time, but when you suspect that the airway obstruction is due to an excessive palatal drape, it might prove useful as a diagnostic tool. Simply have the patient wear it to sleep. If it clears the airway enough for the patient to breathe and his spouse tells you that he didn't snore, then this may indicate the need for a UPPP surgery. This appliance is rarely used and is shown here to give a historical perspective on the evolution of appliance design.

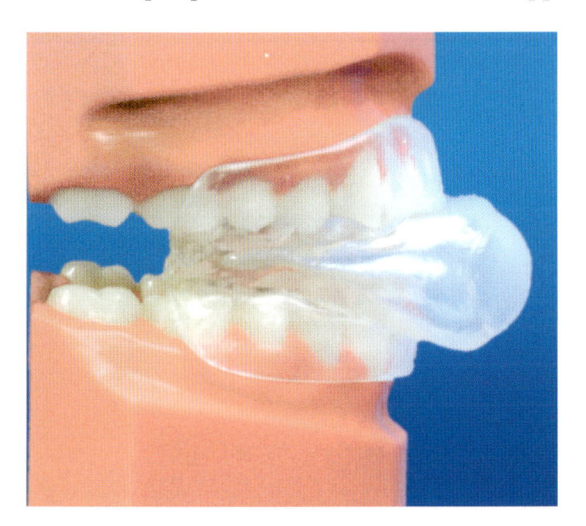

5512 The Tongue Retaining Device (TRD)

In this appliance, the tongue goes into the anterior bulb. Pushing the tongue forward and giving the bulb a little squeeze creates a suction that holds the tongue in a forward position. It is a lab fabricated appliance and is made out of a flexible polyvinyl material. This appliance has excellent sleep studies to support its use.

Most of the other appliances that are used to clear the airway in the hypopharyngeal region work by bringing the mandible forward, but not everyone can bring his or her mandible forward. For these patients, bringing the tongue forward with an appliance like this may be the best way to clear the airway. Patients who are edentulous or periodontally compromised may also benefit from this appliance.

6332X The Snor-X

Developed by Dr. Alvarez in the San Francisco area, the Snor-X can be used as a test appliance or as a training device to see if the patient can wear the TRD. It can also be used as a treatment appliance. Just like the TRD, it holds the tongue forward so it can't drop back. The Snor-X is not retained on the teeth in any manner and allows total freedom of movement of the mandible.

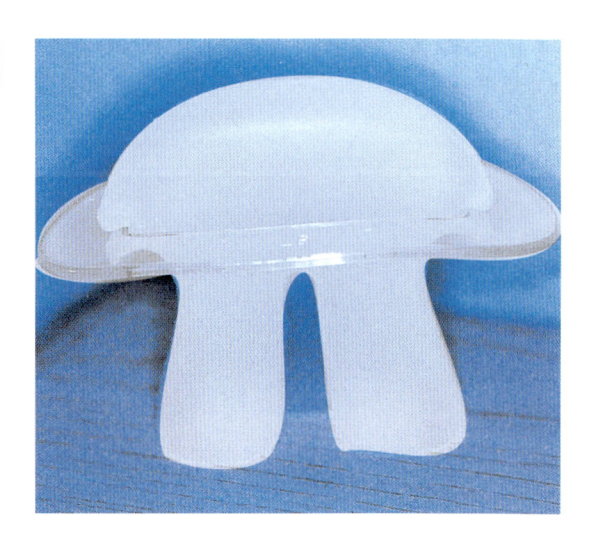

18.1

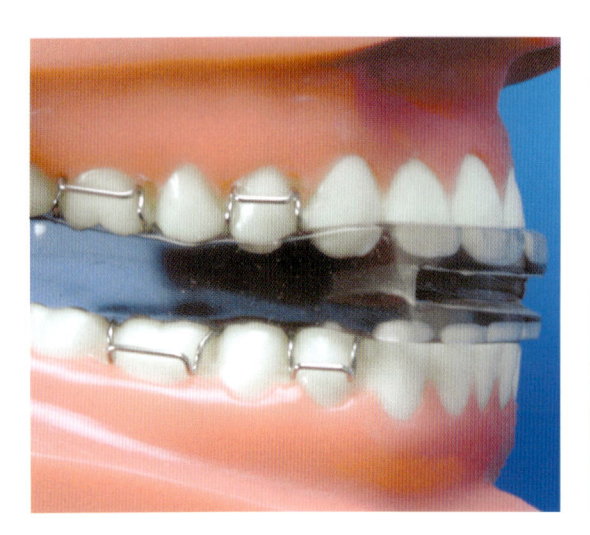

OBSTRUCTIVE SLEEP APNEA & SNORING

6323 The Clasp Retained Mandibular Repositioner

CT scans taken with this device in place show that the tongue is more superiorly placed with a narrowing of the dorsal aspect. There is also an enlargement of the airway. This appliance uses multiple clasps to positively lock the mandible into the appliance and prevent it from retruding. There is also a larger airway cut into the acrylic in this design. The position of the mandible must be predetermined and accurately produced in a construction bite for proper appliance fabrication. Typically, the mandible must be advanced to only 75% of its maximum protrusion with the anterior/vertical separation of 4mm. This prevents excessive strain on the TMJ and facial musculature.

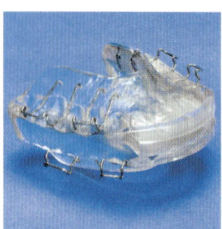

6322 The Mandibular Inclined Repositioning Splint

An open airway is maintained with this appliance by directly holding the mandible in a forward position. An incline flange is used to direct the mandible forward and prevent it from dropping back upon opening. This flange is made out of a thermoplastic material that softens at body temperature making it more comfortable and greatly reducing the possibility of soreness to the anterior teeth and tissues.

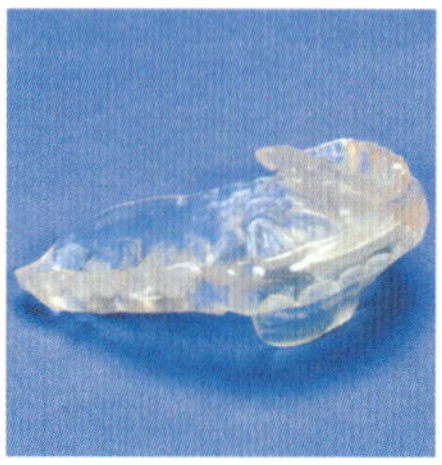

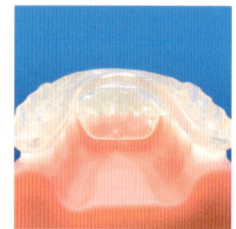

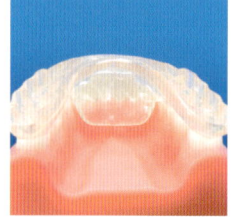

The body of the appliance is fabricated from hard clear acrylic and snap fits to the maxillary arch. The lower dentition is deeply indexed into the occlusal surface of the appliance to hold the mandible in the forward position. A breathing hole is placed in the anterior portion of the appliance to allow for easy breathing throughout the night.

The position of the mandible must be predetermined and accurately produced in a construction bite for proper appliance fabrication. Typically, the mandible must be advanced to only 75% of its maximum protrusion with the anterior/vertical separation of 4mm. This prevents excessive strain on the TMJ and facial musculature.

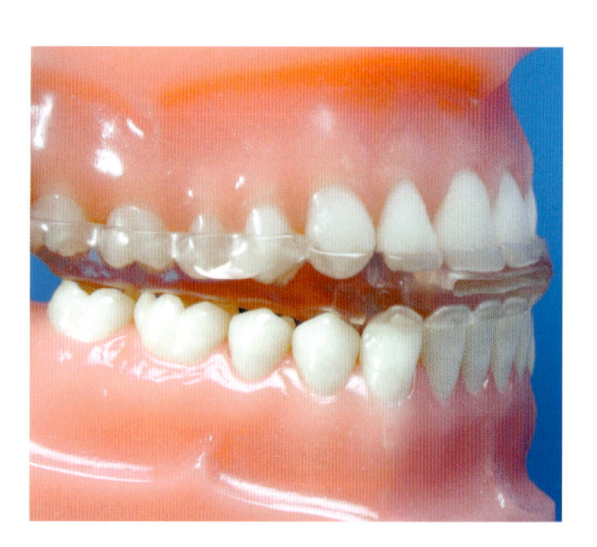

OBSTRUCTIVE SLEEP APNEA & SNORING

6326 The Silent Night Appliance

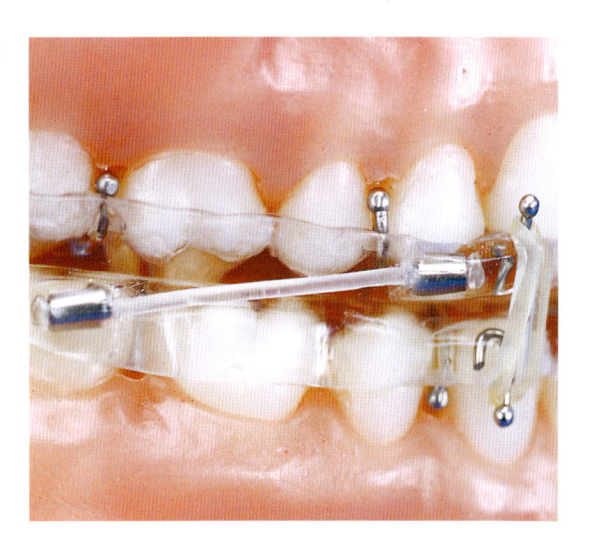

This appliance utilizes precision milled upper and lower occlusal splints to open the vertical relationship while holding the mandible in the desired forward position with highly resilient nylon fibers. The nylon is placed in stainless tubes and processed into the acrylic in the upper cuspid and lower molar areas.

Like the Modified Herbst designs, this appliance allows the mandible to move freely. The vertical elastics in the cuspid region encourage a lip-together posture. The use of the nylon fibers makes this appliance less bulky. The smooth buccal finish is an advantage if your patient has extremely sensitive intra-oral tissues.

Note - A carefully taken construction bite indicating the amount of mandibular advancement required is essential for fabrication of this appliance since it is not adjustable in the AP direction once completed.

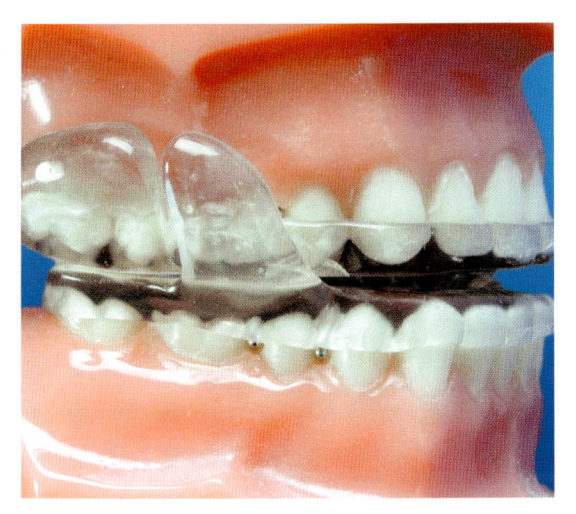

6322D The Dorsal Appliance

The Dorsal Appliance utilizes precision milled upper and lower occlusal splints to open the vertical relationship while holding the mandible in the desired forward position by the use of interlocking buccal inclines. The inclines are milled in such a way that they allow a degree of mandibular lateral movement alleviating the occurrence of any muscle trismus. The inclines also aid in keeping the mandible from dropping open during sleep.

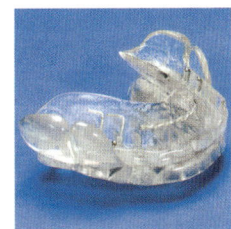

18.3

OBSTRUCTIVE SLEEP APNEA & SNORING

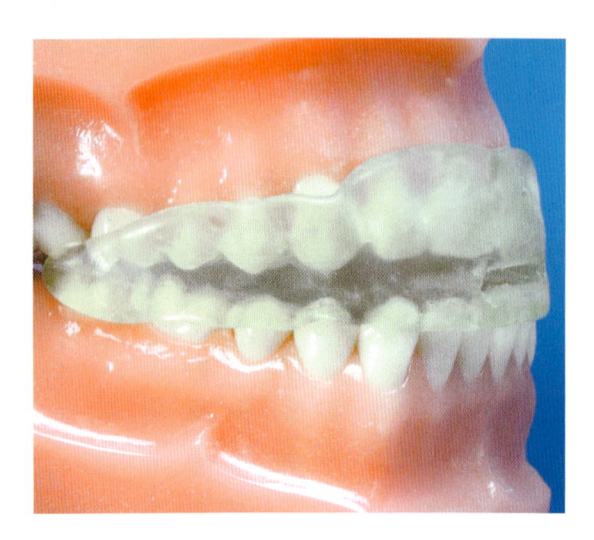

6710 The SnoreFree™ Appliance

The SnoreFree™ is a one-piece thermoplastic mandibular repositioning appliance that is made chair side. It comes in a kit that contains complete instructions and all the forms necessary to screen your patients for snoring and apnea.

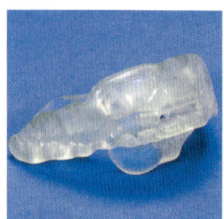

When treating obstructive sleep apnea with a dental appliance, the SnoreFree™ is often used as an initial or test appliance. This allows the dentist to inexpensively evaluate whether a mandibular repositioning appliance will work for that patient. If necessary, it is possible to alter the mandibular position after initial appliance fabrication; however, this needs to be done very carefully.

Design Notes:

OBSTRUCTIVE SLEEP APNEA & SNORING

6324 The Garry-Prior Modified Herbst

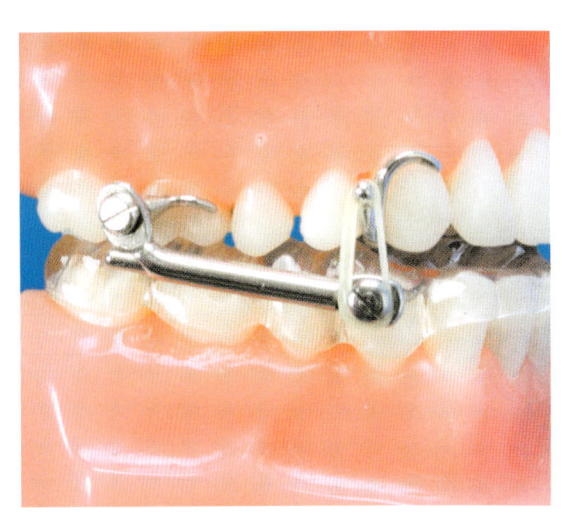

Through the combined use of a mandibular occlusal splint attached to an upper cast framework by a bilateral Herbst tube assembly, the Garry-Prior appliance positively postures the mandible in a down and forward position. The utilization of Herbst tubes allows the mandible to move freely in both a vertical and lateral direction. This is extremely helpful since EMG studies have shown that locking the mandible to the maxilla and preventing its normal function can induce muscle tension.

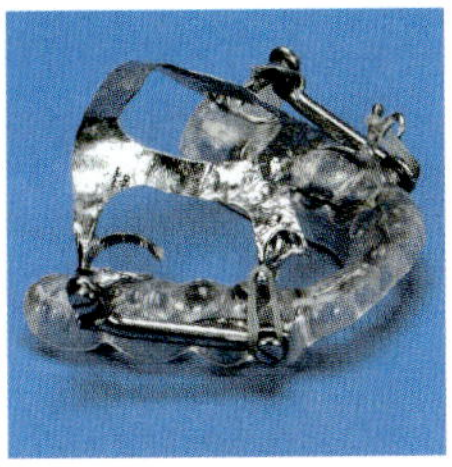

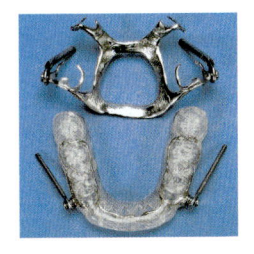

Drs. Garry and Prior, the developers of this appliance, use a low frequency T.E.N.S. unit to determine an optimal neuromuscular mandibular position. It is in this position that a construction bite is taken. This will eliminate the possibility of loading the TMJ and inducing myalgia.

The mandibular portion of this appliance is typically finished to a cusp-fossa relationship with the maxillary dentition. The maxillary portion of the appliance is a thin, cast framework that allows for maximum tongue volume. The purpose of the vertical elastics in the cuspid area encourages a lip-together posture that will enhance nasal respiration without locking the mandible to the maxilla. Since the appliance allows the mandible to translate and rotate, patients find this design extremely comfortable. Patients report that they can converse normally and even drink liquids without removing the appliance from their mouth.

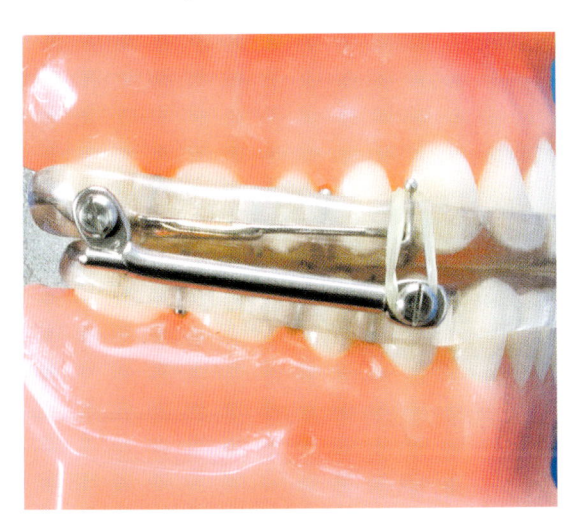

6325 The Clark (UCLA) Modified Herbst Appliance

This appliance consists of two occlusal splints held together by a bilateral Herbst tube assembly. This set-up allows the mandible to positively be postured forward. Posturing the mandible forward brings the tongue anteriorly to open up the airway. This unique design allows the mandible to move freely in both a vertical and a lateral direction while at the same time preventing the mandible from dropping back during sleep. Because the Herbst tubes are placed buccally to the teeth, there is nothing to interfere with the patient's tongue position and patients find this design extremely comfortable.

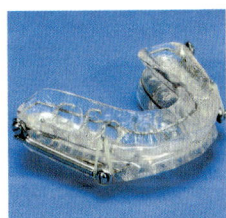

Users of this appliance typically provide a construction bite taken with the mandible positioned 75% of the way from maximum intercuspation to maximum protrusive with a 4mm vertical opening in the anteriors. This appliance can also be titrated forward from its initial position by adding shims in 1mm, 2mm, and 3mm increments.

The occlusal surfaces of the upper and lower portions of this appliance are carefully milled into full contact. Vertical elastics are used in the cuspid region to create a proprioceptive response that encourages a lip together posture. Maximum retention is achieved through multiple ball clasps on both the upper and the lower portions of the appliance.

18.5

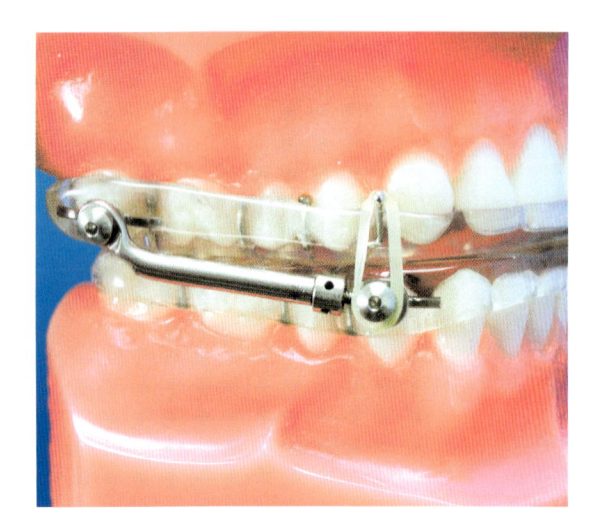

OBSTRUCTIVE SLEEP APNEA & SNORING

6325A The Adjustable Herbst Sleep Appliance

Having the ability to easily bring the mandible forward in small measurable increments is often the difference between success and failure when using a sleep appliance to treat apnea.

Although this can be accomplished with the original U.C.L.A. design by adding shims to the Herbst assembly, this new Herbst design allows you to incrementally bring the mandible forward with greater ease and adjustability.

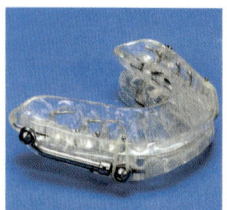

As with its predecessor, the palate is clear of any obstruction that would encourage the posterior placement of the tongue. In all other aspects this appliance is identical to the original design.

6332E The EMA (Elastic Mandibular Advancement)

This appliance consists of upper and lower custom pressure-molded clear trays that are joined together by flexible elastic bands. These elastic bands come in various lengths and degrees of flexibility allowing the dentist to regulate the precise amount of mandibular advancement and lateral movement desired. These parameters will be different for every patient.

Because the bands are easily changed, you will be able to quickly find the right set of bands that provide your patient with optimum results.

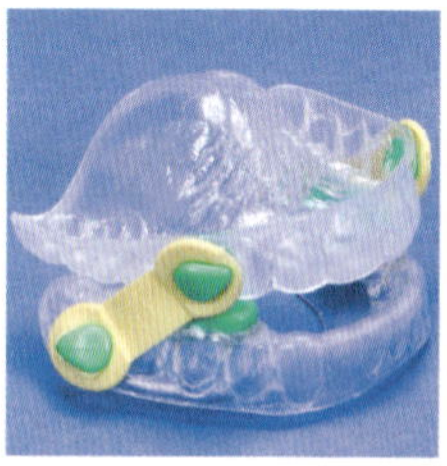

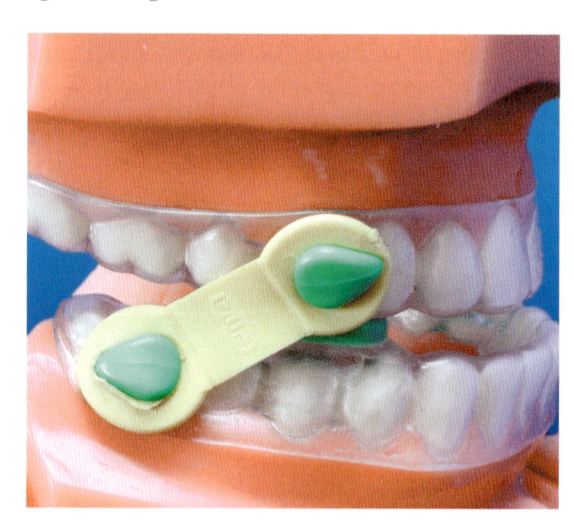

Design Notes:

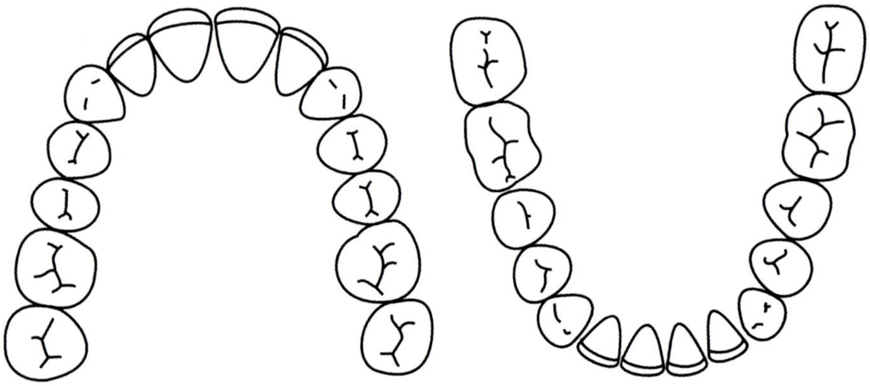

OBSTRUCTIVE SLEEP APNEA & SNORING

6330 The Original TAP® Appliance

This appliance incorporates two hard outer polycarbonate shells that are lined with a unique thermoplastic polymer blend, called ThermAcryl™. ThermAcryl™ has the right balance of flexibility and rigidity to give the TAP® excellent retention without tooth movement. Although initial fabrication of the appliance is accomplished on stone casts of your patient's arches, an even more precise fit is accomplished at delivery by heating the ThermAcryl™ and molding it to the patient's dentition.

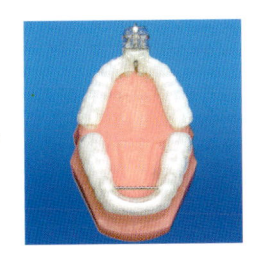

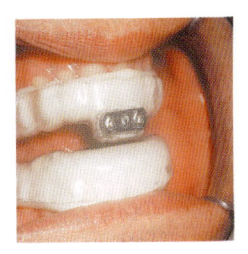

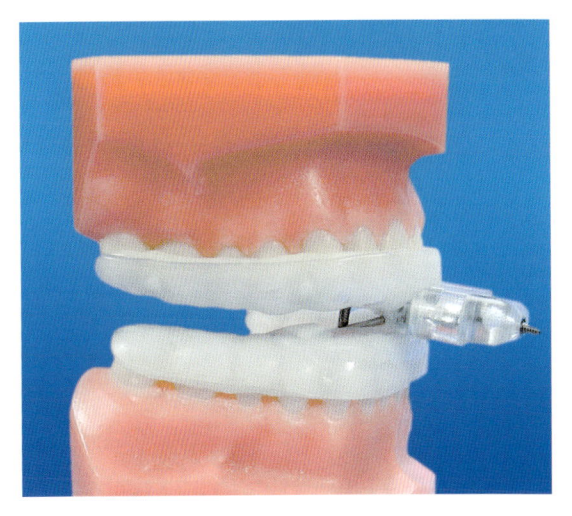

Attached to the upper and lower dual laminate thermoplastic trays is a unique hook and screw device that is used to bring the jaw forward to maintain an open airway. This hook and screw provides 8 mm of vertical adjustment, a minimum of 25 mm of lateral freedom and is infinitely adjustable anterior-posteriorly.

Although the initial trial position of the appliance is set at delivery, the dentist is not limited to a range of predetermined positions with the TAP®. An adjustment knob is used to advance the mandible .25 mm with each turn. The patient can vary the position precisely by counting the turns. This allows both the dentist and the patient to confidently maintain the proper treatment position and yet be able to vary it depending on the patient's symptoms. This feature also allows titration of the appliance in the sleep lab by a technician or the adjustment at home by the bed partner if the patient's symptoms return while the patient is asleep.

Once the ideal treatment position has been determined, the dentist or patient can elect to remove the adjustable device as shown in the accompanying inset photo. In such a case a locking nut is then applied to fix the hook in one location. If adjustment again becomes necessary, the change can easily be reversed.

Another unique feature of the TAP® is that it has a unique universal mount for a CPAP mask that attaches to the adjustment mechanism. For the severe apneic, the TAP® reduces the required pressure while providing a leak free, stable, "strapless" mask system.

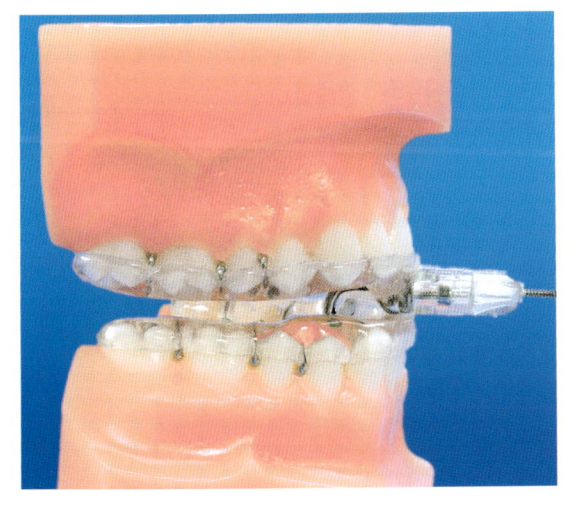

6331 The Clasp Retained Hard Acrylic TAP®

Although the ThermAcryl™ material used in the original TAP® has the benefit of allowing you to improve the retention of the appliance chairside, regardless of the accuracy of the models, if the appliance is not meticulously maintained it can delaminate and/or become difficult to keep clean. To eliminate the possibility of delamination, and provide a cleansable appliance, a hard acrylic clasp retained TAP® was designed.

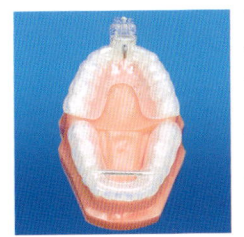

The clasps can be easily adjusted throughout treatment to maintain retention. In all other aspects, this appliance is identical to the original design.

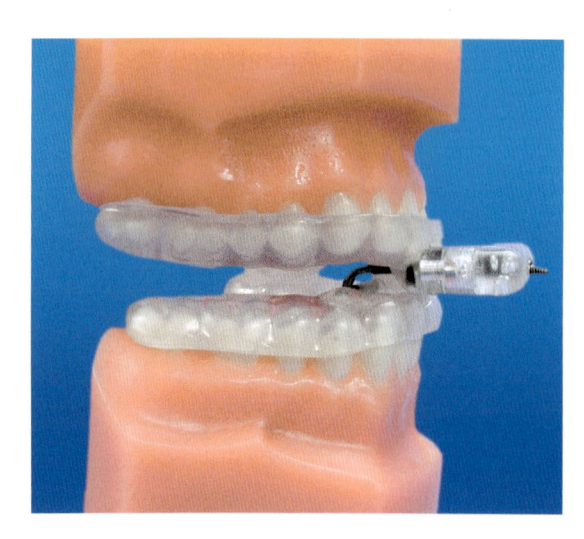

OBSTRUCTIVE SLEEP APNEA & SNORING

6331TL The Multi-Laminate TAP®

Many patients prefer the comfort of a soft material against their teeth. To accomplish this, a layer of soft ethyl vinyl acetate has been incorporated into the design of the TAP®. This is accomplished by laminating three separate layers together under high heat and pressure. What is created is a clasp-free appliance that uses the buccal and lingual undercuts for retention.

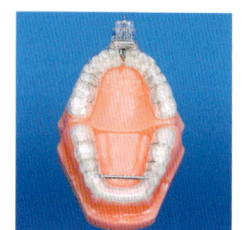

6322S The Snore-Aid®

The Snore-Aid® appliance is designed to open the upper airway by mandibular repositioning and antero-superior reposturing of the tongue. It combines a single mandibular bite plate, which has a flat occlusal surface, with an external lip shield. The appliance is titrated by manually adjusting the shield in a rearward direction upon a calibrated anterior extension off of the dental plate. This action advances the lower plate relative to the lip shield, thus advancing the mandible. Titration of this appliance can be made immediately and it can be done even while it is being worn. The adjustment is also easily reversible.

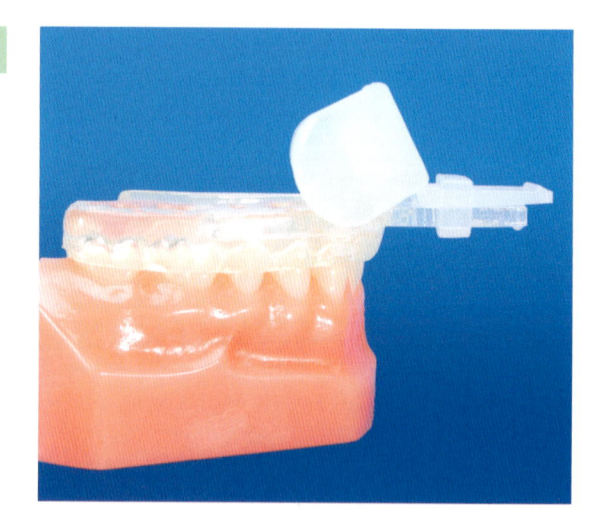

Some of the benefits of this design are that it has no palatal structure to interfere with an ideal antero-superior tongue position. In fact, the mandibular plate is wide enough that it actually helps to elevate the tongue as the mandible is advanced. This supports the genioglossus muscle and prevents it from settling posteriorly and inferiorly into the pharynx.

The occlusal surface of the appliance is designed so that the maxillary dentition contacts uniformly. This gives the mandible complete freedom to function laterally and vertically. The bite plate surface can also be customized to alter the vertical dimension. This makes this appliance ideal for nocturnal bruxers and for patients undergoing diurnal splint therapy for TMJ dysfunction. The appliance itself can be made out of hard acrylic with Ball clasps for retention or with a thermoplastic material bi-laminate splint like our Talon™ splints.

OBSTRUCTIVE SLEEP APNEA & SNORING

The Klearway Appliance

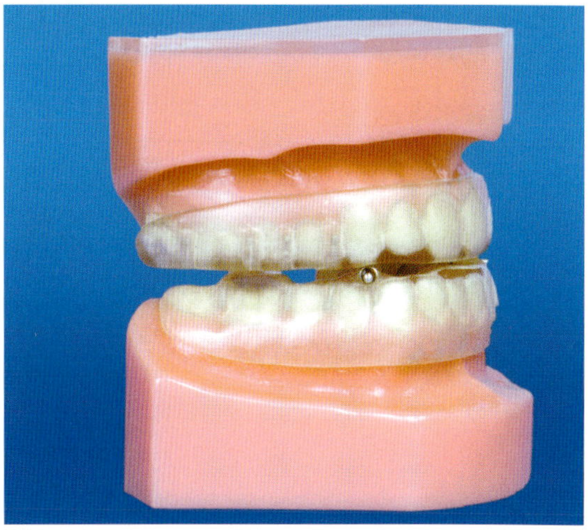

This appliance is a mandibular repositioning appliance. It is fabricated with a thermo active acrylic, giving it excellent rentention and comfort for the patient It has an expansion screw in the palate that allows you to adjust the mandibular position in 0.25mm increments. Lateral and vertical jaw movements are sufficient to allow the patient to yawn, swallow and drink water without dislodging the appliance. Its adjustability makes it a very good appliance. Data from a large clinical trial, funded by the Canadian government, indicates a 78% success rate for the treatment of sleep apnea.

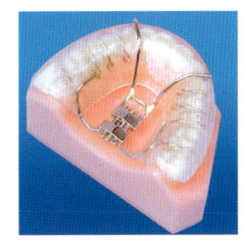

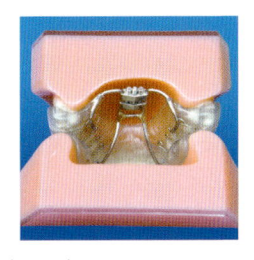

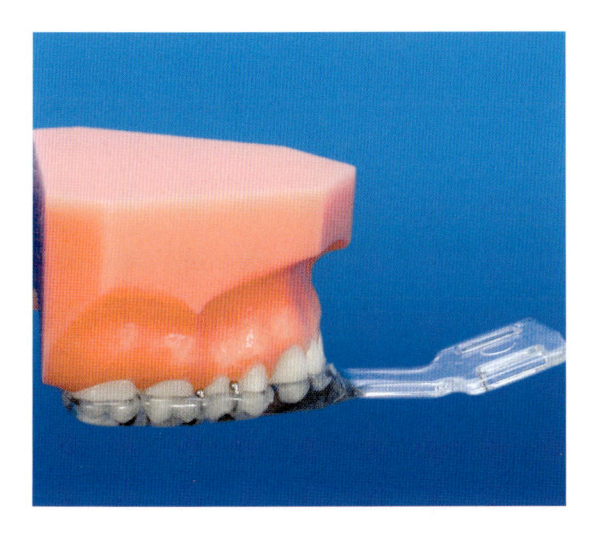

6603 The CPAP/PRO

CPAP has a 50% failure rate because patients find most masks unbearable to wear. But, nightly CPAP doesn't have to be torture. A new CPAP interface called the CPAP/PRO may be the answer to a better night's sleep. Unlike all other masks and nasal devices that require straps and/or headgear to keep them in place, the CPAP/PRO typically utilizes a simple customized dental mouthpiece that easily snaps onto the upper teeth. A small thin bracket is attached to the dental mouthpiece and extends outward through the lips to support the fully adjustable CPAP/PRO.

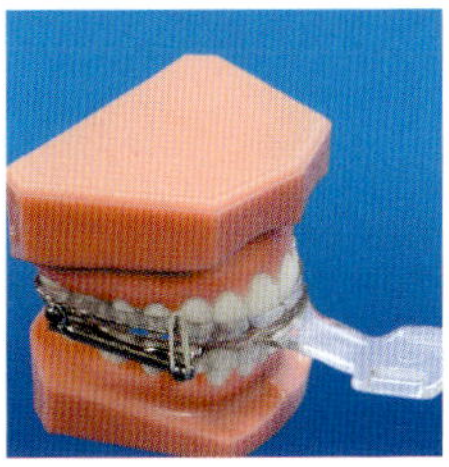

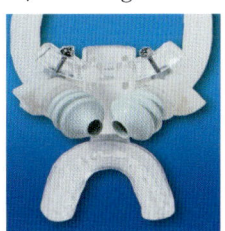

Two highly flexible tubes convey the CPAP air to the nostrils. Unique nasal inserts, which are foam filled and inflate slightly during use from the CPAP pressure, provide excellent nasal sealing with just feather-light pressure applied to the nostrils. Regardless of all the twisting and turning done throughout the night, the CPAP/PRO stays in positive position with the nose.

As illustrated in the above insert photo, the CPAP/PRO assembly can also be added to mandibular advancement appliances.

Design Notes

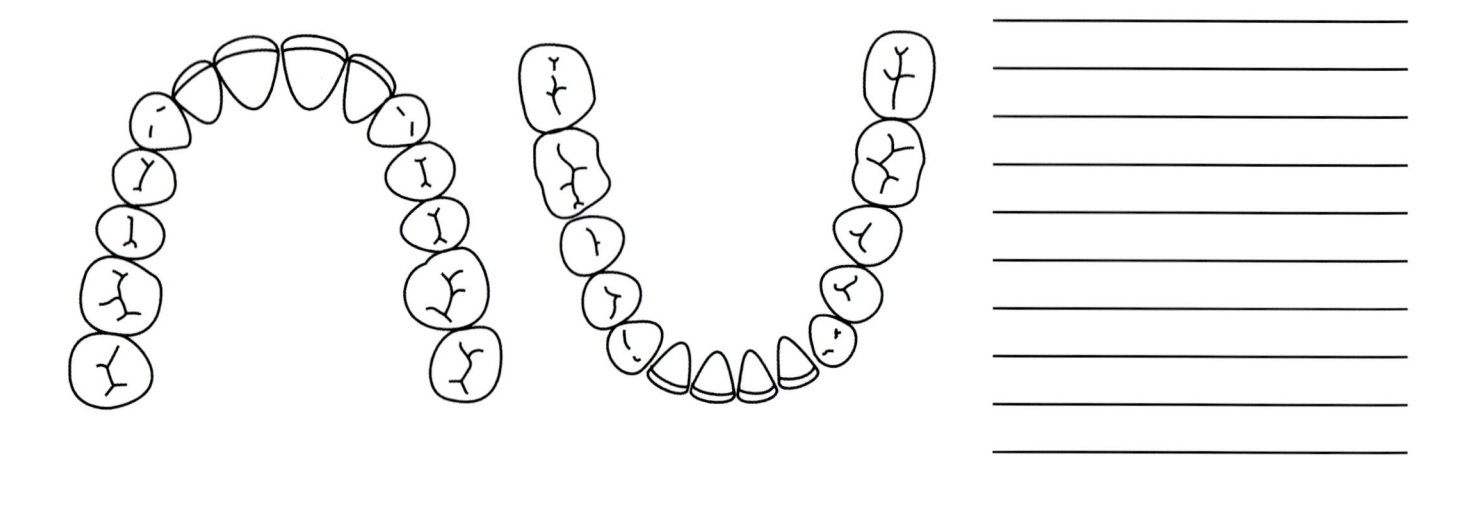

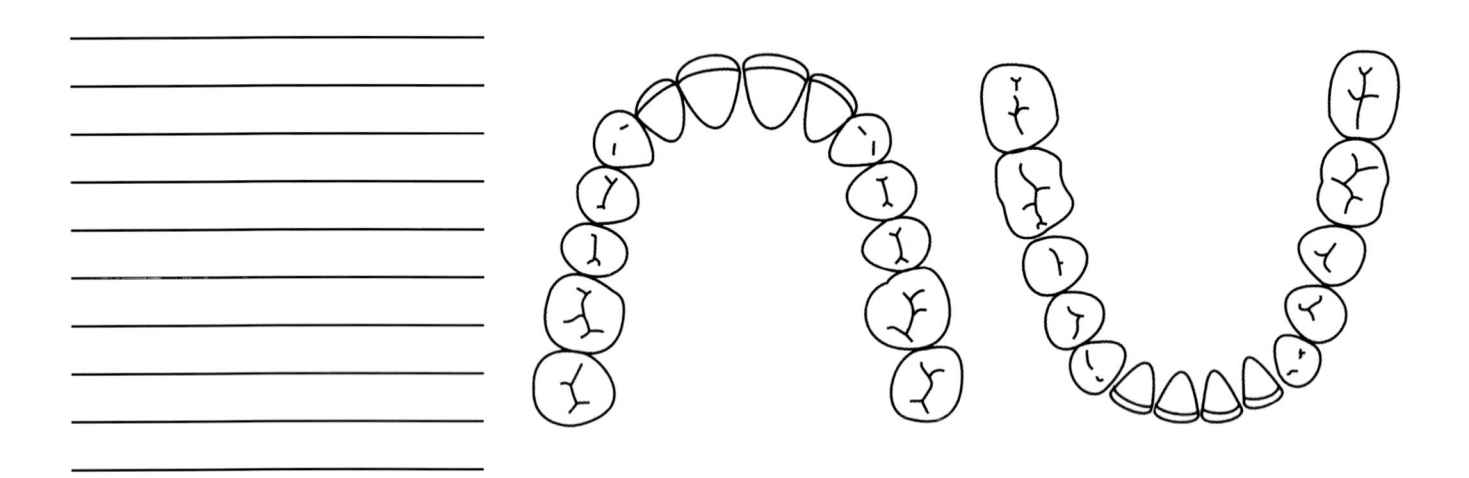

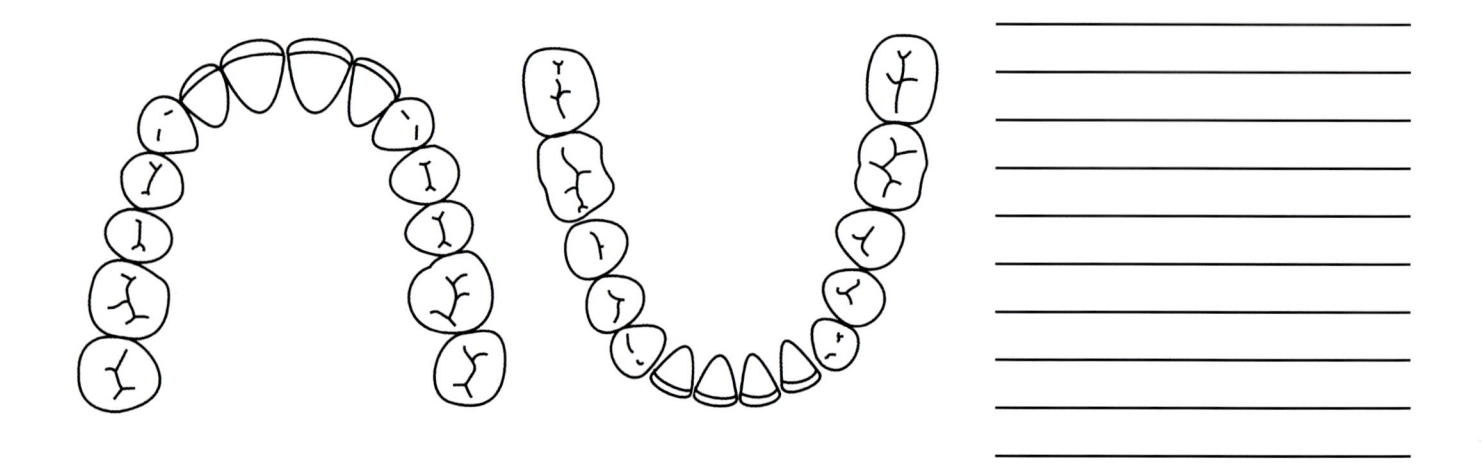

General Index of Appliances and Procedures

Abutment Tooth
   When not fully erupted (2012B) [2]
   When stainless steel crown is needed (2021, 2021R) [2]
Adaptor™ (1332) [11]
Adjustable Herbst Sleep Appliance (6325A) [18]
A.L.F. Appliance (3106) [8]
Alternative Lightwire Functional Appliance (3106) [8]
Anterior/Posterior
   Arch Development
      Fixed Appliances [8-4.1 thru 8-4.2]
      Removable Appliances [8-3.1 thru 8-3.4]
   Lateral Development
      Combination, Removable Appliances [8-5.1]
      Combination, Fixed [8-6.1 thru 8-6.5]
Anteriors
   Aligning prior to Veneers (1076, 2053) [14]
   Bicuspid (unerupted), creating space for (1042) [14]
   Crowding (1091, 1103, 1333, 4182) [14]
   Flared (1122B, 2211B) [14]
   Moving (1073, 2031, 2133, 2044) [4]
   Retracting (1122B, 2211B) [14]
Appliances
   Fixed (2027, 2028, 2031, 2032, 2033, 2035, 2037, 2038, 2041, 2041G, 2044, 2045, 2045M, 2133, 2142, 2502M, 2511) [4]
   Removable (1042, 1042D, 1043, 1044, 1073) [4]
Arch
   Expanding Temporary Partial (4183E) [8]
   Development for Mixed Dentition (1094, 1094B 1095) [8]
Arnold Expander (2092) [8]
Bicuspid, moving mesially (2031, 2032, 2035, 2038, 2041G) [4]
Bio Finisher (3032) [9]
Bionators [9]
   Balters Appliance (3021, 3022, 3023) [9]
   Neutral Bionators (3013, 3023) [9]
   To Close an Open Bite (3012, 3022) [9]
   To Open a Closed Bite (3011, 3021) [9]
Bleaching Trays (6111B) [14]
Bloore Aligner (1076F) [6, 11]
Bluegrass Appliance (2113) [3]
Bowbeer Appliance (1162E) [8]
CD Distalizer (20454) [4, 8] (2045M) [4]
Chan LV I Orthodic (6205C) [13]

Clark
   (UCLA) Modified Herbst Appliance (6325) [18]
   Trombone Appliance (2511) [4], 10 (2521) [10]
Clasp Retained Hard Acrylic TAP (6331) [18]
Class II, Division II, Correction (1105) [8]
Closing
   Diastema (1076, 1121, 2051, 2053) [5]
Excess Space (1122, 1122B, 2211B) [17]
   Posterior
      Space (1125, 2052) [5]
      Open Bites (1141, 1706, 2705, 2706, 3032, 3701, 3706) [9]
Construction Bites for Bionators [9-9.1]
CPAP Appliances (6603) [18]
Creating Space for Bridge or Implant (1037, 1042, 1042D, 4182, 2034, 4184) [14]
Crossbite Correction
   Anterior (1073, 1074, 1075, 1091, 3504) [7]
   Bicuspid region (2154) [7]
   Bilateral (1095, 1343, 2154, 2155) [7]
   Posterior (1076E, 1082, 1082A, 1083, 1084, 1095, 1334, 1343, 2081, 2082, 2154, 2155) [7]
   Single tooth (1075, 1076E, 1084, 1091, 1334, 2081, 2082) [7]
   Unilateral (1082, 1082A, 1083, 1084, 1334, 2081, 2082) [7]
Crozat Appliance (3101, 3102, 3103, 3104, 3800, 3801) [8]
CT Scan Appliances (6520A, 6520B) [16]
Diastema Closing (2053) [14]
Differential Lateral Development
   Fixed Appliance [8-8.1 thru 8-8.4]
   Removable Appliance [8-7.1 thru 8-7.5]
Dillingham Habit Expansion Appliance (2150H) [3, 8]
Distalizing
   First and Second Molar (1042D) [4]
   Six-Year Molar Erupted (1042, 1043, 1044, 2027, 2028, 2035, 2037, 2038, 2041, 2045, 2045M, 2142) [4]
   Six-Year Molar Unerupted (2033) [4]
Distribution of Abnormal Forces [17]
"Dorsal" Appliance (6322D) [18]
E Arch (2092) [8]
Ectopically Erupting Molar, correcting (1044, 2027, 2028) [4]
Encouraging Eruption (1063, 1072B, 1076C) [6]
Essix Retainer (1116E) [11]

(Appliance number in parentheses)   Superscripts = Chapter Numbers

General Index of Appliances and Procedures

Excess Mobility [17.1 thru 17.7]
Extra Coronal Splints
    Removable (1116P, 1165, 6191, 6192, 6193) [17]
    Fixed (2013, 2014, 2023, 2165, 2167, 2212, 4022, 4023, 6401, 6402) [17]
Extrusion (1072B, 1078, 1079, 2211) [17]
Face Mask (2444, 2444E) [9]
F.A.C.T. Appliance (6203F) [13]
Final Retainers
    Removable (1115, 1116, 1161, 1162, 1164, 1165, 1169A) [11]
    Fixed (2164, 2165, 2166, 2167, 2212) [11]
Fixed
    Holding Arches (2502, 2507) [10]
    Molar Distilization (2501) [10]
F.L.E.A. (Fixed Lingual Expansion Appliance) (2155F) [8]
Fluoride
    Delivery (6111) [17]
    Protection (6111) [14]
    Tray (6111) [14]
Forced Eruption (1078, 1079, 2211) [14]
Frankel
    Appliances [Chapter 9]
    Frankel III Appliance (3503) [9]
Gary-Prior Modified Herbst Appliance (6324) [18]
Gingival Grafting Stent (6510) [17]
Groper Appliance (4310, 4310C) [2]
Grumrax Appliance (2085F) [8]
Habits
    Cheek Biting (1117) [3]
    Finger Biting (1113, 2111, 2112, 2113, 2114, 2115, 2150) [3]
    Lip Biting (2118) [3]
    Lateral Tongue Thrust (1119) [3]
    Tongue Biting (1113, 1114, 2110, 2111, 2112, 2114, 2115, 2150) [3]
Halterman Appliance (2027) [4]
Han Appliance (3504) [7]
Haas
    Appliance (2153) [8]
    Memory Appliance (2153M) [8]
    Modified Haas expander (2153CD) [8]
Herbst Appliance (2443, 2443C) [9]
Herbst, Cantilevered (2443C) [10]

Hydrax
    Appliance (2154, 2155R) [8]
    Multi-action (2154CD) [8]
Implant
    Site Protectors (2013, 2014, 2023, 4021, 4022, 4023, 4024, 4025, 4181, 4185, 4191, 4602) [16]
    Stent (6520D) [17]
Incisal Blocks (1400) [10]
Indirect Banding and Bonding [Chapter 10]
Interim Partials/Bridges [Chapter 15]
Intra Coronal Splints (2320, 4602, 4603) [17]
Jackson Appliance (1096, 1098) [8]
Labial Arch Wires [Chapter 11]
Lateral
    Arch Development
        Fixed Appliance (8-2.1 thru 8-2.6) [8]
        Removable Appliance (8-1.1 thru 8-1.5) [8]
        Expansion, Fixed (2503) [10]
Levandoski Stabilization Prosthesis (6209) [13]
Magill Sagittal (2046A) [8]
Mahony Twin Block (3616) [9]
Mandibular
    Arch Development (2504) [10]
    Clasp Retained Repositioner (6323) [18]
    EMA Elastic Mandibular Advancement (6332E) [18]
    Inclined Repositioning Splint (6322) [18]
    Repositioning (1706, 2443, 2443C, 2640, 2705, 3023, 2706, 2708, 3011, 3012, 3013, 3021, 3022, 3026, 3610, 3610BC, 3615, 3616, 3706, 3804, 3907) [9] (6322, 6322D, 6322S, 6323, 6324, 6325, 6325A, 6326, 6330, 6331, 6331TL, 6332E, 6710) [18]
Multi-laminate TAP (6331TL) [18]
M.A.R.A. Appliance (2708) [9]
Maryland Bridge, temporary (4021) [15]
Maxillary
    Anchorage (2507) [10]
    Protrusion (2444, 2444E) [9]
Midline
    Correction (1094C) [8]
    Shift, prevention (2016, 2133) [2]
Minor Tooth Movement
    Prior to placing Veneers (1121, 1176, 2051, 2053) [5]
    Minor Tooth Movement (4182) [14]

(Appliance number in parentheses)   Superscripts = Chapter Numbers

General Index of Appliances and Procedures

Molars
    Crossbites (1334, 2081, 2082) [14]
    Inclined, Distalizing Mesially (1042, 1042D) [14]
    Uprighting (1037, 1076E, 1084, 2027, 2028, 2034, 4184) [14]
Moving teeth
    Buccally (1072E, 1076D, 1076E, 1334) [6]
    Labially (1071, 1072, 1076B, 1076C, 1076F, 1091, 2061) [6]
    Lingually (1054, 1076B) [6]
    Mesially/Distally (1054, 1063, 1072, 1076B, 1076C, 1076D, 1076F, 2061) [6]
Molar Distalization (1251, 1252) [8]
Mouthguards
    Boxer's (62080, pro mouthguard 61409) [12]
    Intact (youth 61401/adult 61402/professional 61403) [12]
    Marshall Arts (61404) [12]
    Multi-laminated, Heat Pressurized (61401, 61402, 61403, 61404, 61409) [12]
    Vacuum-formed, "Proform" (62010, 62020, 62023) [12]
Pendex Appliance (2085MX) [8]
M Pendulum Appliance (2085M) [8]
Myofunctional Therapy (1114, 2110) [3]
Nance Appliance (2025) [2]
Natanium Palatal Expander (2157) [8]
Neuromuscular Orthodics (6205) [13]
Night Guards [Chapter 13]
Occlusal Trauma Protection (1116P, 1165, 6191, 6192, 6193) [17]
Orthopedic Corrector (3026) [9]
Orthodics [Chapter 13]
Partials
    Active (4182, 4183B, 4184) [14, 15] (4183C) [15]
    Controlling vertical dimension (4187) [15]
    Essix temporary (4191) [15]
    Fixed Pedo (4210, 4310, 4310C, 4172, 4173A, 4173B) [2]
    Interim (4180, 4181, 4185H, 4025) [15]
    Kidie Pedo (4173A, 4173B) [2]
    Transitional (4185H, 4186) [15]
    Treatment (4182, 4183, 4183B, 4184, 4187) [15]
Pendex/Hilgers Pendulum Appliance (2085E) [8]

Periodontal Disease
    Flared Anteriors (1122, 1122B, 2211B) [17]
    Surgical Site Protection (4021, 4024, 4025, 4181, 4185H, 4191, 4602) [17]
Porter Appliance (2101) [8]
Positioners (5551) [10, 11]
Posterior Bite Collapse (1122, 1122B, 2211B) [17]
Premaxilla, underdeveloped (1073B, 1105, 1261, 1263, 1265) [8]
Primary Posterior Tooth, early loss [Chapter 2]
Pseudo Class III Corrections (3503, 3504) [9]
Quad Helix (2084) [8]
Rapid Palatial Expanders (2150H, 2153, 2153M, 2154, 2154S, 2155R, 1343, 1343LS, 1343SR) [8]
Removable Temporary Partials (4024, 4025, 4180, 4181, 4182, 4183B, 4183C, 4184, 4185, 4185H, 4186, 4187, 4191) [15]
Retainers
    EZ Bond Retainer (2212) [11]
    Finishing (1065, 1076F, 1333, 1332, 5511) [11]
    RAM (1164) [11]
    San Antonio (1165) [11]
    Spring (1065, 1333) [11]
Retracting
    Anteriors (1121, 1122, 1123, 1124) [5]
    Cuspids (1076C, 1076D, 1054, 1054B) [6]
Retroclined Anteriors (1073B, 1105, 1261, 1263, 1265) [8]
Reverse Pull Headgear (2444, 2444E) [9]
Rick-a-Nator (1706, 2705, 2706, 3706) [9]
R.P.E.
    Appliances (1343, 1343LS, 1343SR, 2150H, 2153, 2153M, 2154, 2154S, 2155R) [8]
    Bonded (1343, 1343LS, 1343SR) [8]
    Fixed "fan-screw" (2154F) [8]
Rotating Teeth (1063) [6]
Sagittal
    Anterior (1073B, 1105, 1261, 1263, 1265, 2046A, 2158) [8]
    To Distalize (1105D, 1105L, 1251, 1252, 2046B) [8]
Schwarz Appliances (1093, 1094, 1094A, 1094B, 1094C, 1095, 1097, 1231) [8]
"Silent Night" Appliance (6326) [18]

(Appliance number in parentheses)   Superscripts = Chapter Numbers

General Index of Appliances and Procedures

Six-year Molar
    Guiding the eruption (2022) [2]
    Prevent Mesial Drifting (various i.e. 2016 lower, 2025 upper, 2026 upper, 2027 lower) [2]
Skeletal
    Class II Correction (1141, 1706, 2443, 2443C, 2640, 2705, 2706, 2708, 3011, 3012, 3013, 3021, 3022, 3023, 3026, 3610, 3610BC, 3615, 3616, 3706, 3804, 3907) [9]
    Class III Corrections (3503, 3504) [9]
Sleep Appliances, Prefabricated (6710) [18]
Snodgrass Appliance (2085G) [8]
SnoreFree™ Appliance (6710) [18]
Snore-Aid® (6322S) [18]
Snor-X (6332X) [18]
Soft Palatal Lift Appliance (6321) [18]
Space Maintainers
    Adjustable (2013, 2016, 2026A, 2133, 2502) [2]
    Anterior (4210, 4310, 4310C, 4172) [2]
    Band and loop (2011, 2012) [2]
    Crown and loop (2021, 2021R) [2]
    Lingual Arch (2016, 2032, 2072, 2502) [2]
    Removable (1116E, 1161, 1162) [2]
Space Management (4182) [14]
Spahal Split Vertical Appliance (3701) [9]
Splints
    Bruxism (1163, 6191, 6191N, 6192, 6193, 6194, 6196) [13]
    Gelb (6203, 6205) [13]
    May (6204) [13]
    M.O.R.A. (6203) [13]
    Occlusal (1163, 6191, 6191N, 6192, 6193, 6194, 6196) [13]
    Oakes (1163) [13]
    Repositioning (6203, 6203F, 6203W, 6204, 6205, 6205C, 6206, 6207, 6209) [13]
    Talon (6196) [13]
    Witzig (6203W) [13]
Straight Wire Technique [Chapter 10]
Super Screw Appliance (2154S) [8]

Surgical Stents (6520A, 6520B, 6520C) [16]
Suture Expanding Appliances (1343, 1343LS, 1343SR, 2153M, 2150H, 2153, 2154, 2155R, 2154S) [8]
Swallowing, Abnormal (1113, 1114, 2110, 2111, 2112, 2114, 2115, 2150) [3]
Swing Lock Appliance (1103) [8]
TAP Appliance, original (6330) [18]
Temporary Fixed Bridges (2013, 2014, 2023, 4021, 4022, 4023, 4024, 4172, 4602) [15]
Titratable Appliances (6322S, 6324, 6325, 6325A, 6330, 6331, 6331TL, 6332E) [18]
TMJ Appliances (6203, 6203F, 6203W, 6204, 6205, 6205C, 6206, 6207, 6209) [13]
Tongue
    Positioners (5512, 6332X) [18]
    Retaining Device (TRD) (5512) [18]
Transfer Trays (2619) [10]
Transpalatal Appliance (2026, 2026A) [2]
Trauma Kits [Chapter 10]
Twin Block
    Appliances (2640, 3610, 3610BC, 3616, 3804, 3907) [9]
    Evans Twin Block (3610BC) [9]
    Fixed (2640) [9]
    Truax (3804) [9]
Vertical
    Defects/Correcting (1037, 1072B, 1078, 1079, 2027, 2028, 2034, 2211, 4184) [17]
    Eruption (1141, 1706, 2705, 2706, 3032, 3701, 3706) [9]
Williams Expander (2156) [8]
Wilson
    Expansion Appliances [Chapter 8]
    Lingual Arch, Fixed (2502) [10]
    Multi-action Palatal Appliance (2505) [8, 10]
    Nance Button (2507) [10]
    Quad Helix Appliance (2503) [8, 10]
    Quad-action Mandibular Appliance (2504) [8, 10]
    3D® Modular Orthodontic System (2501, 2502, 2503, 2504, 2505, 2507) [10]
Wipla Swivel Appliance (1104) [8]
Witzig Crossbite Appliance (1082A) [7]

(Appliance number in parentheses)   Superscripts = Chapter Numbers

The following is a list of text and videos used for reference in the preparation of this manual. They are suggested reading for complete information on the topics presented.

The Appliance Adjustment Video, Space Maintainers Laboratory, 1987.

Bell, W.: Orofacial Pains: Classification, Diagnosis, Management, St. Louis, C.V. Mosby Co., 1985.

Bell, W.: Temporomandibular Disorders: Classification, Diagnosis, Management, St. Louis, C.V. Mosby Co., 1985.

Christianson, G.J.: Fluoride Professionally Applied and Home Use, Practical Clinical Courses Video V-40.

Clark, G.: OSA and Dental Appliances, Use of Dental Appliances to Treat Sleep Disorders, CDA Journal, Oct. 1988.

Clark, W.: The Clark Twin Block Technique, Dr. Clark's course manual, 1991.

Clinical Protocol for Dental Appliance Therapy for Snoring and Obstructive Sleep Apnea, Sleep Disorders Dental Society, 11676 Perry Hwy. Bldg., Wesford, PA 15090.

Clinical Research Associates Newsletter, Fluoride Update Review, Vol. 14, Issue 5, may 1990.

Dierks, Keller: Obstructive Sleep Apnea Syndrome; Correction by Mandibular Advancement, So. Medical Journal, Vol. 83, April 1990.

Enlow: Facial Growth, Philadelphia, W.B. Saunders Co., 1990.

Garguilo, Weintz, Orban: Dimensions and Relations of the Dentinogingival Junction in Humans, J. Periodontal, 1961.

Garry, J.: The Role of a Dentist in Sleep Apnea, Dr. James Garry,* 1321 No. Harbor Blvd., #201, Fullerton, CA 92635.

Gelb, H.: Clinical Management of Head, Neck and TMJ Pain and Dysfunction, Philadelphia, W.B. Saunders, 1985.

Graber, Neumann: Removable Orthodontic Appliances, Philadelphia, W.B. Saunders Co., 1990.

Graber, Rakos, Petrovic: Dentofacial Orthopedics with Functional Appliances, St. Louis, C.V. Mosby Co., 1985.

Henderson, D.: McCracken's Removable Partial Prosthodontics, 6th Edition, St. Louis, C.V. Mosby Co., 1981.

Isaacson, Reed & Stephens: Functional Orthodontic Appliances, Oxford, Blackwell Scientific Publications, 1990.

Johnson: Airway Changes in Relationship to Mandibular Posturing, Otolaryngol Head Neck Surgery, Vol. 106, 1992.

Khouw, Norton: The Mechanism of Fixed Molar Uprighting Appliances, J. Prosthetic Dent., April 1972.

Lamberg, L.: Sleep Apnea-Symptoms, Causes, Evaluation, Treatment, Rochester, MN, America Sleep Apnea Disorders Association, 1988.

Lee-Knight, C.T.: Protective Mouthguards in Sports Injuries, Journal of Canadian Dental Association, Vol. 57, number 1, Jan. 1991.

Mandel, Binzer, Withers: Forced Eruption in Restoring Severely Fractured Teeth Using Removable Orthodontic Appliances, J. Prosthetic Dentistry, March 1982.

Marks, Corn: Atlas of Adult Orthodontics, Philadelphia, Lea & Febiger, 1989.

McCarthy, M.: Sports and Mouth Protection, Vol. 38, number 5, Sept./Oct. 1990.

Miller, Grasso: Removable Partial Prosthodontics, 2nd Edition, Baltimore, Williams & Wilkins, 1979.

Moyers, R.: Handbook of Orthodontics, Chicago, Yearbook Medical Publishers, 1980.

Okeson, J.P.: Fundamentals of Occlusion and Temporomandibular Disorders, St. Louis, C.V. Mosby Co., 1985.

Pfitzinger, W.: Banding and Bracketing Video, Space Maintainers Laboratory, 1992.

Prichard, J.: The Diagnosis and Treatment of Periodontal Disease in General Practice, Philadelphia, W.B. Saunders Co., 1979.

Profit, Wm.: Contemporary Orthodontics, St. Louis, C.V. Mosby Co., 1986.

Ramford, Ash: Occlusion, Philadelphia, W.B. Saunders Co., 1983.

Reitz, Weiner: The Fabrication of Interim Acrylic Resin Removable Partial Dentures with Clasps, J. Prosthetic Dent., 1978.

Starr, C.: Management of Periodontal Tissues for Restorative Dentistry, J. Esthetic Dentistry, Nov./Dec. 1991.

Starvo, Jenkins, Watson: Restorative Treatment Utilizing Forced Eruption, Ontario Dentist, December 1985.

Stewart, K.: Clinical Removable Partial Prosthodontics, St. Louis, C.V. Mosby Co., 1983.

Vanarsdall, Swartz: Adjunctive Orthodontics for the General Practitioner Molar Uprighting, California, Ormco, 1987.

Wilson, Wilson: Enhanced Orthodontics with 3D Modular 1st Phase Fixed/Removable, RMO, 1988.

Witzig, Spahal: The Clinical Management of Basic Maxillofacial Orthopedic Appliances, Vol. I, Chicago, Yearbook Medical Publishers, Inc., 1987.